Baillière's
# CLINICAL
# ONCOLOGY
INTERNATIONAL PRACTICE AND RESEARCH

Baillière's

# CLINICAL
# ONCOLOGY

INTERNATIONAL PRACTICE AND RESEARCH

Volume 1/Number 1
March 1987

# Bone Tumours

ROBERT SOUHAMI MD, BSc, FRCP
*Guest Editor*

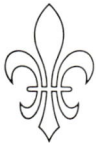

Baillière Tindall
**London Philadelphia Toronto Sydney Tokyo**

Baillière Tindall    24–28 Oval Road
W.B. Saunders    London NW1 7DX, UK

West Washington Square
Philadelphia, PA 19105, USA

1 Goldthorne Avenue
Toronto, Ontario M8Z 5T9, Canada

Harcourt Brace Jovanovich Group (Australia) Pty Ltd
Post Office Box 300, North Ryde, NSW 2113, Australia

Exclusive Agent in Japan:
Maruzen Co. Ltd. (Journals Division)
3–10 Nihonbashi 2-chome, Chuo-ku, Tokyo 103, Japan

ISSN 0950–3560

ISBN 0–7020–1226–2 (single copy)

*Baillière's Clinical Oncology* is published three times each year by Baillière Tindall.
Annual subscription prices are:

| TERRITORY | ANNUAL SUBSCRIPTION | SINGLE ISSUE |
| --- | --- | --- |
| 1. UK & Republic of Ireland | £29.50 post free | £17.50 post free |
| 2. USA & Canada | US $55.00 post free | US $28.00 post free |
| 3. All other countries | £37.50 post free | £19.50 post free |

The editor of this publication is Seán Duggan, Baillière Tindall, 24–28 Oval Road,
London NW1 7DX, UK.

*Baillière's Clinical Oncology* was published from 1982 to 1986 as
*Clinics in Oncology*.

Typeset by Phoenix Photosetting, Chatham.
Printed and bound in Great Britain by Mackays of Chatham Ltd.

# Contributors to this issue

**VIVIEN H. C. BRAMWELL** PhD, MBBS, FRCP, Head of Medical Oncology, London Regional Cancer Centre, 391 South Street, London, Ontario N6A 4G5, Canada.

**ALAN W. CRAFT** MD, FRCP, Department of Child Health, Royal Victoria Infirmary, Newcastle upon Tyne NE1 4LP, UK.

**HELENA M. EARL** MBBS, MRCP, Senior Registrar in Medical Oncology, University College Hospital, Gower Street, London WC1E 6AU, UK.

**WILLIAM F. ENNEKING** MD, Distinguished Service Professor, University of Florida School of Medicine, Gainesville, Florida, USA.

**HUGH KEMP** MS, FRCS, Orthopaedic Surgeon, Royal National Orthopaedic Hospitals, London and Stanmore, UK.

**JEAN A. S. PRINGLE** MB, ChB, Senior Lecturer, Department of Morbid Anatomy, Institute of Orthopaedics, Brockley Hill, Stanmore, Middlesex HA7 4LP, UK; Honorary Consultant, Royal National Orthopaedic Hospital.

**HERBERT S. SCHWARTZ** MD, Resident in Orthopedics, Mayo Graduate School of Medicine, 200 First Street SW, Rochester, Minnesota 55905, USA.

**FRANKLIN H. SIM** MD, Consultant, Department of Orthopedics, Mayo Clinic and Mayo Foundation; Professor of Orthopedic Surgery, Mayo Medical School, 200 First Street SW, Rochester, Minnesota 55905, USA.

**ROBERT SOUHAMI** MD, BSc, FRCP, Kathleen Ferrier Professor of Clinical Oncology, University College and Middlesex School of Medicine, Faculty of Clinical Sciences, Gower Street, London WC1E 6AU, UK.

**D. SPOONER** BSc, MRCP, FRCR, Consultant Radiotherapist, Woodlands Orthopaedic Hospital, Bristol Road South, Birmingham; Consultant Radiotherapist, Queen Elizabeth Hospital, Edgbaston, Birmingham B15 2TH, UK.

**DENNIS J. STOKER** FRCP, FRCR, Consultant Radiologist, Royal National Orthopaedic Hospital, 45–51 Bolsover Street, London W1P 8AQ, UK.

**LESTER E. WOLD** MD, Consultant, Section of Surgical Pathology, Mayo Clinic and Mayo Foundation; Assistant Professor of Pathology, Mayo Medical School, 200 First Street SW, Rochester, Minnesota 55905, USA.

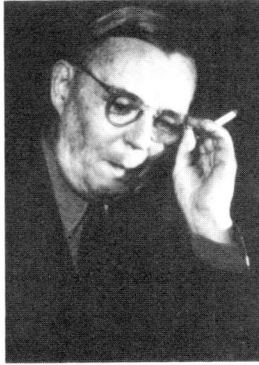

**Dedication**

This volume is dedicated to the memory of Dr Harrison S. Martland (1883–1954) whose researches defined the major effects of internally deposited radium and who first noticed the association between skeletal radium deposition and the development of osteosarcoma in radium dial painters. These observations were made while he was Chief Medical Examiner at Newark City Hospital, New Jersey, USA.

# Table of contents

## FORTHCOMING ISSUES

July 1987
**Contemporary Palliation of Difficult Symptoms**
T. D. BATES

November 1987
**Metastases**
M. SLEVIN

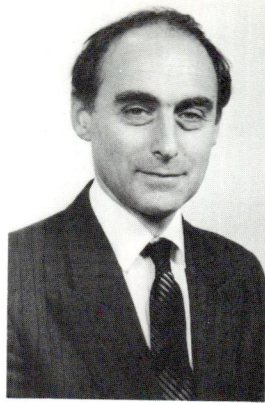

# Foreword

The last ten years have seen several major advances in the management of malignant and benign bone tumours. In osteosarcoma the prognosis has improved as a result of combination chemotherapy, with the prospect of further advances to come. We have seen new agents introduced into the treatment of Ewing's sarcoma and the roles of radiation and surgery are being reconsidered in this tumour. Several studies have shown that other high grade sarcomas, such as malignant fibrous histiocytoma, are drug-sensitive neoplasms. The use of endoprosthetic replacement for benign and malignant limb tumours has been widely adopted in place of amputation, and this has greatly improved the quality of life of many patients.

In this volume we have been fortunate in obtaining the opinions of those with experience and authority in the diagnosis and management of these complex tumours. The practical management of bone tumours has now become a matter of teamwork between radiologist, pathologist, surgeon and oncologist. For this reason and because of the rarity of some of the diseases, management is increasingly concentrated in a few larger clinical departments. However, the principles of management concern every orthopaedic surgeon and oncologist and this volume aims to review some of the growing areas which will be of importance to clinicians in these fields.

ROBERT SOUHAMI

# 1

# Incidence and aetiology of malignant primary bone tumours

## ROBERT SOUHAMI

Although rare, primary malignant tumours of bone account for a significant proportion of cancers occurring in childhood and adolescence. Figure 1 shows the average annual incidence of cancer per million children taken from the data of Kramer et al (1983) for American children aged 0–14 years. Similar data have been published by Birch et al (1980) from the Manchester Children's Tumour Registry. After the age of 14 years the relative incidence of bone sarcomas rises (because of the rarity of neuroblastoma and Wilms' tumour at this age) so that malignant bone tumours become the fifth commonest neoplasm at this age (after leukaemia, CNS tumours, lymphomas and soft tissue sarcoma). The relative frequency of the major histological types of malignant bone tumour is shown in Table 1.

## AGE AND SEX INCIDENCE

The age and sex incidence for osteosarcoma and Ewing's sarcoma for white American children are shown in Figure 2. There is a slight male prepon- derance which becomes more marked in late adolescence for both tumours. It is noticeable that the period of greatest risk is earlier (10–14 years) for girls than for boys (15–17 years). The incidence falls in the age range of 20–40 years, but then rises due to the development of osteosarcoma in Paget's disease and post-radiation sarcomas, which constitute 25% and 5–10% respectively of all bone sarcomas seen at large institutions. Price (1955) claims that the incidence of osteosarcoma is at its highest at the age of 60–80 years but that

**Table 1.** The relative overall frequency of the three major histological types of bone sarcoma in black and white residents of New York State (1975–1980).

| Sarcoma | White population | | Black population | |
|---|---|---|---|---|
| | No. | % | No. | % |
| Osteosarcoma | 219 | 43.4 | 47 | 72.3 |
| Chondrosarcoma | 162 | 32.1 | 13 | 20 |
| Ewing's sarcoma | 124 | 24.5 | 5 | 7.7 |
| | 505 | | 65 | |

From Polednak (1985a), with permission.

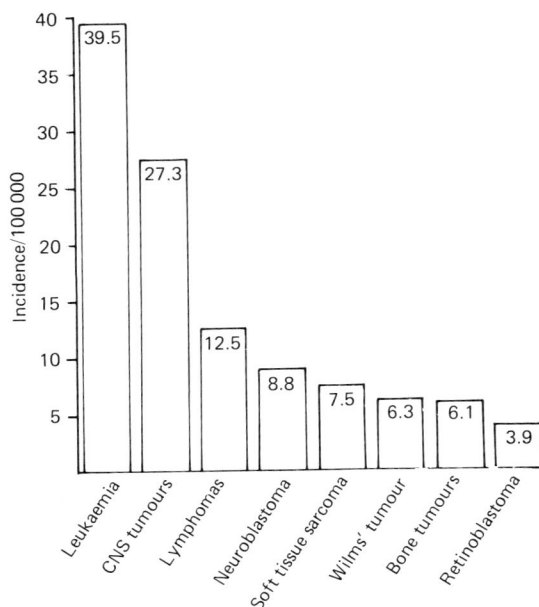

**Figure 1.** Average annual cancer incidence per million white children, aged 0–14 years, in the USA, 1970–1979. From Kramer et al (1983).

these cases are under-reported since they are often not referred to specialist centres. The position is not completely clear since the precise histological categorization of Paget's sarcoma and irradiation sarcoma is not clearly established, especially in the earlier literature. Fibrosarcoma (including malignant fibrous histiocytoma) and chondrosarcoma are uncommon in the young and increase in frequency with age.

The increase in frequency of primary bone tumours in adolescence has led to several studies examining the relationship of tumour development to skeletal growth. Osteosarcomas in the humerus tend to arise earlier than those in the femur (Price, 1958), possibly related to the relatively greater increase in bone length in the humerus in early life. Both Price (1958) and Weinfeld and Dudley (1962) noted a tendency for osteosarcoma of the flat bones to arise somewhat later. In the study of Fraumeni (1967), the distribution of heights at diagnosis of children with osteosarcoma and Ewing's sarcoma was compared with age-matched children with non-osseous cancers. With both tumours there was a significant, but small, difference in height, the children with both types of bone tumour tending to be taller than the controls. Polednak (1985b) calculated the relative risks for osteosarcoma and Ewing's sarcoma, related to height percentile. He found that there was a significant increase in risk for children above the ninety-seventh percentile for both tumours ($\times 7.97$ and $\times 6.25$ for osteosarcoma and

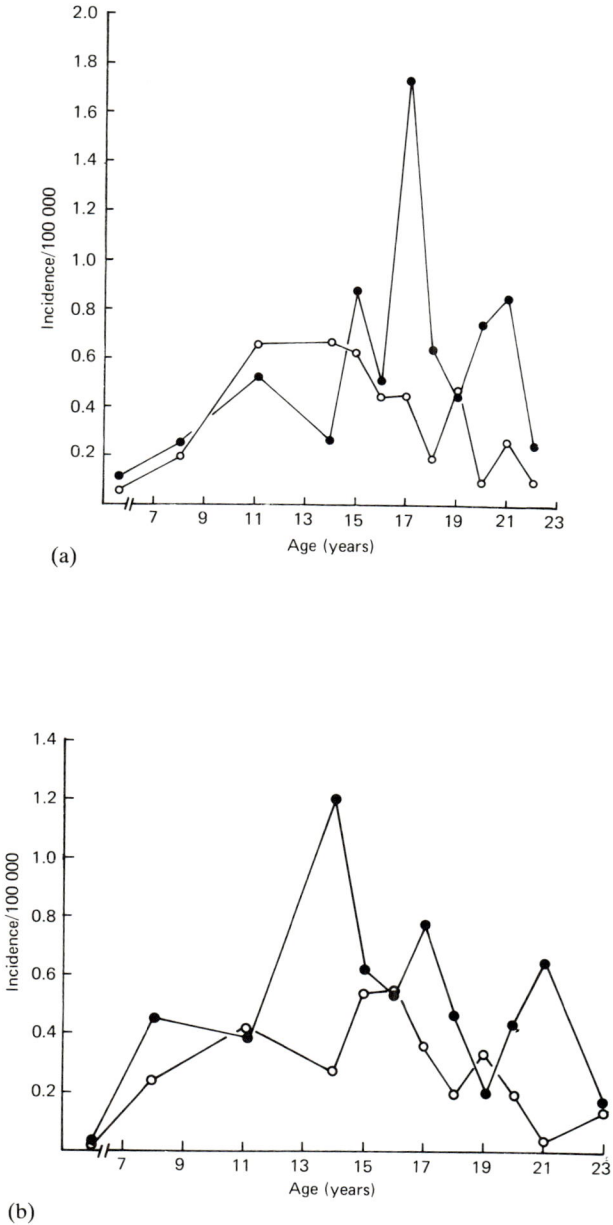

**Figure 2.** Annual incidence rates per 100000 by age and sex, for (a) osteosarcoma and (b) Ewing's sarcoma in New York residents, 1974–1980 (closed circles = males, open circles = females). From Polednak (1985b).

Ewing's sarcoma respectively). The increase in risk is particularly noticeable in males aged 12–17 years, which is the period of peak incidence in boys.

Miller (1981) studied this phenomenon in a slightly different way. He noted no sex difference in the incidence of bone cancer *mortality* between boys and girls until the age of 13 years, when there was a clear difference, that of boys exceeding girls. At this age the difference in height also became apparent—the boys growing more than the girls. It is of interest that in dogs, osteosarcoma is much more common in very large breeds than in large or small ones (risk ratio 185:13:1, Tjalma, 1966).

It can be postulated therefore that the phase of rapid linear bone growth is in some way related to the origin of bone sarcoma and that this is manifest as an increased incidence in tumours during adolescence and in taller children. Similar factors may be operating in Paget's disease (see below) and in the aetiology of tumours arising in areas of previous bone trauma and old bone infarcts.

## RACE

The most striking racial difference in incidence is in the extreme rarity of Ewing's sarcoma in blacks compared with whites (Figure 3). This was first reported by Glass and Fraumeni (1970) and by Jensen and Drake (1970) and has since been amply confirmed in the USA and other countries. In Uganda, data from the cancer registry in Kampala revealed 56 cases of skeletal tumours (Burkitt's lymphoma was excluded) of which 22 were osteosarcoma and none were Ewing's sarcoma. Chinese children have a similarly low incidence (Li et al, 1980). Whites and blacks have very similar incidence rates for osteosarcoma (Miller, 1976, 1981; Polednak, 1985a). Huvos et al (1983b), at the Memorial Sloan-Kettering Hospital, noticed an increasing referral of cases of osteosarcoma in black Americans and wondered if this represented an increase in its incidence. There are at present no firm epidemiological data to support this. In their report the authors noticed little difference in histological type, age of onset, or outcome between black and white patients, but there was an increased proportion of upper tibia tumours in blacks. Polednak (1985a) noticed a suggestive, but not conclusive, increased incidence of chondrosarcoma in whites compared with blacks. The data are shown in Figure 4. The basis of these racial differences is not understood.

## GENETIC AND FAMILIAL FACTORS

Patients cured of retinoblastoma have an increased risk of developing other cancers, especially sarcomas (Jensen and Miller, 1971; Kitchin and Ellsworth, 1974). Since the early report of Sagerman et al (1969) there have been many reports of osteosarcoma of the orbit in patients with retinoblastoma who have been irradiated. Other sarcomatous orbital neoplasms occur as well (Francois, 1977). It seems that the incidence of this complication has

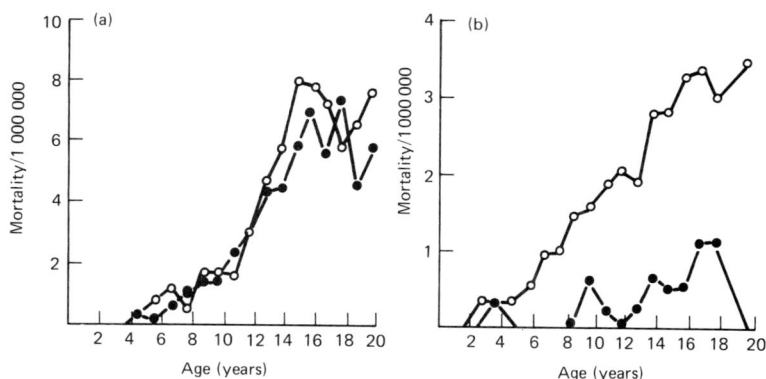

**Figure 3.** Mortality per million for (a) osteosarcoma and (b) Ewing's sarcoma in US whites (open circles) and blacks (closed circles). The figures are taken from Miller (1981) with permission. They span the years 1960–1964 for ages of less than 15 years, and 1965–1968 for ages of over 15 years. During this time period, mortality was a reasonable reflection of incidence.

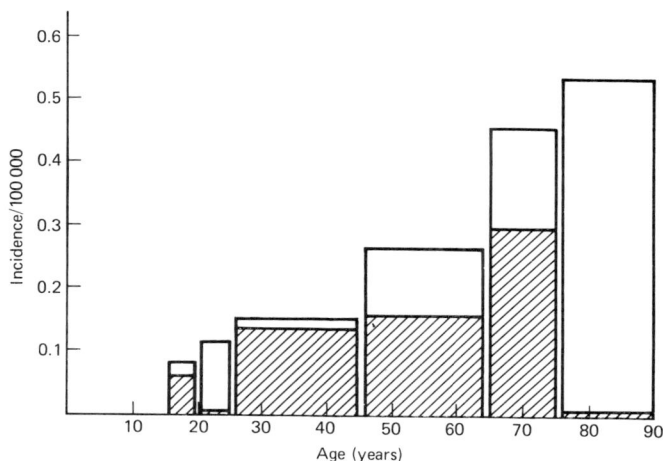

**Figure 4.** Annual age-specific incidence per 100000 of chondrosarcoma in white (open bars) and black (hatched bars) residents of New York State, 1975–1980. Data from Polednak (1985b).

fallen as the dose of radiation has been reduced, and is now estimated at 1–2% (Kitchin and Ellsworth, 1974).

Sarcomas also develop in non-irradiated retinoblastoma patients, and at unirradiated sites in patients who have been treated with radiotherapy. These cases almost always occur in patients with bilateral retinoblastoma (Vogel, 1979) in whom the risk of second tumours may be as high as 20% (Kitchin, 1976). A wide variety of second cancers may occur, carcinomas and sarcomas, but osteosarcoma is the commonest tumour. The cancers usually affect the long bones and the latent period (the period between the onset of retinoblastoma and the diagnosis of the second tumour) is about 10 years (Berg and Weiland, 1978). About 30% of retinoblastomas are bilateral and, of these, 20% are familial (6% of the total) and 80% are not familial. It appears that the retinoblastoma gene confers a general susceptibility to cancer, especially sarcomas, and that orbital irradiation acts to promote the appearance of the second orbital primary. The gene has been localized to the q14 band on the long arm of chromosome 13 (13q14) (Sparkes et al, 1980; Ward et al, 1984). Mutations affecting this gene can be inherited or may arise somatically. A recent report (Friend et al, 1986) has suggested that absence or inactivation of the gene or part of the gene is a feature of retinoblastoma and osteosarcoma. Recently there has also been a report of Ewing's sarcoma of the ulna in a 9-year-old girl who had her eyes removed 9 and 7 years previously (Schifter et al, 1983).

In a survey of first- and second-degree relatives of patients with bilateral (hereditary) retinoblastoma, there was an excess of cancer deaths, but this did not include excess deaths from bone sarcoma (Strong et al, 1984). Nevertheless, there have been reports of osteosarcoma in first-degree relatives of children with bilateral retinoblastoma (Schimke et al, 1974; Francois, 1977). It will be necessary to develop molecular probes for the retinoblastoma gene, or the closely associated esterase D locus, before the risk of osteosarcoma in carriers of the gene can be determined accurately.

Bone tumours may develop as part of other inherited syndromes which involve the bones. The best known syndrome is the sarcomatous change which occurs in Ollier's disease (multiple enchondromatosis). The tumour is almost always a chondrosarcoma and malignant change occurred in 10 out of 36 patients described by Unni and Dahlin (1979). In this disease multiple sarcomas may arise synchronously (Goodman et al, 1984). Osteosarcoma has been described in osteogenesis imperfecta (Klenerman et al, 1967) and is well recognized in Maffucci's syndrome. This is a syndrome of endochondromatosis and deep, cutaneous haemangiomas, occasionally with skin pigmentary changes. The progression to neoplasia occurs in adult life. The bone tumours are cartilaginous, but osteosarcoma may occur and sarcomas may develop in the skin lesions (Lewis and Ketcham, 1973). Malignant sarcomatous change may rarely occur (0.4% of cases) in fibrous dysplasia, usually when it is polyostotic (Schwartz and Alpert, 1964). Mulvihill et al (1977) have described an American Indian family in which three out of nine siblings had osteogenic sarcoma, nine of the family had erythrocyte macrocytosis, and one child had abnormalities of the limb.

Family aggregation of osteosarcoma has been reported and, in some of these cases, other tumours have occurred (including carcinoma of the adrenal cortex and glioma). In the families the usual relationship is that the tumour arises in siblings (Miller, 1981). Ewing's sarcoma has been reported in siblings twice (Hutter et al, 1964).

In 1983 there were two reports of a chromossoal abnormality in cultured fresh Ewing's tumour cells (Aurias et al, 1983) and cell lines (Turc-Carel et al, 1983). In the first study, reciprocal translocations were found in band q12 of chromosome 22. In two cases the translocation was t(11:22) (q24:q12).

In the second study, five cell lines were examined and a reciprocal translocation between chromosomes 11 and 22 was found in four of the cell lines, and the translocation in each case was t(11:22) (q24:q12). In three lines every cell showed the translocation, and 21% of cells showed it in the fourth line. It is of interest that the human homologue of the simian sarcoma virus oncogene (c-sis) has been located on the long arm of chromosome 22. It is possible that this cytogenetic abnormality may play a role in initiating malignant transformation or in maintaining cell growth after transformation has occurred.

## IONIZING IRRADIATION

Malignant bone tumours in humans can be caused by ionizing irradiation. There are two situations in which this has been clearly shown to occur. In the first the sarcomas arise in women who paint watch dials with radioactive paint, and in the second sarcomas develop when the bone has been included in a radiation field used to treat a previous malignancy.

### Radium-induced bone sarcoma

The history of the discovery of the association between bone tumours and the ingestion of radioactive paint by women working in a watch factory is remarkable in many respects. The definition of the problem was the work of an outstanding man—Harrison S. Martland—and his papers describing the conditions of employment, the chemistry of the paint, and the skeletal and haematological consequences to the workers make fascinating reading. In 1903 Sir William Crookes had discovered that when alpha rays (helium nuclei) impinged on a zinc sulphide screen, scintillations were produced. Using radium and zinc sulphide, luminous paints were developed in the USA from 1913 onwards, and in 1917 there were many small companies in the USA employing women to paint figures on military instruments, watches and clocks. Part of the impetus for the development of the industry had come from the USA entry into the first world war, and partly from the novelty of luminous watches. From 1913 to 1919 the output of radium dial watches rose from 8500 to 2 200 000. The conditions of employment were deplorable, with poor ventilation, dust everywhere and cans of radioactive mixtures lying about. The US Department of Labor (1929) reported that in some factories the walls and the employees' clothes were luminous in the dark. In the years 1917 to 1924 approximately 800 women were employed at a single factory in New Jersey, USA, painting watch and clock dials with luminous paint. The formula for the paint had been devised by the chemist, Dr Sabin A. von Sochocky of the United States Radium Corporation. It consisted of zinc sulphide crystals to which were added radium ($^{226}$Ra) and mesothorium ($^{228}$Ra) in the form of insoluble sulphates in varying and probably inconstant proportions. These crystals decayed, emitting alpha particles and causing disintegration of the zinc sulphide. Dr von Sochocky devised almost all of the compound used by the industry. Von Sochocky was said to have been fascinated by the qualities of radium, to have played with it, watching the scintillations in the dark, and to have plunged his arms up to the elbow in solutions of radium or mesothorium (Bureau of Labor Statistics, 1929). Many of the records of his formulae have never been found. The girls pointed the brushes on their lips before painting the dial. No protective precautions were taken in the factory until 1925.

The first sign of trouble was in 1922 when a 20-year-old woman developed osteomyelitis of the jaw after a tooth extraction. She was reported as a case of 'phosphorus necrosis' on 26 December of that year, but Dr Szamatolski, the consulting chemist for the New Jersey Department of Labor, doubted this and suggested, for the first time, that this was due to the 'serious influence of radium'. Two other deaths were then discovered and the fifth case—a 24-year-old woman—developed anaemia and jaw necrosis and died. Her case was reported in 1924 by a dentist, Theodore Blum, at a meeting of the American Dental Association (Blum, 1924). A further report by F. L. Hoffman (1925) described 17 cases of anaemia and jaw lesions. Castle et al (1925) also described aseptic jaw necrosis. Harrison Martland was the county medical examiner for Essex County, New Jersey, and a pathologist at the City Hospital, Newark. As medical examiner he had a function 'to prevent the wastage of human life in industry' (Martland, 1929). He first showed the deposition of radioactivity in the bones at the autopsy of a patient with jaw necrosis and anaemia by a remarkable use of 'auto historadiography' which has only just been invented by Lacassagne in 1925. The deposition was in both the mandible and in bones remote from the site of ingestion, such as the femur (Martland, 1926). The necrosis of the mandible was correctly recognized as osteoradionecrosis by Martland and was presumably due to paint penetrating between the gum and the teeth. The aplastic anaemia was due to marrow irradiation and the aetiology of the aplasia was also correctly recognized by Martland. Later he described a case of osteosarcoma of the scapula in an employee (Martland and Humphries, 1929) and referred to another case of which he had heard. The occurrence of two cases in 15 affected workers was 'too high to be mere coincidence', he wrote.

In 1931 Martland reported a total of five cases of osteosarcoma which had occurred from 1924 to 1931 in the women at this one factory (an annual incidence of 1 in 1000, which is 100 times greater than spontaneous osteosarcoma). By this time the radionecrosis of the jaw had stopped appearing and there were no further deaths from aplastic anaemia. Martland developed further techniques to demonstrate the radon gas which was being exhaled in the breath of the workers (Martland, 1929), and he developed a detailed theory of the deposition of the insoluble paint particles, after absorption through the gut, into the phagocytic cells of the bone marrow, liver and spleen. Here, persistent, highly damaging, alpha particle irradiation continued for the lifetime of the victims. Dr von Sochocky died of aplastic anaemia, 'a horrible death' according to Martland (1929), but before he died he helped Martland with his investigations and his understanding of the chemistry of the production of the paint.

Studies and follow-up of these women were undertaken at the New Jersey

State Board of Health, the Argonne National Laboratory and the Massachusetts Institute of Technology, and have given valuable and detailed information on the oncogenic properties of ionizing irradiation and of bone-seeking isotopes in particular. From 1969 these studies were centralized at the Centre for Human Radiobiology in Argonne. A detailed account is given by Woodard (1980). The first comprehensive report, of 30 heavily exposed patients, was provided by Aub et al (1952, with Martland as co-author). This series is very selective and therefore gives no estimate of incidence, but provides a comprehensive account of dosimetry, measurement techniques and clinical details. It is also the first description of the carcinomas of the mastoid air cells and paranasal sinuses which also developed in these women.

Following ingestion or intravenous injection, $^{226}$Ra and $^{228}$Ra [mesothorium (MsTh) which is isotopic with $^{226}$Ra] are rapidly lost from the soft tissues and, in man, over 90% of the retained dose is found in the bones. The highest concentrations are found, in growing rats, in the epiphyses and trabecular bone, and the lowest concentrations are found in the metaphysis. Bone-seeking isotopes such as $^{228}$Ra (mesothorium), strontium and plutonium are taken into the bone (in the case of radium this is on the surface of the trabeculae) and thence into new bone crystals as they are formed. The diffuse deposition of radium in bone is a slow process. The osteoblasts, which are the probable progenitors of osteosarcoma, lie on the trabecular surface and are thus most heavily exposed to the alpha particle emission from $^{226}$Ra. The sequence of radioactive decay of $^{226}$Ra and $^{228}$Ra is shown in Table 2. While $^{226}$Ra is deposited in bone in a manner similar to calcium, radiothorium—a decay product of $^{228}$Ra—has the same atomic number as thorium and will be handled like that element. Aub et al (1952) claimed that radiothorium is deposited in the periosteum and endosteum of the bone rather than in the bone crystals. They considered that $^{228}$Ra may have been as important as $^{226}$Ra in the induction of the cancers, but there is little evidence to support this.

**Table 2.** The radioactive decay of $^{226}$Ra and $^{228}$Ra (mesothorium). The reader is reminded that the atomic mass number is the number of protons plus the number of neutrons. Alpha emission is two protons and two neutrons (a helium nucleus, fall in mass no. of 4) and beta emission is a neutron decaying to a proton and an electron (no change in mass no.).

| | Isotope | Mass no. | t1/2 | Emission | Product |
|---|---|---|---|---|---|
| A | Radium | 226 | 1600 yr | α | Radon (gas) |
| | Radon | 222 | 3.8 days | α | RaA |
| | RaA to RaD | 218–210 | 33 min | 2α 2β | RaD |
| | RaD | 210 | 22 yr | β | RaE |
| | RaE to RaG | 210–206 | 145 days | 1α 1β | RaG |
| | | | | | |
| B | $^{228}$Ra (mesothorium) | 228 | 6.7 yr | β | MsTh$_2$ |
| | MsTh$_2$ | 228 | 6 h | β | RdTh |
| | RdTh | 228 | 1.9 yr | α | $^{224}$Ra (ThX) |
| | $^{224}$Ra ThX | 224–208 | 3.65 days | 4α 1β | ThD ($^{208}$Pb) |

RaA–G = radium A–G, MsTh = mesothorium, RdTh = radiothorium, ThX = thorium X, ThD = thorium D.

Over the next 20 years, cases of osteosarcoma and fibrosarcoma of bone occurred in these dial workers and were reported occasionally. Woodard and Higinbotham (1962) reported a case of a 54-year-old woman who in 1954 developed the first symptoms of osteosarcoma of the left knee 37 years after she had worked in the watch factory in Newark. She died of the tumour. The authors were able to calculate that the accumulated dose to the areas of high radioactivity in the bone (demonstrated by autoradiography) was 88000 rads, while to the 'diffuse' areas away from the focal sites the dose was 1400 rads. They expressed the view that the cancer would arise from the intermediate areas since cell death would occur at the regions of high radioactivity. Interestingly, although the patient was 16 years old when she started work, the radioactivity was concentrated at the epiphyseal plate—presumably still the site of active bone remodelling at that age.

The US Bureau of Labor Statistics (1929) estimated that up to 2000 people had been employed from 1913. Of these, 1400 were identified and 1250 were located. From the mid-1950s up to 1975, no less than 751 of these women had been examined and the body radium burden measured and calculated. In 20 cases the radium content of exhumed skeletons was measured. The results of this enquiry, insofar as it relates to bone cancer, were described by Dr A. P. Polednak, then also working at the Centre for Human Radiobiology in Argonne (Polednak, 1978). He pointed out the great difficulty of making reliable calculations of the latent interval between exposure and the development of the tumour in a situation in which people are being followed over a long period of time, because death occurs from other causes. Nevertheless, a striking cumulative risk of developing bone cancer was shown for those receiving 200–749 µCi and 750 µCi or greater (Figure 5). Below 200 µCi, no cases of bone cancer occurred. This dose appeared to be a biological threshold in that no tumours developed within the lifespan of the individual. There was a tendency for this risk to be greater in those below the age of 18 years at the time of the first exposure. The details of the histology of the 58 bone cancers were not available. The results of a more detailed analysis of the dose–response relationship for both the osteosarcoma and the mastoid and paranasal carcinomas ('head cancers') was presented by Rowland et al (1978). They calculated that $^{226}$Ra was 2.5 times as effective as $^{228}$Ra in producing bone sarcomas. In the case of the head cancers, they followed the suggestion of Evans (1966) that the noble gas, radon, would be the main aetiological factor. This is liberated from $^{226}$Ra but not from $^{228}$Ra so this isotope can be ignored for this tumour. The doses and exposures were calculated back from actual measurements in 759 women using a retention function developed by Norris et al (1955). They developed a curve-fitting programme which was able to define precisely the equation of the line which best fitted the observed incidence of osteosarcoma (Figure 6) and head cancer. Interestingly, the function for osteosarcoma was a dose-squared exponential, while the best fit for head cancer was linear.

From 1920 in the USA it was common practice for solutions of radium to be taken by mouth, or given intravenously, as a tonic, as a treatment for arthritis or tuberculosis. One such remedy was called 'Radiothor', made and sold by the Bailey Radium Laboratories between 1925 and 1930. Each bottle

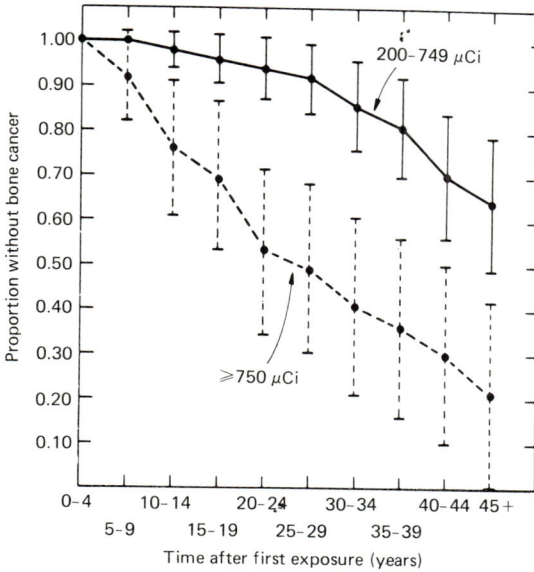

**Figure 5.** The probability of *not* developing bone cancer at the end of each stated time period in two groups of intake-dose. The bars represent 95% confidence limits and it is assumed that there have been no deaths from causes other than from bone cancer. From Polednak (1978), with permission.

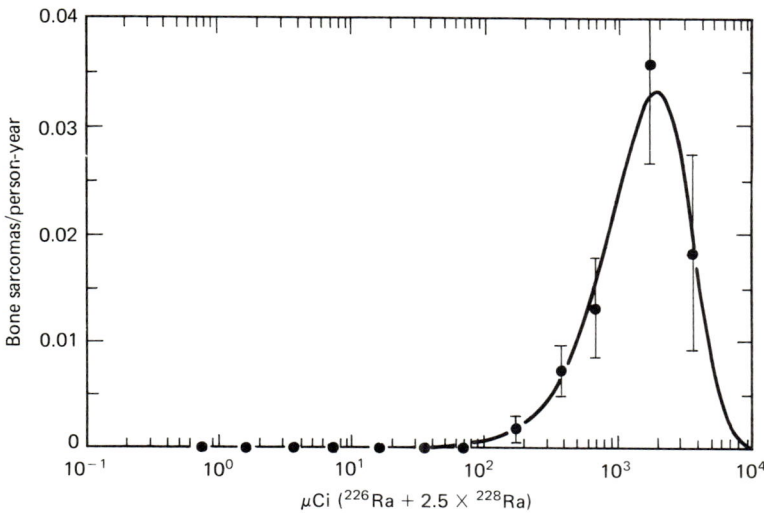

**Figure 6.** Bone sarcomas per person/year at risk as a function of systemic intake of $^{226}$Ra plus $2.5 \times {}^{228}$Ra, in microcuries, for female dial workers exposed before 1930. From Rowland et al (1978), with permission. The reference gives details of the fitted equation from which the line is derived.

had 1 µg of $^{226}$Ra and 1 µg $^{228}$Ra in 0.5 oz of water, and one bottle was recommended with each meal. Many victims drank over 1000 bottles (Gettler and Norris, 1933). Ampoules of 2 ml containing 5–100 µg of radium were used for intravenous injection. These patients have added to the information obtained from the radium dial painters. Further experience of radium carcinogenesis in man came from Germany, where about 2000 children and adults were treated by intravenous $^{224}$Ra between 1944 and 1957. Fifty-one per cent had tuberculosis and most of the rest had ankylosing spondylitis. They were aged from 1 to 70 years, and the doses ranged from 40–5000 µCi over periods from 2 to 72 months. The adverse results of this therapy have been described (Spiess and Mays, 1970, 1973; Mays et al, 1978). Bone sarcomas were induced in 53 out of 897 traceable patients. The short half-life of $^{224}$Ra (Table 2) means that exposure to radioactivity ceased within a few weeks of the last injection (which was, of course, not the case with long-lived $^{226}$Ra and $^{228}$Ra). This enabled Spiess and Mays (1973) to calculate the effect of protraction of the dose on the induction of bone sarcomas. The intravenous $^{224}$Ra was often given weekly, with the duration of treatment ranging from a few weeks to years. Spiess and Mays (1973) interpret the data as showing that, for $^{224}$Ra, the likelihood of developing bone sarcoma increased with increasing length of the period over which injections were given. Although larger doses tended to be given over a longer time period, the association of sarcoma with increasing duration of exposure appeared to be independent of the dose.

Osteogenic sarcomas have been produced experimentally in dogs, rats and other species by a variety of radioactive isotopes in addition to radium, including $^{45}$calcium and $^{90}$strontium. In most of these animal models the number of cancers increases with the administered dose and the time of administration, and there is a latent period for the induction of the tumour. This accords with the human data.

The damaging effects of long-lived, bone-seeking radioisotopes have been demonstrated and emphasized by these unfortunate events. Great care must be taken to protect workers and the general population from contact with such substances. In this context it is reassuring that no increased risk of cancer appears to apply to employees in the Atomic Energy Authority of the UK. In a survey conducted in 1985, Beral et al showed that in 39 546 employees working with the authority from 1946 to 1979 there was no increase in bone cancer (and no significant increase in standardized mortality in ratio for any tumour).

**Post-radiation sarcoma**

External beam irradiation can also cause bone cancer. In 1945, Hatcher reported three cases, and Cahan et al added a further 11 in 1948. Since then, the subject has been extensively reviewed (Arlen et al, 1971; Weatherby et al, 1981; Huvos et al, 1985).

At the time when Hatcher (1945) described three cases, there had been 24 case reports of sarcoma of bone arising in an irradiated field dating back to the first report by Beck in 1922. Of these cases, 17 had received external beam radiotherapy for tuberculous arthritis, and six had received radium treatment. The mean latent period was 6 years. (In this context 'latent period' means the time interval between the irradiation and the clinical appearance of cancer.) Hatcher's cases were a sarcoma arising 6 years after a giant cell tumour of bone had been irradiated at the age of 17 years, a 22-year-old irradiated for benign giant cell tumour who developed fibro-sarcoma 11 years later, and a rib chondrosarcoma arising 12 years after irradiation for breast cancer. The first two cases raised the difficult question of the nature of a second bone tumour after irradiation for a primary, but presumed benign, bone lesion.

In order to establish that there is a connection between the development of a sarcoma and previous radiotherapy, Cahan et al (1948) laid down certain guidelines which have usually been followed. These are: (1) that the sarcoma occurred in the radiation field, (2) that the histology of the pre-existing bone lesion, if present, was known, or that there was radiological evidence of its existence, (3) that there was histological proof of the sarcoma, and (4) that there was a latent period between radiation and the development of the sarcoma.

In the series described by Huvos et al (1985), different selection criteria were employed. They reviewed all their cases of osteosarcoma from 1921–1983 and found 66 cases (5.5%) which were post-radiation ones. In 42 cases the bone had been normal at the time of treatment, and in 24 the radiation was for a bone tumour or 'tumour-like lesion'. They excluded 23 other malignant bone lesions because they were not osteosarcoma. These were 15 malignant fibrous histiocytomas, four chondrosarcomas and four fibro-sarcomas. The age distribution is shown (for men and women) in Figure 7. The higher frequency in women aged 51–60 years is in part due to six cases who were previously irradiated for breast cancer.

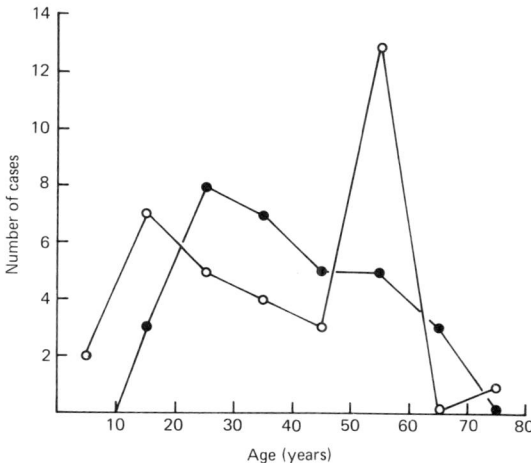

**Figure 7.** Age and sex distribution of post-radiation bone sarcoma. Data from Huvos et al (1985). ○, females; ●, males.

The sites of involvement (from various series) are shown in Table 3 and the histological subtypes in Huvos's series in Table 4. This report emphasized, as have other reviews, the high frequency of axial skeletal lesions, the preponderance of fibrohistiocytomatous lesions and the relative frequency of giant cell tumour and aneurysmal bone cysts as an underlying benign lesion on which the sarcoma develops. The mean radiation dose and latent period were similar in both groups (where the bone had previously either been normal or the site of a benign tumour) and values are shown in Table 5. These cases were chosen as being examples of radiation-induced osteosarcoma, but it is clear that a variety of histological types of bone sarcoma may be induced by radiation, and classification is not easy when there is overlap between histological appearances.

Radiotherapy of malignant bone tumours may itself give rise to second malignant bone neoplasms. Strong et al (1979) estimated the risk of a second malignant bone tumour in patients treated with radiotherapy and chemotherapy for Ewing's sarcoma to be 2600 times that of the normal childhood population. In a series of 23 cases studied more than 3 years after the completion of treatment, four cases had developed osteosarcoma and one other a cutaneous malignant fibrous histocytoma. These sobering findings are of great importance in the design of future treatment protocols in Ewing's tumour. Greene et al (1979) reported a similar, but less striking, association. In their series of 31 long-term survivors, one patient developed a bone fibrosarcoma at the irradiated site, and another a renal medullary

**Table 3.** Sites of post-radiation bone sarcoma compiled from various series.

| Site of sarcoma | % |
| --- | --- |
| Scapula, clavicle, humerus | 21 |
| Femur | 18 |
| Pelvis | 15 |
| Skull and jaw | 13.5 |
| Extraosseus | 10.5 |
| Cervical vertebrae | 3 |
| Tibia | 3 |
| Metacarpal | 1.5 |
| Ulna | 1.5 |

**Table 4.** Histological types of post-radiation osteosarcoma.

| Osteosarcoma | % |
| --- | --- |
| Fibrohistiocytomatous | 38 |
| Osteoblastic | 18 |
| Mixed pattern | 14 |
| Chondrosarcomatous | 12 |
| Fibrosarcomatous | 7.5 |
| Other | 7.5 |
| Telangiectatic | 3 |

From Huvos et al (1985), with permission.

**Table 5.** Dose of radiation and latent period in the induction of bone sarcoma in normal bone and after radiation of a prior bone lesion.

| | Induction of bone sarcoma | |
|---|---|---|
| | In normal bone | After radiation of a prior bone lesion |
| Radiation dose (rads) —mean and range | 4500 (2500–11 000) | 5900 (1660–11 500) |
| Latent period (yr) —mean and range | 10.5 (4–30) | 10.5 (3–33) |

From Huvos et al (1985), with permission.

neuroblastoma. Although the relative risk was not as high as in the report of Strong et al, the duration of follow-up was not as long.

## BONE TUMOURS AFTER TREATMENT OF CHILDHOOD CANCER

In the report of the Late Effects Study Group (Mike et al, 1982), 14 610 children diagnosed as having cancer were followed for a minimum observation period, from diagnosis, of 9 years. Known hereditary causes of cancer were excluded (xeroderma pigmentosum, retinoblastoma). In the survivors, 113 cases of second neoplasm were seen, with a cumulative probability of the development of a second cancer of 3.3% at 20 years and a ten-fold risk. Interestingly, eight out of the 1066 bone tumour cases developed a second cancer, and four of these were bone tumour. Overall, bone and soft tissue sarcomas were the commonest second cancer (20 cases out of 113). No details of the site of the bone cancers in relation to any irradiation were given. One interpretation of these data is that radiation and chemotherapy in childhood carry a small, but not insignificant, risk of causing bone cancer and other malignant tumours.

## PAGET'S SARCOMA

A variety of malignant bone tumours can arise in bones which are the site of Paget's disease. Paget himself reported five cases of sarcoma out of 23 patients with osteitis deformans (Paget, 1889) and since that time there have been several comprehensive reviews (Price and Goldie, 1969; Greditzer et al, 1983; Huvos et al, 1983a; Haibach et al, 1985). Paget's sarcoma is a disease of late middle age onwards. The age distribution in the series of Price and Goldie is shown in Figure 8. The highest frequency is in the sixth and seventh decades and, in many series, men are more commonly affected than women. The histology of the tumour is variable but osteosarcoma and fibrosarcoma are the commonest types (Table 6). The frequency of the different histological types is subject to variation in classification; in particular, some fibrosarcomatous forms of osteosarcoma are probably classified as fibrosarcomas in earlier series.

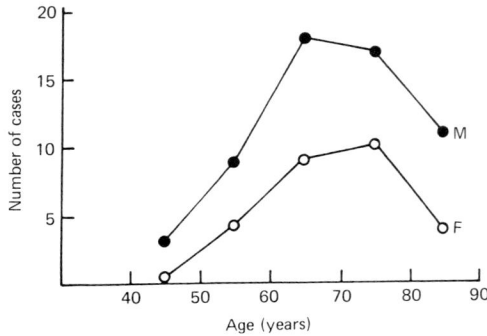

**Figure 8.** Age and sex distribution of Paget's sarcoma. Data from Price and Goldie (1969).

**Table 6.** Histological types of bone sarcoma in Paget's disease. Note that there may be considerable overlap between, for example, 'fibrosarcoma' and 'fibrosarcomatous osteosarcoma'.

| Sarcoma | Frequency (%) |
| --- | --- |
| Osteosarcoma | 58 |
| Chondrosarcomatous | 8.7 |
| Fibrosarcomatous | 10 |
| Fibrohistiocytomatous | 15 |
| Telangiectatic | 4 |
| Osteoblastic | 13 |
| Mixed | 8 |
| Fibrosarcoma | 25 |
| Lymphoma | 3 |
| Giant cell sarcoma | 5 |
| Other | 9 |

About 25% of all osteogenic sarcomas arise in bones affected by Paget's disease. The frequency with which this complication arises is not known for certain because the true incidence of Paget's disease is unknown. Price and Goldie (1969) give an annual incidence of Paget's sarcoma of 0.17 in 100000 in Bristol and Leeds, with an incidence of 0.38 in 100000 over the age of 40 years. Since Paget's disease is found in 3.7% of autopsies, the authors estimate that the risk of sarcomatous change is about 1 in 500 cases. It contrast, an estimate of 1% is given by Wick et al (1981) but this seems far too high for such a common disease as Paget's. Curiously, the sarcomas do not completely reflect the sites of Paget's disease itself. Table 7 shows the frequency with which different bones are affected by Paget's disease, primary osteosarcoma and Paget's sarcoma. While the vertebral bodies are frequently the site of Paget's disease, it is extremely rare for a Paget's

**Table 7.** Frequency of Paget's disease, primary osteosarcoma and Paget's sarcoma at different sites (data compiled from several large studies).

| | Paget's disease (%) | Osteosarcoma (%) | Paget's sarcoma (%) |
|---|---|---|---|
| Humerus | 7 | 17 | 22 |
| Femur | 8 | 44 | 24 |
| Skull | 13 | 2 | 9 |
| Pelvis | 30 | 6 | 22 |
| Tibia | 5 | 16 | 10 |
| Vertebra | 32 | 1 | 1 |
| Jaw | 0 | 5 | 3 |
| Sacrum | 2 | 1 | 3 |
| Other | 3 | 8 | 5 |

sarcoma to arise at this site (Campbell and Whitfield, 1943; Shannon and Hopkins, 1977). Paget's sarcoma appears to develop more frequently in the humerus and femur than would be expected from the frequency of Paget's disease at these sites. Rarely, Paget's sarcoma may arise synchronously at multiple sites.

Paget's disease itself commonly causes pain, and sarcomatous change is usually manifested by increasingly severe pain, later accompanied by swelling. The symptoms of sarcomatous transformation may be present for up to 5 years before diagnosis, but usually for less than a year. About one-quarter of all patients experience a fracture at the site of the sarcoma. The bone X-ray usually shows a lytic lesion (65% of cases) but sclerotic changes may occur, or a mixture of the two. The fibrohistiocytic form of osteosarcoma is particularly likely to cause a lytic bone lesion, and the predominance of this type and 'fibrosarcoma' probably explains the frequency of the lytic lesion and fracture.

The age of patients and the site of the tumours makes treatment difficult. Surgical excision is the mainstay of treatment, but this is not feasible in many patients. There has been almost no examination of the role of chemotherapy, probably because of the difficulty in treating this predominantly elderly population with the intensive regimens which appear to be necessary in the young patient with osteosarcoma. At inoperable sites, current management consists of combination chemotherapy as for operable osteosarcoma, if the patient's age and condition allows it, and radiotherapy. The latter must be given at a high dose (see chapter 10) to have any chance of local control. Debulking surgery may sometimes be feasible prior to chemotherapy and radiation.

Results of treatment, in reported series, are poor. Huvos et al (1983a) reported only 3 out of 65 patients surviving at 5 years, with a median survival of 8 months and a 2-year survival of approximately 17%. Almost identical data were reported by Price and Goldie in 1969 in the era before chemotherapy.

## SUMMARY

A great deal is known about aetiological factors in bone sarcoma, especially osteosarcoma. The tragedy of the ingestion of radium by the dial painters has given valuable information on dose and latency in bone cancer. The association of the tumours with the phase of rapid bone growth in adolescence and in Paget's disease suggests that increased rate of cell division in bone is an associated causal factor perhaps acting in association with environmental and hormonal stimuli. Constitutional and acquired genetic abnormalities have been shown to be associated with osteosarcoma and Ewing's sarcoma respectively. As with many human cancers, multiple steps are probably necessary for oncogenesis and subsequent tumour and growth development.

## Acknowledgements

I would like to thank the following for their great help in providing me with information about the radium dial workers and for biographical details of Dr Martland: Dr Samuel Berg, Dr Anthony Polednak, Dr William Sharpe, Dr James Stebbings, Dr Helen Woodard.

## REFERENCES

Arlen M, Higinbotham NL, Huvos AG et al (1971) Radiation-induced sarcomas of bone. *Cancer* **28:** 1087–1099.

Aub JC, Evans RD, Hempelmann LH & Martland HS (1952) Late effects of internally-deposited radioactive materials in man. *Medicine* **31:** 221–329.

Aurias A, Rimbaut C, Buffe D, Dubousset J & Mazabraud A (1983) Chromosomal translocations in Ewing's sarcoma. *New England Journal of Medicine* **309:** 496–497.

Beck A, (1922) Zur Farge des Rontagensarkoms, zugleich ein Beitrag zur Pathogenese des sarkomas. *Munchener Medicale Wehnschrift* **LXIX:** 623.

Beral V, Inskip H, Fraser P et al (1985) Mortality of employers of the United Kingdom Atomic Energy Authority, 1946–1979. *British Medical Journal* **291:** 440–447.

Berg HL & Weiland AJ (1978) Multiple osteogenic sarcoma following bilateral retinoblastoma. *Journal of Bone and Joint Surgery* **60A:** 251–253.

Birch JM, Marsden HB & Swindell R (1980) Incidence of malignant disease in childhood: a 24 year review of the Manchester Children's Tumour Registry data. *British Journal of Cancer* **42:** 215–223.

Blum T (1924) Osteomyelitis of the mandible and maxilla. *Journal of the American Dental Association* **11:** 802–805.

Cahan WG, Woodard HQ, Higinbotham NL, Stewart FW & Coley BL (1948) Sarcoma arising in irradiated bone: report of eleven cases. *Cancer* **1:** 3–29.

Campbell E & Whitfield RD (1943) Osteogenic sarcoma of vertebrae secondary to Paget's disease: report of three cases with compression of spinal cord and cauda equina. *New York State Journal of Medicine* **43:** 931–938.

Castle WB, Drinker KR & Drinker CK (1925) Necrosis of the jaw in workers employed in applying a luminous paint containing radium. *Journal of Industrial Hygiene* **7:** 371–382.

Evans RD (1966) The effect of skeletally deposited alpha-ray emitters in man. *British Journal of Radiology* **39:** 881–895.

Francois J (1977) Retinoblastoma and osteogenic sarcoma. *Ophthalmologica* **175:** 185–191.

Fraumeni JF (1967) Stature and malignant tumours of bone in childhood and adolescence. *Cancer* **20:** 967–973.

Friend SH, Bernards R, Rogel JS et al (1986) A human DNA segment with properties of the gene that predisposes to retinoblastoma and osteosarcoma. *Nature* **323:** 643–646.

Gettler AO & Norris C (1933) Poisoning from drinking radium water. *Journal of the American Medical Association* **100:** 400–407.

Glass AC & Fraumeni JF (1970) Epidemiology of bone cancer in children. *Journal of the National Cancer Institute* **44:** 187–190.

Goodman SB, Bell RS, Fornasier VL, de Demeter D & Bateman JE (1984) Ollier's disease with multiple sarcomatous transformations. *Human Pathology* **15:** 91–93.

Greditzer HG, McLeod RA, Unni KK et al (1983) Bone sarcomas in Paget's disease. *Radiology* **146:** 327–333.

Greene, MH, Glaubiger DL, Mead GD & Fraumeni JF (1979) Subsequent cancer in patients with Ewing's sarcoma. *Cancer Treatment Reports* **63:** 2043–2046.

Haibach H, Carrell C & Dittrich FJ (1985) Neoplasms arising in Paget's disease of bone: a study of 82 cases. *American Journal of Clinical Pathology* **83:** 594–600.

Hatcher CH (1945) The development of sarcoma in bone subjected to roentgen or radium irradiation. *Journal of Bone and Joint Surgery* **27:** 179–195.

Hoffman FL (1925) Radium (mesothorium) necrosis. *Journal of the American Medical Association* **85:** 961.

Hutter RV, Francis KC & Foote FW Jr (1964) Ewing's sarcoma in siblings. Report of the second known occurrence. *American Journal of Surgery* **107:** 598–603.

Huvos AG, Butler A & Bretsky SS (1983a) Osteogenic sarcoma associated with Paget's disease of bone. A clinicopathologic study of 65 patients. *Cancer* **52:** 1489–1495.

Huvos AG, Butler A & Bretsky SS (1983b) Osteogenic sarcoma in the American black. *Cancer* **52:** 1959–1965.

Huvos AG, Woodard HQ, Cahan WG et al (1985) Postradiation osteogenic sarcoma of bone and soft tissues: a clinicopathologic study of 66 patients. *Cancer* **55:** 1244–1255.

Jensen RD & Drake RM (1970) Rarity of Ewing's sarcoma in Negroes. *Lancet* **i:** 777–779.

Jensen RD & Miller RW (1971) Retinoblastoma: epidemiologic characteristics. *New England Journal of Medicine* **285:** 307–311.

Kitchin FD (1976) genetics of retinoblastoma. In Rees AE (ed.) *Tumors of the Eye*, pp 90–132. Harper and Row: Hagerstown, Maryland.

Kitchin FD & Ellsworth RM (1974) Pleiotropic effects of the gene for retinoblastoma. *Journal of Medical Genetics* **11:** 244–246.

Klenerman L, Ockenden BG & Townsend AC (1967) Osteosarcoma occurring in osteogenesis imperfecta. Report of 2 cases. *Journal of Bone and Joint Surgery* **49B:** 314–323.

Kramer S, Meadows AT, Jarrett P & Evans AE (1983) Incidence of childhood cancer: experience of a decade in a population-based registry. *Journal of the National Cancer Institute* **70:** 49–55.

Lewis RJ & Ketcham AD (1973) Maffucci's syndrome, functional and neoplastic significance, case report and review of the literature. *Journal of Bone and Joint Surgery* **55A:** 1465–1479.

Li FP, Tu J, Liu F & Shiang E (1980) Rarity of Ewing's sarcoma in China. *Lancet* **i:** 1255–1257.

Martland HS (1926) Microscopic changes of certain anaemias due to radioactivity. *Archives of Pathology* **2:** 465–472.

Martland HS (1929) Occupational poisoning in manufacture of luminous watch dials. *Journal of the American Medical Association* **92:** 466–473.

Martland HS (1931) The occurrence of malignancy in radioactive persons. *American Journal of Cancer* **15:** 2435–2516.

Martland HS & Humphries RE (1929) Osteogenic sarcoma in dial painters using luminous paint. *Archives of Pathology* **7:** 406–417.

Mays CW, Spiess H & Gerspach A (1978) Skeletal effects following Ra 224 infections into humans. *Health Physics* **35:** 83–90.

Mike V, Meadows AT & D'Angio GJ (1982) Incidence of second malignant neoplasms in children: results of an international study. *Lancet* **ii:** 1326–1331.

Miller RW (1976) Aetiology of childhood bone cancer: epidemiologic observations. *Recent Results Cancer Research* **54:** 50–62.

Miller RW (1981) Contrasting epidemiology of childhood osteosarcoma, Ewing's tumor and rhabdomyosarcoma. *National Cancer Institute Monograph* **56:** 9–14.

Mulvihill JJ, Gralnick HR, Whang-Peng J & Leventhal BE (1977) Multiple childhood osteosarcomas in an American Indian Family with erythroid macrocytosis and skeletal anomalies. *Cancer* **40:** 3115–3122.

Norris WP, Speckman TW & Gustafson PF (1955) Studies on the metabolism of radium in man. *American Journal of Roentgenology, Radiation Therapy and Nuclear Medicine* **73:** 785–802.

Paget J (1889) Remarks on osteitis deformans. *Illustrated Medical News* **2**: 181–182.

Polednak AP (1978) Bone cancer among female radium dial workers. Latency periods and incidence rates by time after exposure. *Journal of the National Cancer Institute* **60**: 77–82.

Polednak AP (1985a) Primary bone cancer incidence in blacks and whites in New York State. *Cancer* **55**: 2883–2890.

Polednak AP (1985b) Human biology and epidemiology of childhood bone cancers: a review. *Human Biology* **57**: 1–26.

Price CHG (1955) Osteogenic sarcoma: an analysis of the age and sex incidence. *British Journal of Cancer* **9**: 558–574.

Price CHG (1958) Primary bone-forming tumours and their relationship and skeletal growth. *Journal of Bone and Joint Surgery* **40B**: 574–593.

Price CHG & Goldie W (1969) Paget's sarcoma of bone. A study of 80 cases from the Bristol and Leeds Bone Tumour Registries. *Journal of Bone and Joint Surgery* **51B**: 205–224.

Rowland RE, Stehney AF & Lucas HF (1978) Dose–response relationships for female radium dial workers. *Radiation Research* **76**: 368–383.

Sagerman RH, Cassady JW, Tretter P & Ellsworth RM (1969) Radiation induced neoplasia following external beam therapy for children with retinoblastoma. *American Journal of Roentgenology* **105**: 529–535.

Schifter S, Vendelbo L, Jensen OM & Kaae S (1983) Ewing's tumour following bilateral retinoblastoma. *Cancer* **51**: 1746–1749.

Schimke RN, Lowmann JT & Cowan GA (1974) Retinoblastoma and osteogenic sarcoma in siblings. *Cancer* **34**: 2077–2079.

Schwartz DT & Alpert HR (1964) The malignant transformation of fibrous dysplasia. *American Journal of Medical Science* **247**: 1–20.

Shannon FT & Hopkins JS (1977) Paget's sarcoma of the vertebral column with neurological complications. *Acta Orthopaedica Scandinavica* **48**: 385–390.

Sparkes RS, Sparkes MC, Wilson MG et al (1980) Regional assessment of genes for human esterase D and retinoblastoma to chromosome band 13q14. *Science* **208**: 1042–1044.

Spiess H & Mays CW (1970) Bone cancers induced by Ra 224 (ThX) in children and adults. *Health Physics* **19**: 713–729.

Spiess H & Mays CW (1973) Protraction effect of bone sarcoma induction of $^{224}$Ra in children and adults. In Saunders CL (ed.) *Radionuclide Carcinogenesis*, pp 437–450. US Atomic Energy Commission.

Strong LC, Henderson J, Osbourne BM & Sutow WW (1979) Risk of radiation-related subsequent malignant tumours in survivors of Ewing's sarcoma. *Journal of the National Cancer Institute* **62**: 1401–1405.

Strong LC, Herson J, Haas C et al (1984) Cancer mortality in relatives of retinoblastoma patients. *Journal of the National Cancer Institute* **73**: 303–311.

Tjalma RA (1966) Canine bone sarcoma: estimation of relative risk as a function of body size. *Journal of the National Cancer Institute* **36**: 1137–1150.

Turc-Carel C, Philip I, Berger M-P, Philip J & Lenoir G (1983) Chromosomal translocations in Ewing's sarcoma. *New England Journal of Medicine* **309**: 497–498.

Unni KK & Dahlin DC (1979) Premalignant tumours and conditions of bone. *American Journal of Surgical Pathology* **3**: 47–58.

US Bureau of Labor Statistics (1929) Radium poisoning. *Monthly Labor Review* **28**: 1200–1275.

Vogel F (1979) Genetics of retinoblastoma. *Human Genetics* **52**: 1–54.

Ward PS, Packman PS, Loughman W et al (1984) Location of the retinoblastoma susceptibility gene(s) and the human esterase D locus. *Journal of Medical Genetics* **21**: 92–95.

Weatherby RP, Dahlin DC & Ivins JC (1981) Post-radiation sarcoma of bone: review of 78 Mayo Clinic cases. *Mayo Clinic Proceedings* **56**: 294–306.

Weinfeld MS & Dudley HR (1962) Osteogenic sarcoma. *Journal of Bone and Joint Surgery* **44A**: 269–276.

Wick MR, McLeod RA, Siegal GP et al (1981) Sarcomas of bone complicating osteitis deformans (Paget's disease): fifty years experience. *American Journal of Surgery and Pathology* **5**: 47–59.

Woodard HQ (1980) Radiation carcinogenesis in man: a critical review. USA: Department of Energy.

Woodard HQ & Higinbotham NL (1962) Development of osteogenic sarcoma in a radium dial painter 37 years after the exposure. *American Journal of Medicine* **32**: 96–102.

**2**

# Pathology of bone tumours

## JEAN A. S. PRINGLE

Changing methods in the treatment of primary bone tumours, in particular adjuvant chemotherapy and conservative surgery, have increased the contribution of the histopathologist to the management of bone tumour cases. In addition to establishing the diagnosis, confirmation of clearance at the time of local resection is required, together with evaluation of histological response to preoperative chemotherapy.

## BONE BIOPSY

With few exceptions, lesions where a bone tumour is considered in the differential diagnosis are biopsied. Biopsy should be carried out only when all other aspects of the case have been thoroughly examined and appropriate X-rays have been performed. At this stage a differential diagnosis has evolved, enabling the pathologist to decide prior to biopsy what particular techniques might be appropriate in handling the tissue. Frozen sections are rarely used at the Institute of Orthopaedics. They are often technically difficult and may be unsatisfactory or frankly misleading. In our experience the use of touch/imprint preparations can often establish or confirm a diagnosis. This technique is also of great value in assessing clearance during local resection of tumours. The technique is simple and the imprints can be made by the surgeon or radiologist performing the biopsy if the pathologist is not at hand to deal with the fresh tissue. A small piece of tumour is prepared with a scalpel to give a fresh cut surface. If very bloody, excess blood is carefully blotted off and then holding the tumour gently with forceps, the fresh cut surface is placed in contact with the surface of a dry, clean glass slide and lifted off. This is done four to six times in a circular area near the centre of the slide. The slides are air dried and either stained immediately or stored. Conventional and special stains, enzyme histochemistry and immunocytochemistry can all be performed on these imprint preparations. There is often great pressure on the pathologist to produce an answer rapidly, and this is particularly so in the case of a suspected bone tumour. Unfortunately, inadequate fixation and over-rapid or incomplete decalcification can contribute to sections of poor quality, making diagnosis difficult. The use of the imprint preparation in addition to conventional histology can often provide a very rapid diagnosis. Discussion of the case by the surgeon and the pathologist is of particular importance in assessing clearance at the time of prosthetic replacement. However, the use of touch preparations is not advisable in hospitals where only very occasional bone tumours are seen, and even in specialist centres, these preparations should not be used without adequate knowledge of all aspects of the case.

Surgical aspects of bone biopsy are discussed in Chapter 5.

## CLASSIFICATION OF BONE TUMOURS

The major primary bone tumours are derived from the specialized skeletal connective tissue that comprises bone. This connective tissue has the ability to produce different matrices—collagen, osteoid, bone and cartilage. Tumours are named according to the pattern of differentiation they show. Within any one pattern of differentiation there are benign and malignant tumours and often a group of lesions of intermediate malignancy.

Other primary bone tumours are of unknown histogenesis, such as Ewing's sarcoma, while another group is derived from tissues within bone but not peculiar to bone, including tumours of vascular, smooth muscle, nerve and fat origin. Myeloma and lymphoma may be confined to bone at the time of presentation. Rarely, malignant change may occur in a pre-existing benign bone lesion. A small number of tumours are associated with abnormal bone. Finally, a small group arises from tissue rests within bone.

## TUMOURS OF OSTEOBLASTIC DIFFERENTIATION (Table 1)

### Osteoid osteoma and benign osteoblastoma

Although histologically they may be indistinguishable, these two tumours fully justify separate names as their clinical, radiological and gross patho-logical features are very different (Schajowicz and Lemos, 1970). Both tend to occur in children, adolescents and young adults (see Chapter 6). Both comprise regular trabeculae of osteoid with a varying amount of mineral-ization arising from a background of vascular, moderately cellular tissue containing osteoblasts and osteoclasts (Figure 1). The osteoid osteoma measures less than 1 cm in diameter (Byers, 1968) and is surrounded by a zone of dense reactive bone (Figure 2). Fine detail X-rays are helpful in locating the lesional tissue.

### Aggressive osteoblastoma

Benign osteoblastoma may recur locally if removal is incomplete, without any histological evidence of aggression (Jackson, 1978). A few cases have been reported where a lesion that was initially entirely acceptable as a benign osteoblastoma has, over a period of time, undergone malignant transformation (Merryweather et al, 1980). In 1976, Schajowicz and Lemos

**Table 1.** Tumours of osteoblastic differentiation.

*Benign*
Osteoma
Osteoid osteoma
Benign osteoblastoma

*Intermediate*
Aggressive osteoblastoma

*Malignant*
Osteosarcoma, high grade, conventional, central or rarely juxtacortical. Histological subtypes:
    osteoblastic
    fibroblastic
    chondroblastic
    osteoclast-rich
    teleangiectatic
Parosteal osteosarcoma
Periosteal osteosarcoma
Multicentric osteosarcoma
Osteoblastoma-like osteosarcoma
Low-grade central osteosarcoma

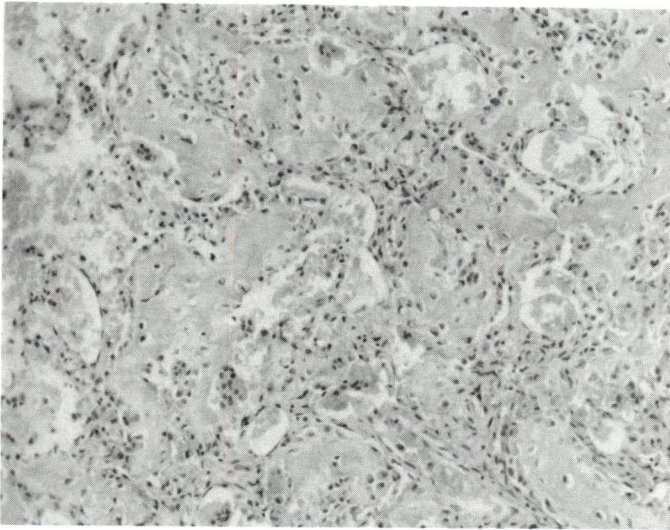

**Figure 1.** Benign osteoblastoma. Regular trabeculae of osteoid are set in a background of vascular tissue containing osteoblasts of fairly uniform size which are rimming many trabeculae. Osteoclasts are also present. Original magnification × 200.

described eight osteoblastic tumours of intermediate malignancy which they called 'malignant osteoblastoma'. Other labels applied to this group of tumours include 'aggressive osteoblastoma' (Revell and Scholtz, 1979), and more recently 'osteoblastoma-like osteosarcoma' (Bertoni et al, 1985). They are exceedingly rare and have a predilection for the axial skeleton.

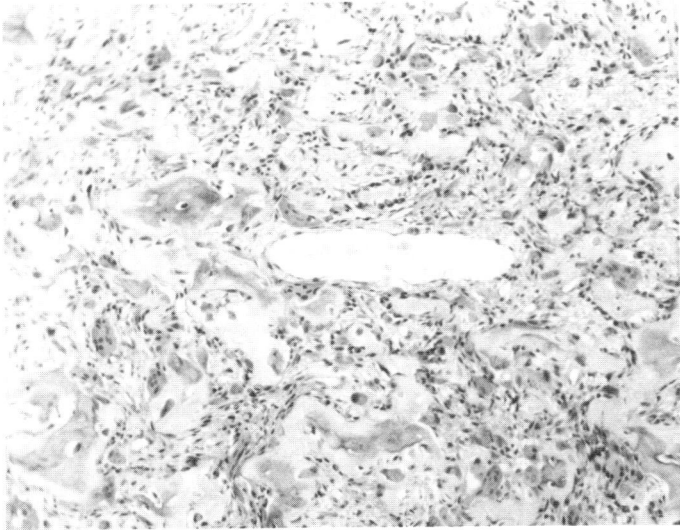

**Figure 2.** Osteoid osteoma. Similar features to benign osteoblastoma. In this case there is mineralization of the central core of many osteoid trabeculae. Original magnification × 200.

Death is often due to repeated local recurrence and involvement of vital structures. Contrary to the original description by Schajowicz, metastases can occur. A variety of histological features are seen, including epithelioid osteoblasts with numerous but normal mitoses, sheets or stubby trabeculae of osteoid, spiculated blue bone, and large numbers of osteoclasts (Figure 3). In contrast to frank osteosarcoma, permeation of the pre-existing bone trabeculae does not occur, and some aggressive osteoblastomas are surrounded by a shell of reactive bone.

**Conventional high-grade osteosarcoma**

Osteosarcoma is the commonest primary malignant bone tumour, usually occurring in the metaphysis of long bones during the period of maximum skeletal growth. In order of frequency the common sites affected are the distal femur, proximal tibia and proximal humerus. The tumour arises in the medulla, grows, permeates or destroys the overlying cortex, and escapes into the subperiosteal space. Here its growth is restricted by the confines of the tough, fibrous periosteum (provided it is intact). This restriction of direction of growth leads to the sun-ray pattern of tumour bone formation perpendicular to the underlying cortex. The tumour bulk strips the periosteum off the cortex beyond the margin of the tumour mass, and in this area the periosteum responds by laying down a wedge of reactive bone referred to as Codman's triangle. Once beyond the confines of the periosteum, the tumour is free to grow in any direction, resulting in an irregular pattern of tumour bone formation in soft tissue (Figure 4). In many cases the clinical

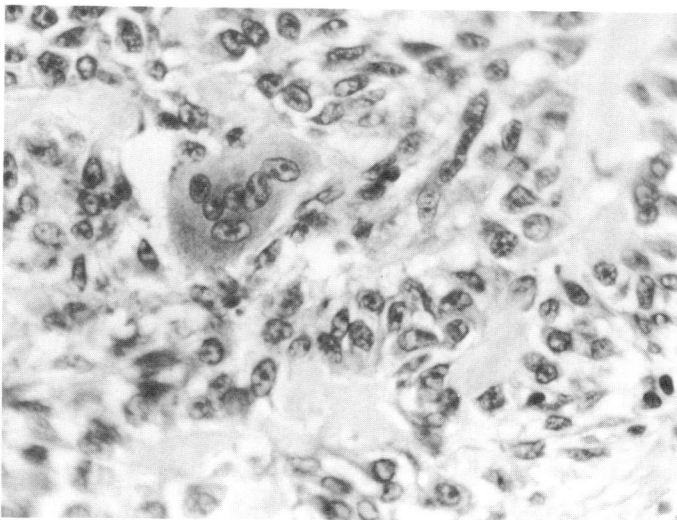

**Figure 3.** Aggressive osteoblastoma. Solitary pulmonary metastasis from primary tumour in proximal fibula; plump epithelioid osteoblasts with prominent nucleoli are producing delicate trabeculae of osteoid. Osteoclasts are numerous. Original magnification × 800.

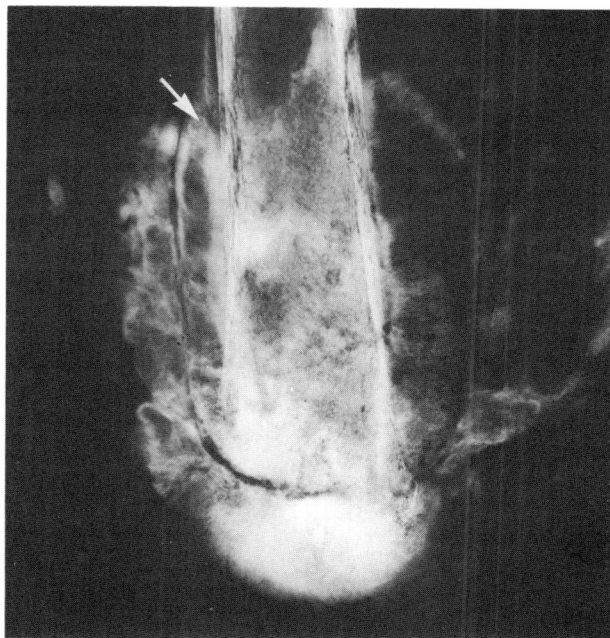

**Figure 4.** Fine detail X-ray of a longitudinal slab of an osteosarcoma of distal femur. The tumour is at an advanced stage and has extended into soft tissue beyond the periosteum. The original Codman's triangle can be seen ( ↑ ).

and radiological features are so typical that the diagnosis is not in doubt, but biopsy is always carried out for confirmation. However, in other cases the X-ray appearance may be atypical and the diagnosis depends entirely on the pathology.

Rarely, a high-grade osteosarcoma may arise on the outer aspect of the bone, referred to as *juxtacortical high-grade osteosarcoma*. Until recently the presence of tumour osteoid or bone was required to establish the diagnosis, but the use of frozen sections or imprint preparations stained with alkaline phosphatase enables a definite diagnosis to be established in a small biopsy sample, where no tumour osteoid or bone is present, provided that alkaline phosphatase can be demonstrated in the tumour cells (Sanerkin, 1980b). At present, unfixed tissue is required to demonstrate alkaline phosphatase. This technique should be used only in cases where the other aspects have been well investigated. It is of particular value in confirming that the fibroblastic, chondroblastic, osteoclast-rich and telangiectatic types are truly osteosarcoma, as they may contain little or no tumour osteoid or bone.

Although the most common type of high-grade osteosarcoma shows a mixed histological pattern, with fibroblastic, osteoblastic and chondroblastic areas, a number of tumours have a preponderance of one of the five histological patterns listed in Table 1.

## Osteoblastic osteosarcoma

This type of tumour shows extensive formation of tumour osteoid and bone interspersed with sheets and clumps of malignant osteoblasts (Figure 5). Even within this group, there is considerable variation—the malignant osteoblasts may be spindle shaped, pleomorphic, epithelioid or small cell

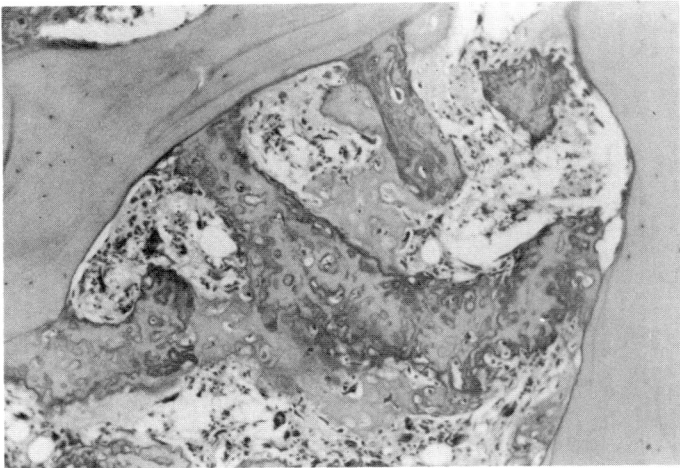

**Figure 5.** Osteoblastic osteosarcoma. Trabeculae of pre-existing bone surrounding a marrow space occupied by osteoblastic osteosarcoma producing dense trabeculae of tumour bone attached in places to the pre-existing bone. Original magnification × 160.

type. The cells do not rim the tumour bone in the manner seen in reactive bone. The trabeculae of tumour bone tend to be delicate (lace-like) and irregularly arranged. In some cases the trabecular pattern is not very obvious and the osteoid may be laid down in sheets. The use of polarized light or a reticulin stain may help to demonstrate a trabecular pattern. Some osteoblastic osteosarcomas have a dense mineralized trabecular pattern of tumour bone formation. The marrow spaces may be entirely occupied by this dense tumour bone, leading to a sclerotic pattern on X-ray. The differential diagnosis is from reactive bone formation and benign and intermediate osteoblastic tumours. All are positive for alkaline phosphatase. A regular pattern of woven bone with rimming of the trabeculae by regular osteoblasts is typical of reactive bone as seen in myositis ossificans, fracture callus and periosteal reaction. In reactive lesions the intertrabecular tissue is loose vascular connective tissue and skeletal mesenchymal cells. In an early lesion a worrying number of (normal) mitoses may be present. However, this cellular tissue can often be seen merging into more mature reactive bone. The clinical and radiological features may be helpful in difficult cases (see Chapter 3).

## Fibroblastic osteosarcoma

In this category the tumour cells are spindle shaped or rather pleomorphic, and a varying amount of collagen is produced by the tumour cells (Figure 6).

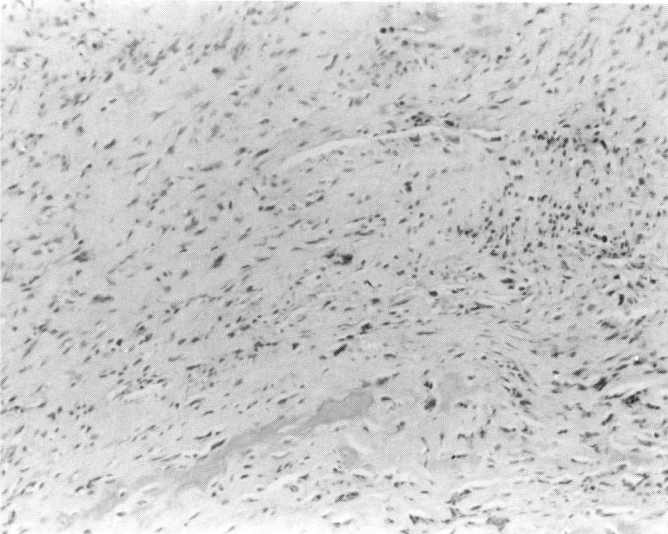

**Figure 6.** Fibroblastic osteosarcoma. Tumour comprising spindle cells showing some pleomorphism and producing collagen, with sparse tumour bone formation. A trabecula of tumour bone is seen towards the lower margin of the field. Original magnification × 160.

Tumour osteoid and bone are sparse or absent. The differential diagnosis includes malignant fibrous histiocytoma and fibrosarcoma. If fresh tissue is available and the tumour cells are shown to contain alkaline phosphatase, the diagnosis of osteosarcoma is confirmed. Fibrosarcoma and malignant fibrous histiocytoma do not contain alkaline phosphatase. If no fresh tumour is available, the age, site and X-ray appearance must be taken into consideration. If all are in keeping with a diagnosis of osteosarcoma, then that should be the working diagnosis. Fibrosarcoma and malignant fibrous histiocytoma are exceedingly rare in children, adolescents and young adults.

**Chondroblastic osteosarcoma**

This histological type of tumour may cause diagnostic problems unless biopsied in a specialist centre. The tumour tends to be aggressive with a large extraosseous component at the time of presentation. Histological examination shows lobules of malignant chondroid tumour. The tumour cells usually show more cellular atypia than is seen in well-differentiated chondrosarcoma (Figure 7). In some cases there are areas of spindle cell tumour, and there may be scattered foci of osteoid or tumour bone. Alkaline phosphatase is present in the tumour cells of chondroblastic osteosarcoma, even in the absence of tumour bone and osteoid. This is in contrast to chondrosarcoma where the tumour cells do not contain alkaline phosphatase. Chondrosarcoma is rare in the peak period for osteosarcoma. The distinction from periosteal osteosarcoma may be more difficult. Here the tumour cells are alkaline phosphatase positive. The histological appearance

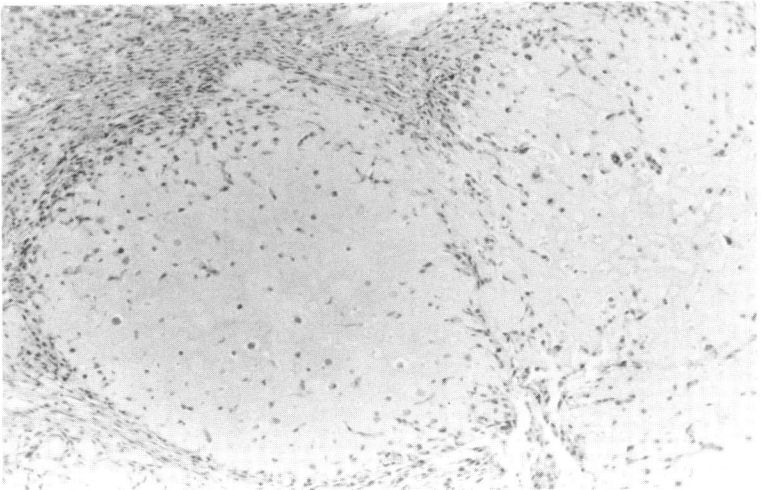

**Figure 7.** Chondroblastic osteosarcoma. Lobules of malignant chondroid are surrounded by closely packed undifferentiated tumour cells. No tumour bone is evident. Alkaline phosphatase was positive. Patient died with pulmonary metastases soon after biopsy. Original magnification × 160.

may be very similar, but appropriate X-rays will demonstrate that the tumour is in a superficial site involving only the outer aspect of the bone.

## Osteoclast-rich osteosarcoma

This is a rare histological type of tumour which often causes problems with diagnosis. On the low power of the microscope, the striking feature is the large number of multinucleate osteoclast giant cells, mimicking the low-power appearance of a giant cell tumour (osteoclastoma). Careful assessment of the mononuclear cells shows a degree of pleomorphism and cellular atypia not seen in giant cell tumour (Figure 8). In addition, abnormal mitoses, not seen in giant cell tumour are frequently present in osteoclast-rich osteosarcoma. Tumour bone formation is sparse or absent. Alkaline phosphatase is present in the tumour cells (but not in the large osteoclasts). Very occasional mononuclear cells are alkaline phosphatase positive in giant cell tumour. Giant cell tumour occurs in a somewhat older age group but it does overlap the upper part of the age group of osteosarcoma. The differential diagnosis also includes malignant fibrous histiocytoma. This tumour usually occurs in adults. There are other histological features which are helpful (p. 53 and Figure 25), and the tumour cells do not contain alkaline phosphatase.

## Telangiectatic osteosarcoma

This is a tumour characterized by large blood-filled cystic spaces. Macroscopically, and on low magnification histologically, it may mimic aneurysmal

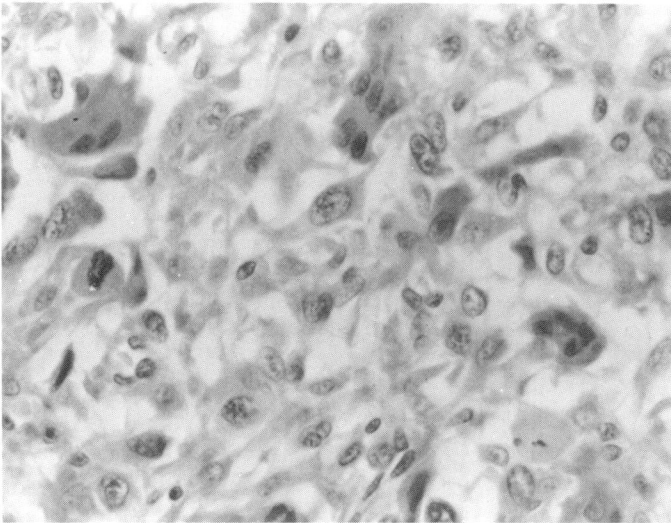

**Figure 8.** Osteoclast-rich osteosarcoma. A cellular tumour containing many osteoclast giant cells. The tumour cells are pleomorphic and abnormal mitoses are seen. No tumour bone or osteoid is present. Original magnification × 640.

bone cyst. Careful histological examination under the high power of the microscope will show a degree of cellular atypia and pleomorphism in the solid septal structures which is not acceptable for aneurysmal bone cyst (Figure 9). Any bone formation, which is usually sparse, will have the lace-like pattern of osteosarcoma rather than the reactive pattern seen in aneurysmal bone cyst. Alkaline phosphatase is positive in both aneurysmal bone cyst and telangiectatic osteosarcoma. Both affect a similar age group. The X-ray appearance may be critical in achieving a diagnosis (see Chapter 3).

## Assessment of adequacy of resection and response to chemotherapy in osteosarcoma

At the time of resection a sample of marrow tissue is taken by the surgeon from the bone beyond the transection point. In patients who undergo surgery 2–3 weeks after chemotherapy, the marrow may appear red and very firm and be a cause of concern to the surgeon. This is due to a period of increased haemopoietic activity as the marrow recovers from transient chemotherapy-induced depression. The marrow sample is examined using the imprint method described and the prosthesis is not fixed into place until the pathologist confirms that the sample is free from tumour (Figure 10). This avoids the necessity for clearance core biopsies done as a separate procedure prior to selecting the transection plane. Any doubtful areas in soft tissue can also be examined during the operation in the same way, with imprints and alkaline phosphatase where required.

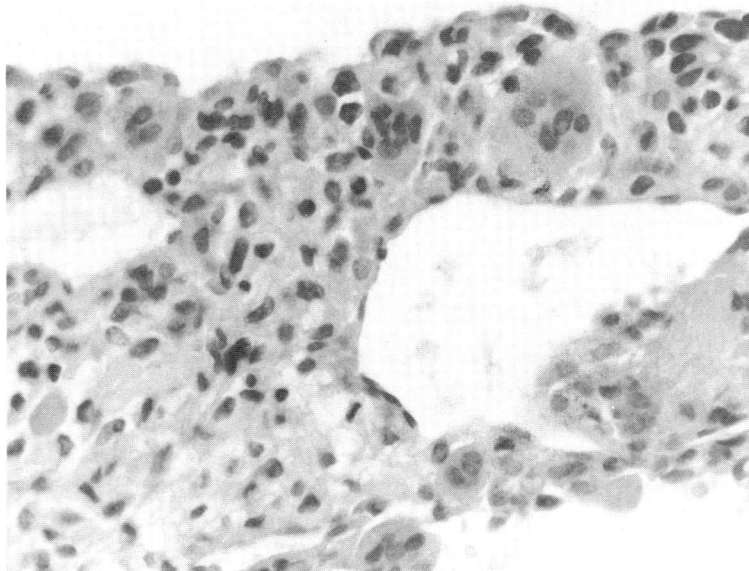

**Figure 9.** Telangiectatic osteosarcoma. Blood-filled spaces are bounded by 'septal' structures which are cellular and contain scattered osteoclast giant cells. The cells are pleomorphic and mitoses are numerous. Original magnification × 800.

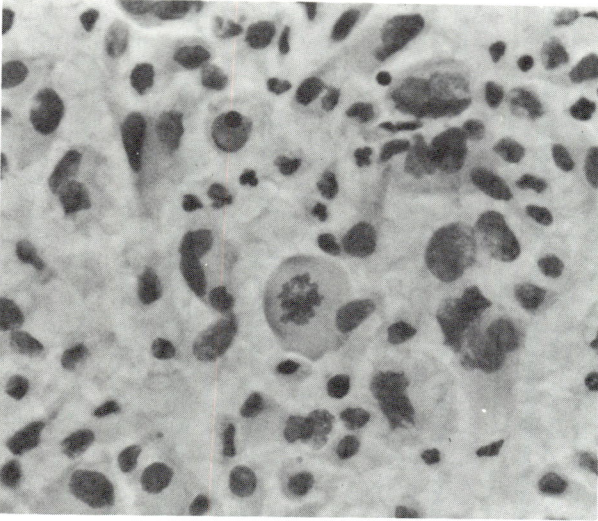

(a)

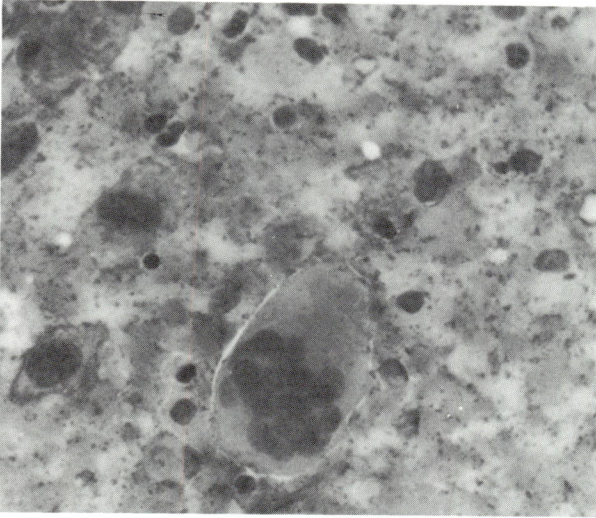

(b)

**Figure 10. (a)** Imprint preparation of osteosarcoma. Many large tumour cells are present with a high nuclear/cytoplasmic ratio. Comparison of size can be made with lymphocytes and poly-morphs included in the preparation. An osteoclast is also present. Original magnification ×  800. **(b)** Imprint of osteosarcoma stained with alkaline phosphatase. Granules of alkaline phosphatase can be seen in tumour cells and also spilled out into the background. A large osteoclast present is devoid of granules. Original magnification × 800.

The resection specimen is examined by cutting a longitudinal slab several millimetres thick in the plane of maximum diameter of the tumour. Photographs and fine detail X-ray are taken to delineate the tumour-bearing area. Histological sections are prepared from the entire slab and the limits of the tumour are compared with those estimated prior to surgery. Histological assessment of response to chemotherapy is made by quantitating all the tumour-bearing areas in the slab. The categories quantitated are necrotic tumour, damaged (altered) tumour and viable tumour (Figure 11). At present the significance of the category referred to as 'damaged' tumour is not known. However, areas of total tumour necrosis and unaffected tumour are relatively easy to assess. It is helpful to have the biopsy for comparison. It is impossible to distinguish histologically between chemotherapy-induced necrosis and naturally occurring necrosis. However, naturally occurring necrosis never exceeds 75% (Misdorp, 1986, personal communication). Some reports seem to indicate that 90% necrosis following chemotherapy is associated with a good prognosis (Huvos et al, 1977), but it is not yet clear if this is a prognostic determinant independent of grade, size and site. The work entailed by the histopathologist in dealing with each case is considerable, but it is only by this meticulous assessment of the tumour tissue that our ability to correlate patterns of histological response with different histological subtypes and with prognosis can be improved.

Some tumours respond to chemotherapy with extensive haemorrhagic necrosis producing large blood-filled cysts. This should not be confused with true telangiectatic osteosarcoma. Another pattern of response is for increased bone formation by the tumour. This is easily identifiable on X-ray. The histological appearance is that of 'increased maturation' and is similar to that described in some childhood tumours. It probably reflects a spectrum of sensitivity where the more primitive tumour cells are most susceptible to chemotherapy. Residual, better differentiated, tumour cells remain and demonstrate their higher degree of differentiation by laying down tumour bone. In the future it is likely that postoperative chemotherapy may be modified or selected on the basis of the histological assessment of response as described by Rosen et al (1982). Current trials conducted by the Medical Research Council are giving a number of pathologists the opportunity to study a large number of these cases and thus to evaluate the spectrum of histological response.

**Parosteal osteosarcoma**

This rare type of osteosarcoma (Unni et al, 1976) has a peak incidence in the third and fourth decades. Because of their slow rate of growth and deceptively bland histological appearance, these tumours are frequently wrongly diagnosed. They may be mistaken for a benign reactive lesion such as myositis ossificans or fibrous dysplasia, fibroma, chondroma and chondrosarcoma. Again, the combination of the clinical features with the radiological and histological appearance is the sure method of achieving a correct diagnosis. This is important because, if correctly diagnosed, these tumours are well suited to local resection, and the incidence of pulmonary metastases

(a)

(b)

(c)

(d)

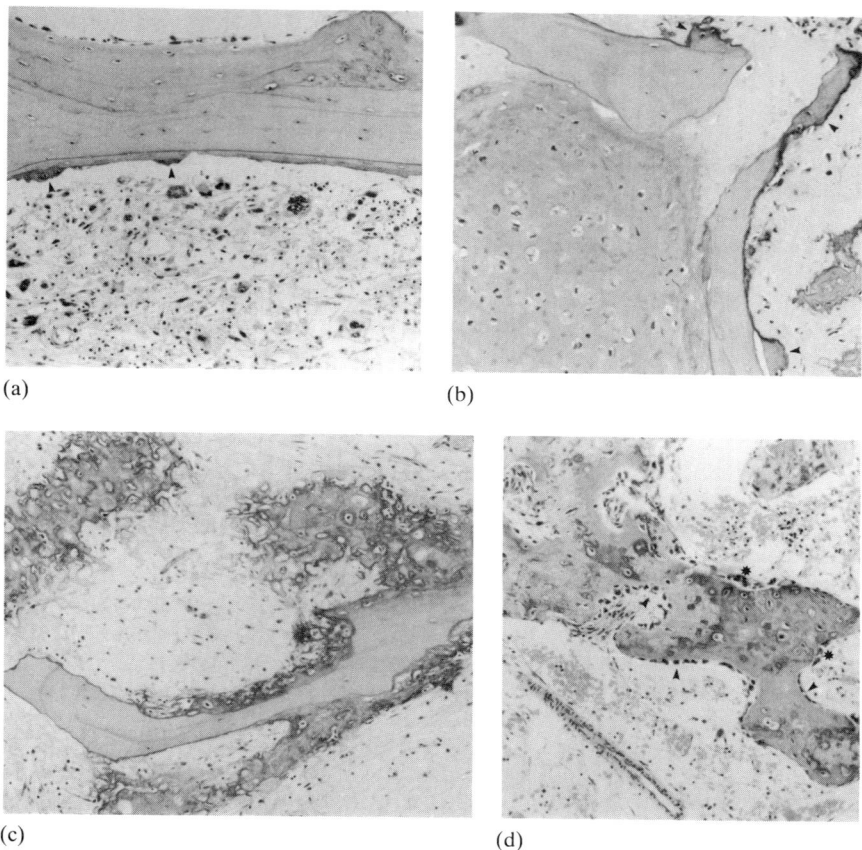

**Figure 11.** The spectrum of appearances in osteosarcoma following chemotherapy. **(a)** Osteosarcoma showing chemotherapy-induced damage in the lower part of the field. Many bizarre multinucleate tumour cells are present. Small foci of mineralized tumour bone ( ↑ ) are attached to the undersurface of the pre-existing bone lying horizontally across the middle of the field. On the upper surface of this bone normal osteoblasts are laying down appositional reactive bone. Original magnification × 200. **(b)** Partially resorbed pre-existing bone divides an area of good response on the right from an area of poor response on the left. The tumour on the right of the field shows severe damage. Acellular areas are present and dense trabeculae of tumour bone contain only scattered tumour cells. Small areas of tumour bone are attached to the pre-existing bone ( ↑ ). In contrast, the left side of the field contains an area of relatively unaffected tumour showing chondroblastic differentiation. The majority of the cells are viable and binucleate forms are present indicating active growth. Original magnification × 200. **(c)** This field shows extensive tumour necrosis, much of the marrow space being occupied by loose connective tissue containing scattered lymphocytes and histiocytes. Dense trabeculae of tumour bone contain small numbers of isolated cells, and tumour bone is attached to a severely eroded trabecula of pre-existing bone. The normal osteocyte lacunae are oval, in contrast to those in tumour bone which are larger, and round or irregular in outline. In addition, the osteocytes are smaller and less hyperchromatic than the enclosed tumour cells. Original magnification × 200. **(d)** In this field much of the tumour has died, leaving areas containing necrotic material and scattered lymphocytes. Residual islands of tumour bone containing scattered tumour cells are showing foci of surface resorption by normal osteoclasts (∗), together with extensive areas of reactive bone formation by normal osteoblasts on the tumour bone surface ( ↑ ). Original magnification × 200.

is low. However, the conventional histological criteria of malignancy are not seen, often leading to underestimation of the true nature of the lesion. The tumour is applied to the outer aspect of the cortex, and tumours of long standing may be wrapped around the shaft of the bone of origin and may at a late stage invade the underlying bone. The histological features are a collagenous spindle-cell stroma with well-defined trabeculae of mainly woven bone, often with irregular cement lines, and a variable amount of well-differentiated cartilage (Figure 12). The outer margin of the tumour may contain little or no bone and cartilage, leading to mistaken diagnoses of fibroma and fibrosarcoma. The deeper zones of the tumour contain an increasing amount of trabecular tumour bone, and close to the underlying cortex the tumour bone becomes very prominent and dense and may be mistaken for a benign reactive lesion. However, in parosteal osteosarcoma the tumour bone appears to emerge directly from the spindle-cell background (Figure 12a). This feature is particularly useful in distinguishing parosteal osteosarcoma from reactive lesions such as periosteal reactive bone, callus and myositis ossificans, where prominent rimming of the bone trabeculae by osteoblasts is usual (Figure 12b). In addition, parosteal osteosarcomas usually have a smooth outer margin, in contrast to myositis, where lobules of reactive tissue are interspersed with skeletal muscle. The thick-walled vessels associated with myositis are not seen adjacent to a parosteal osteosarcoma. A focal, non-specific, inflammatory infiltrate is likely to be more prominent in association with myositis ossificans. On histology alone it may be very difficult to distinguish between parosteal osteosarcoma and fibrous dysplasia, where there is also an absence of osteoblastic rimming of trabeculae. However, the radiological appearance of the two lesions is quite different.

Occasionally there may be a problem in distinguishing parosteal osteosarcoma from a sessile osteochondroma with a growing cartilage cap. Here, the presence of a communication between the medulla of the underlying bone and the stalk, the presence of fatty marrow between the bone trabeculae rather than fibrous tissue, the presence of an outer zone of cartilage rather than fibrous tissue, and evidence of endochondral ossification between the cap and the stalk are all features helpful in recognizing an osteochondroma.

At a late stage in the natural progression of parosteal osteosarcoma, it may permeate the underlying cortex and extend into the medulla. This is associated with an increased risk of pulmonary metastases. Ahuja et al (1977) suggested a system for histological grading of parosteal osteosarcomas. The high-grade areas correspond to more lucent areas on X-ray. Examination of the resected specimen may reveal areas of more high-grade appearance which may also be seen in local recurrence of inadequately treated cases (Figure 13). There is possibly a place for adjuvant chemotherapy in this small group of cases showing a more high-grade histological appearance.

A further late phenomenon is the possibility of dedifferentiation to a high-grade osteosarcoma (Wold et al, 1984). This is rare and tends to occur in cases known to have a long history prior to presentation, or in cases with repeated local recurrence following inadequate surgery. Treatment would then be as for high-grade osteosarcoma.

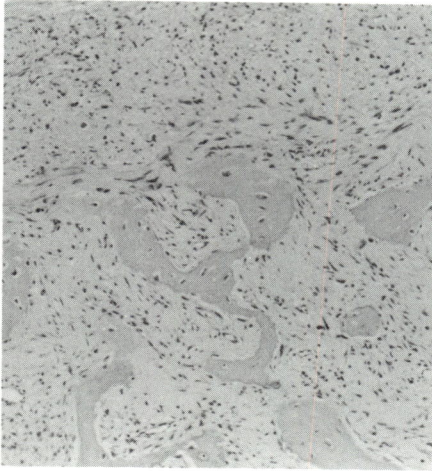

(a)

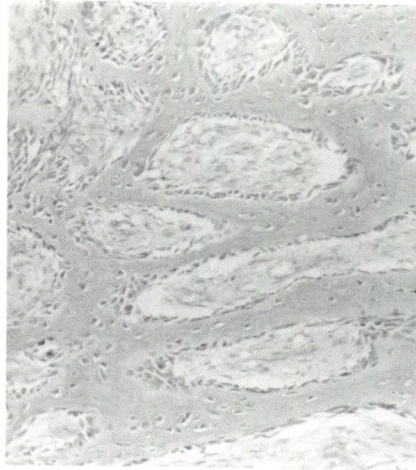

(c)

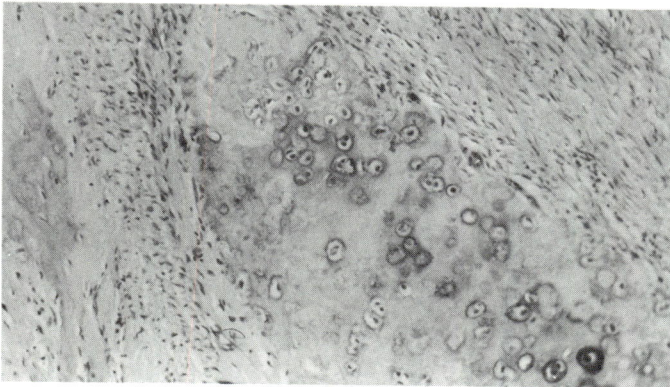

(b)

**Figure 12.** **(a)** Parosteal osteosarcoma. Close to the outer margin (top of field), the tumour comprises only spindle-cell fibroblasts producing collagen. Deeper into the tumour there are irregular trabeculae of tumour bone. There is no rimming of the bone by cells. Where there are curved trabeculae of bone, the appearances resemble fibrous dysplasia. Original magnification × 160. **(b)** Another field from a typical parosteal osteosarcoma shows areas of well-differentiated chondroid tissue set in a bland-looking spindle-cell stroma. A broad area of tumour bone is also present to the left. Original magnification × 800. **(c)** Periosteal reactive bone. The trabecular pattern is regular and there is prominent rimming of the trabecular surfaces by regular osteoblasts. Original magnification × 160.

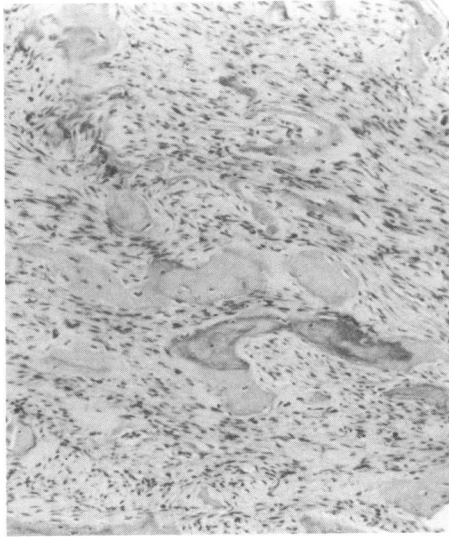

**Figure 13.** Parosteal osteosarcoma of higher grade appearance. The spindle-cell areas are more cellular and the cells are more pleomorphic. The trabeculae of tumour bone are numerous but are small and rather ill defined. Original magnification × 160.

## Periosteal osteosarcoma

This is a rare tumour first described in 1976 when, during a review of all tumours diagnosed as parosteal osteosarcomas in the Mayo Clinic records, it became apparent that a small subset of these superficial tumours showed features that set them apart from the classical parosteal osteosarcoma (Unni et al, 1976). The usual site of these tumours is the proximal tibia. Although commonest in the second decade, the age range is from the very young to the elderly.

Both the macroscopic and histological appearance is of a predominantly chondroid tumour. This fits well with the X-ray appearance. Interpretation of the biopsy may be difficult if the area sampled contains only well-differentiated chondroid tumour tissue. In a typical lesion, however, the peripheral zone contains areas of higher grade pleomorphic tumour tissue, often abutting on thin-walled vascular spaces and containing scattered foci of delicate lace-like osteoid (Figure 14). Imprint preparations are positive for alkaline phosphatase so that a diagnosis may be made in the absence of histological evidence of tumour osteoid and bone formation. The differential diagnosis is from juxtacortical chondrosarcoma, juxtacortical high-grade chondroblastic osteosarcoma and chondromyxoid fibroma. The distinction from periosteal/juxtacortical chondrosarcoma is especially important in planning treatment. Chemotherapy stimulates increased mineralization and maturity in the periosteal osteosarcoma, with the development of thick trabecular tumour bone similar to that seen in par-

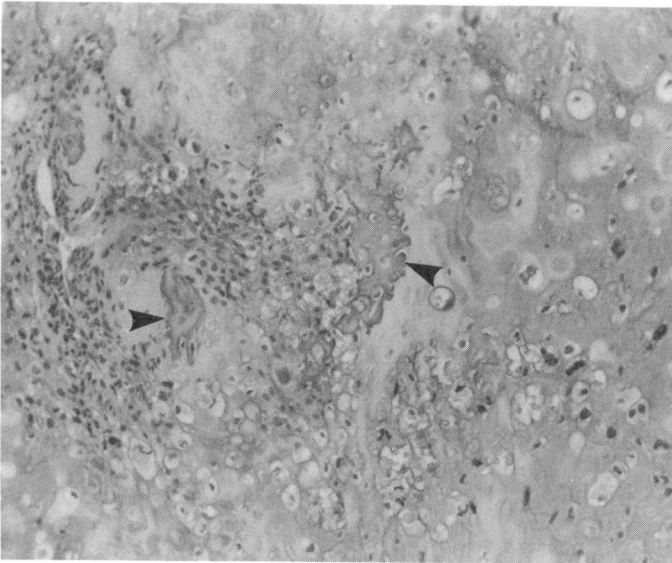

**Figure 14.** Periosteal osteosarcoma. Malignant tumour showing a mixed histological appearance. In some areas the tumour shows chondroid differentiation, while other areas are more high grade and less differentiated. Foci of tumour bone and osteoid can be seen ( ↑ ). Original magnification × 200.

osteal osteosarcoma. Even following chemotherapy, however, the spindle-cell component, seen in parosteal osteosarcoma, is lacking.

The distinction between periosteal osteosarcoma and high-grade chondroblastic osteosarcoma may be difficult. The clinical and radiological features may be helpful, and the histology is that of a more frankly high-grade tumour. Histologically, the chondroid component is less well differentiated and areas of high-grade tumour producing osteoid and tumour bone are more prominent. The problem is an infrequent one and the treatment is similar for both.

Rarely, particularly if the tumour is located in the proximal tibia, chondromyxoid fibroma may be considered in the differential diagnosis. Periosteal osteosarcoma shows more cytological features of malignancy and lacks the characteristic lobulation and interlobular fibrous tissue containing osteoclast giant cells that are so typical of chondromyxoid fibroma. The presence of tumour bone and osteoid are helpful in confirming periosteal osteosarcoma. The radiological features are also helpful in making the distinction between the two tumours.

## TUMOURS OF CHONDROID DIFFERENTIATION (Table 2)

Histological assessment of cartilage tumours should always be made with knowledge of the age of the patient, the site of the lesion, whether there are

**Table 2.** Tumours of chondroid differentiation.

*Benign*
Enchondroma (chondroma)—solitary or multiple
Osteochondroma (cartilage capped exostosis)—solitary or multiple
Chondromyxoid fibroma
Benign chondroblastoma

*Intermediate*
A group of cartilage tumours with evidence of active growth after skeletal maturity is reached.
These lesions recur locally but do not metastasize.

*Malignant*
Chondrosarcoma—grades I, II and III (sometimes subdivided into primary and secondary
chondrosarcomas, the latter arising in a pre-existing benign lesion)
Clear cell chondrosarcoma
Mesenchymal chondrosarcoma
Dedifferentiated chondrosarcoma

symptoms related to the lesion, and whether there is radiological evidence of
active growth in the lesion. A histological appearance regarded as benign in
an enchondroma in a child would justify a diagnosis of chondrosarcoma in
the femoral shaft of an adult.

## Chondroma

The enchondroma in the growing skeleton may be quite cellular and often
lobulated, with crowding of cells at the periphery of the lobules. Evidence of
growth is seen in the presence of numerous binucleate cells. The matrix is
well defined and stains deep blue (particularly with Ehrlich's haemotoxylin).

In children and adolescents affected by Ollier's disease, the degree of
cellularity may cause concern if the pathologist is unfamiliar with the range
of cartilage activity associated with this disease. In solitary or multiple
lesions the cartilage may continue to grow after skeletal maturity. The lesion
then falls into the intermediate category of cartilage tumour. A small
number of enchondromas do undergo frank malignant change to chondrosarcoma (p. 43).

## Osteochondroma

The cartilage-capped exostosis—osteochondroma—has a bony stalk, the
marrow of which communicates with the medulla of the underlying bone. It
is a small fragment of the epiphysis which becomes separated from the main
epiphyseal plate during bone growth. In the growing skeleton a variable
amount of remodelling activity is seen in the cancellous bone of the stalk.
There is active endochondral ossification at the bone/cartilage interface (as
in the epiphyseal plate) and the cartilage cap is usually quite thick with some
binucleate cells, but flat and smooth, rather like a mushroom with a bony
stalk and cartilage cap. Active growth in these tumours usually ceases when
skeletal maturity is reached. However, a small number of the tumours show

evidence of continued growth. The cartilage cap becomes thicker and lobulated. The lobulated cartilage becomes heaped up and spreads outwards, encircling the stalk (Figure 15). The tumour is now like a cauliflower with many 'florets' of lobulated cartilage. At this stage, complete removal is curative, but it is easy for some of the delicate lobules to become detached and remain behind. These will continue to grow slowly and form a local recurrence. Frank malignant change may occur (p. 43).

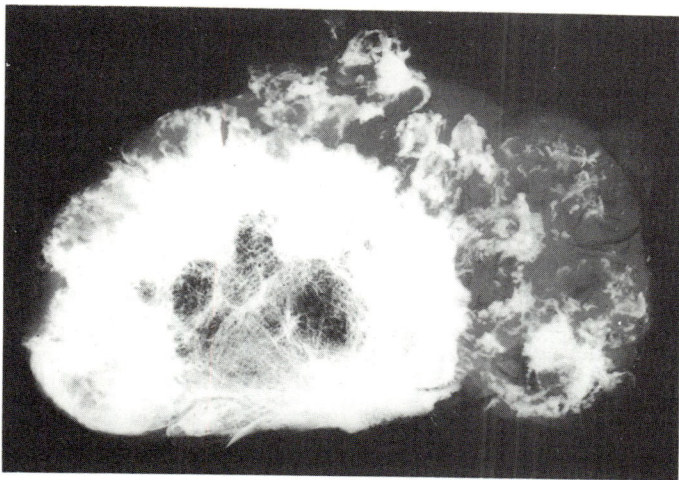

(a)

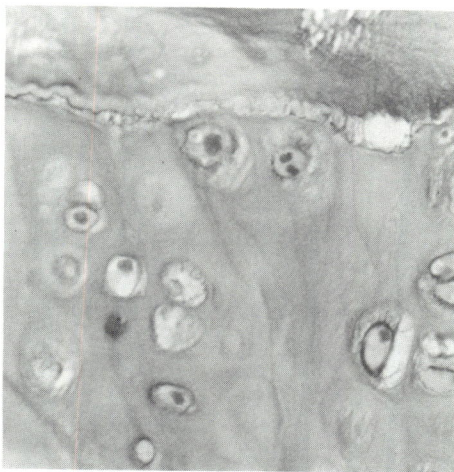

(b)

**Figure 15. (a)** Fine detail X-ray of a large osteochondroma with a growing cartilage cap. The central stalk has a pattern of trabecular bone. Foci of spotty calcification are seen in parts of the cartilage cap. The outer margin contains no mineral. **(b)** Scattered binucleate cells provide histological evidence of growth in the cartilage cap of this osteochondroma. Original magnification × 640.

## Chondromyxoid fibroma

This is a rare tumour affecting adolescents and young adults. It has a characteristic X-ray appearance and usually involves the proximal tibia or proximal humerus. Histologically, it comprises lobules of rather myxoid chondroid tissue, the areas between lobules being vascular, fibroblastic tissue containing a variable number of osteoclast giant cells (Figure 16). In a

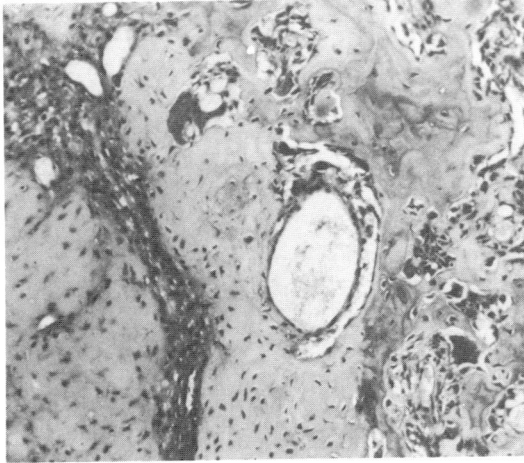

**Figure 16.** Chondromyxoid fibroma. A strikingly lobulated tumour with areas of myxoid chondroid tissue interspersed with cellular fibroblastic areas containing osteoclasts. Original magnification × 200.

few cases, groups of cells may show rather worrying pleomorphism. This feature should be considered in the context of the overall radiological and histological appearance. Occasionally, pathologists with a limited experience of bone tumours will mistakenly diagnose myxoid chondrosarcomas as chondromyxoid fibroma, even when the other histological elements are lacking. This leads to under-treatment on the part of the surgeon, resulting in rapid local recurrence.

## Benign chondroblastoma

This tumour arises centred on the epiphysis in the immature skeleton. Sometimes the distinction of benign chondroblastoma and giant cell tumour may be difficult. In a typical case, islands of chondroid tissue are surrounded by cellular tumour tissue, the cells being more uniformly rounded than in giant cell tumour.

A delicate pattern of calcification may surround individual cells, giving the so-called 'chicken-wire' effect (Figure 17). Local recurrence may follow incomplete removal, and occasionally marked secondary cyst formation mimicking aneurysmal bone cyst may occur.

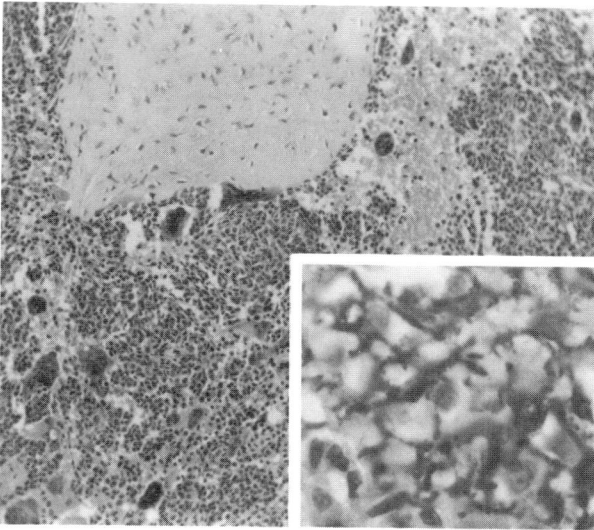

**Figure 17.** Benign chondroblastoma. A background of uniform round chondroblasts containing numerous osteoclast giant cells, with a well-defined island of chondroid tissue (top centre). Original magnification × 160. Inset: area showing classical chicken-wire calcification. Original magnification × 800.

## Chondrosarcoma

The conventional histological criteria for malignancy are not seen in well-differentiated chondrosarcomas. The tumours are therefore under-estimated by the pathologist and inadequately treated by the surgeon, leading to local recurrence. Since chondrosarcomas are insensitive to radio-therapy and chemotherapy, this may have serious and even fatal conse-quences for the patient as there is a tendency for each successive recurrence to show an increase in malignancy. Because chondrosarcoma is a tumour of the mature skeleton which is more common in the middle aged and elderly, and because its progression is usually slow, the patient may have sympto-matic treatment for presumed osteoarthritis and may eventually present with a pathological fracture. Many chondrosarcomas are referred to a specialist centre after the periosteum has been breached both by a fracture and by subsequent surgery. Typically, chondrosarcoma is a very slowly growing tumour, and local recurrence following resection and prosthetic replacement may occur after as long an interval as 12 years (Wilson, 1987). The mode of initial presentation and initial treatment affect the clinical outcome greatly in chondrosarcoma, as does the histological grading (Evans et al, 1977; Sanerkin and Gallagher, 1979; Kriekbergs et al, 1982). Dediffer-entiation is usually a late occurrence but may occasionally be present at the time of initial presentation; it is important to biopsy any atypical areas seen on the X-ray.

Chondrosarcomas of the pelvis and axial skeleton in general have a poor prognosis, not because they are of higher grade malignancy but because of the technical problems in achieving complete surgical removal (Sanerkin, 1980a; Sanerkin and Gallagher, 1979). As with osteosarcoma, the endosteal limit of the chondrosarcoma is of importance in determining the transection plane for the manufacture of a prosthetic replacement. A good guide is to go beyond the zone of periosteal buttressing. If there is any doubt, imprint preparations can be made at the time of prosthetic replacement. In the past, grading of chondrosarcomas was performed as a retrospective study where large areas of tumour were available for assessment (Evans et al, 1977). More complicated techniques such as the estimation of ploidy by flow cytometry are being used at a few centres (Alho et al, 1983). More simply, the use of imprint preparations made from unfixed biopsy tissue allows a good assessment of the cytological features unobscured by matrix. However, the X-ray examination is of extreme importance in assessing the overall appearance of the tumour and highlighting any areas which might be more aggressive in nature.

The histological grade shows good correlation with prognosis. The 5-year survival for grade I tumours is 65–85%, while for grade III it is 15%.

*Grade I chondrosarcoma* has a macroscopic texture and appearance similar to that of benign cartilage, being firm, grey and translucent, with focal areas of calcification and ossification. A bland histological picture is seen, with cells of uniform size evenly spaced in a well-defined matrix. Occasional binucleate forms are present, confirming active growth, and this histological appearance, together with symptoms and an X-ray appearance indicating growth in an adult skeleton, is sufficient to establish a diagnosis of chondrosarcoma. If the biopsy includes the pre-existing bone structure, a very helpful feature in establishing malignancy is the presence of permeation of marrow spaces by the tumour (Figure 18). The use of polarized light will help to distinguish the pre-existing lamellar bone structure, often partially resorbed, from endochondral ossification in a benign cartilage tumour. Sampling can be a problem with cartilage tumours and experience has shown that the most active parts are the growing margin, whether in soft tissue or within bone. Again, the X-ray may be helpful in indicating the best area to biopsy.

*Grade II chondrosarcoma* is softer and more friable in texture, in keeping with a more myxoid histological appearance. In addition, there is increased pleomorphism, more crowding of cells most marked at the periphery of lobules, frequent binucleate forms and a less well-defined matrix.

*Grade III chondrosarcoma* shows more advanced changes than described in grade II. Much of the tumour tissue comprises soft gelatinous pools with little solid tumour tissue. Areas of necrosis and degeneration may be present, and the macroscopic appearance may simulate pus and raise the possibility of osteomyelitis. Histologically, there are extensive myxoid areas, increased cellularity, a greater degree of cellular atypia, numerous binucleate forms and mitoses.

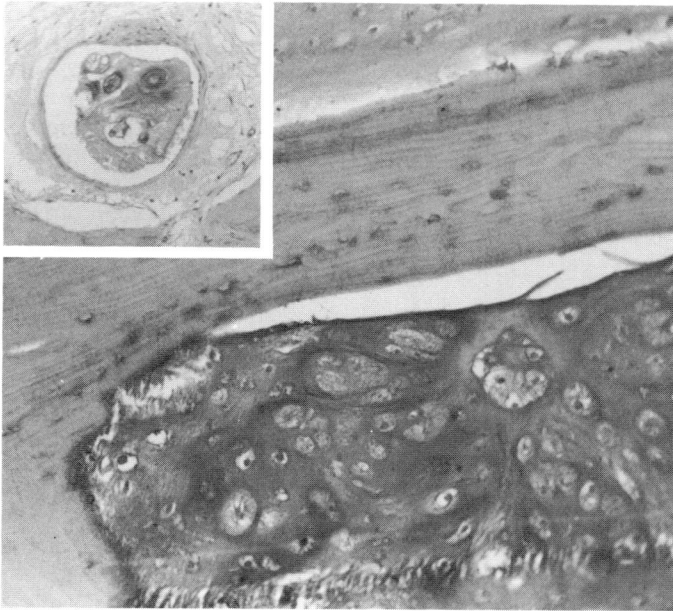

**Figure 18.** Well-differentiated chondrosarcoma. Tumour tissue is permeating the marrow spaces of the pre-existing bone. There is no evidence of 'cytological' malignancy. Original magnification × 200. Inset: vascular plugging by well-differentiated chondrosarcoma. Original magnification × 160.

*Chondrosarcoma arising in a pre-existing benign cartilage tumour.* Secondary chondrosarcomas most commonly arise in the cap of an osteochondroma and particularly if multiple lesions are present (diaphyseal aclasis). The malignant cartilage usually grows outwards, involving adjacent soft tissue but, on occasion, grows inwards, invading the bony stalk and the underlying bone. Rarely they arise in a pre-existing enchondroma, and again this is more likely if there are multiple lesions, as in Ollier's disease. Malignant change most commonly occurs in the middle aged and elderly. However, it occasionally occurs shortly after cessation of skeletal growth. The only distinctive histological feature is that in a small number of cases it is possible to see the original benign lesion remaining in association with the secondary chondrosarcoma, emphasizing the point that techniques employed to assess the degree of malignancy are only valid if the most aggressive area is studied. The radiologist is in a position to advise the surgeon which areas should be biopsied.

## Dedifferentiated chondrosarcoma

Dedifferentiation occurs in around 10% of chondrosarcomas, usually after repeated local recurrence, but occasionally present at the time of initial biopsy (Dahlin and Beabout, 1971; McFarland et al, 1977). Histological examination of these tumours shows classic features of well-differentiated chondrosarcoma in part of the tumour, with a fairly abrupt transition to the dedifferentiated area. The pattern of the dedifferentiated tumour is usually spindle celled (Figure 19b), with features of malignant fibrous histiocytoma or fibrosarcoma; less commonly the dedifferentiated tumour is a high-grade osteosarcoma (Figure 19a).

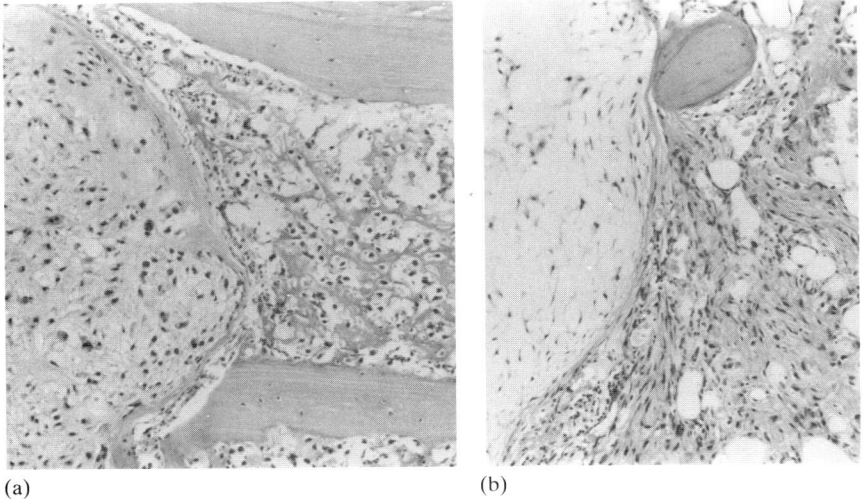

(a)　　　　　　　　　　　　　　　　　　(b)

**Figure 19.** Dedifferentiated chondrosarcoma. (a) On the left of the field is a growing lobule of fairly well-differentiated chondrosarcoma. Numerous binucleate cells are present, indicating active growth, and the tumour has stimulated resorption of the adjacent part of the trabecular cancellous bone in the lower part of the field. Just to the right of the midline there is a transition into a high-grade osteosarcoma. Original magnification × 160. (b) This shows a lobule of myxoid chondrosarcoma on the left, merging into a high-grade spindle-cell sarcoma on the right. A small residual fragment of pre-existing bone is seen towards the top of the field. Original magnification × 160.

*Clear-cell chondrosarcoma*

This tumour, first described by Unni et al (1976), is rare. It usually occurs in the proximal humerus and has some radiological and pathological features of conventional chondrosarcoma. Macroscopic examination shows expansion of the bone with endosteal erosion and thinning of the cortex. A variable amount of the tumour tissue is grey, translucent and somewhat gelatinous, indistinguishable from ordinary chondrosarcoma. Other areas are friable, haemorrhagic and gritty.

Histologically, there is a mixture of chondroid areas with striking clear cells (sometimes raising the possibility of metastatic renal carcinoma), areas of conventional chondrosarcoma, areas resembling benign chondroblastoma, osteoclast giant cells and scattered trabeculae of bone (Figure 20).

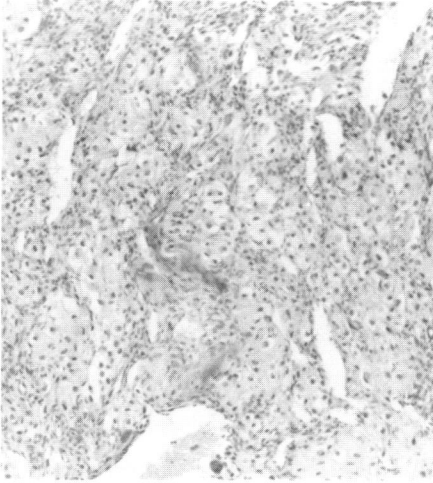

**Figure 20.** Clear cell chondrosarcoma. Solid sheets of tumour cells—some resembling those of benign chondroblastoma, many with striking clear cytoplasm, others showing more distinct chondroid differentiation. A few small osteoclast giant cells are present, as are small trabeculae of bone. Original magnification × 160.

Because of its common site of occurrence and areas resembling chondro-blastoma, it has been suggested that clear-cell chondrosarcoma may develop at the site of a pre-existing benign chondroblastoma, or may be the malignant counterpart of benign chondroblastoma.

*Mesenchymal chondrosarcoma*

This is a tumour of high-grade malignancy (Bertoni et al, 1983; Huvos et al, 1983). Although rare, it is three times more frequent in bone than in soft tissue. The sites most often affected are the jaw and the ribs. It has a distinctive histological appearance, with islands of chondroid tissue sur-rounded by a zone of cellular primitive mesenchymal tumour cells, some-times with a distinctive haemangiopericytoma-like pattern (Figure 21). The chondroid islands are bland in appearance and may have central foci of calcification and ossification. These areas are responsible for the popcorn appearance seen on X-ray. Bone formation is always confined to the centre of the chondroid lobules and the trabeculae of reactive bone at the periphery and separating lobules. In some, the islands of chondroid tissue are large and are sharply demarcated from the mesenchymal component, while in other cases the chondroid areas are less distinct and more diffuse. The differential diagnosis is from dedifferentiated chondrosarcoma and chondroblastic osteosarcoma. In dedifferentiated chondrosarcoma a part of the tumour shows the features of a classical chondrosarcoma, with high-grade dediffer-entiated tumour arising in one area. The dedifferentiated areas most commonly show appearances like malignant fibrous histiocytoma, and less

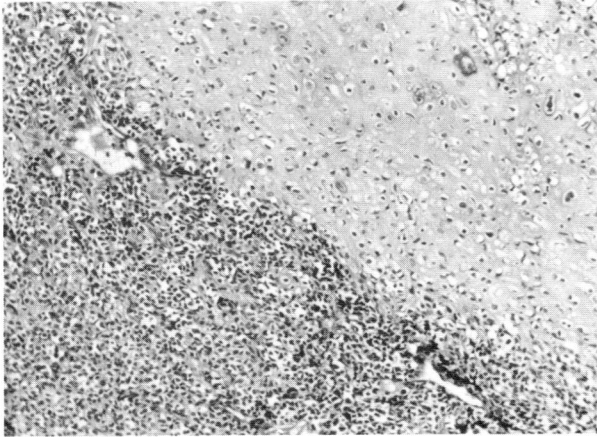

**Figure 21.** Mesenchymal chondrosarcoma. Part of a large island of chondroid tissue (bottom right), with focal calcification towards the centre, is surrounded by a zone of closely packed primitive mesenchymal cells. The interface is well defined.

commonly like osteosarcoma. Chondroblastic osteosarcoma may show small areas of tumour bone and osteoid formation; the tumour cells are not mesenchymal and the chondroid areas have a more malignant appearance. Alkaline phosphatase is negative in mesenchymal chondrosarcoma except in areas of calcification or ossification, but is positive in chondroblastic osteosarcoma.

## FIBROUS TUMOURS (Table 3)

### Non-ossifying fibroma

The classical non-ossifying fibroma (metaphyseal fibrous defect, fibrous cortical defect) is usually small, may be asymptomatic and has a typical radiological appearance (see Chapter 3). Excision or biopsy are rarely necessary unless the case is unusual or the lesion is causing symptoms. The tissue is often macroscopically bright orange-yellow. The typical histological

**Table 3.** Fibrous tumours.

*Benign*
Non-ossifying fibroma
Benign fibrous histiocytoma

*Intermediate*
Desmoplastic fibroma

*Malignant*
Malignant fibrous histiocytoma
Fibrosarcoma

appearance is of spindle-cell fibroblasts arranged in a storiform pattern, producing a variable amount of collagen, and with scattered osteoclast giant cells (Figure 22). Clusters of histiocytes containing haemosiderin and lipid are responsible for the orange-yellow colour. The histological appearance of progressive lesions is identical to the small self-limiting lesions. The current trend is to call these progressive lesions 'benign fibrous histiocytoma' to distinguish them from the classical non-ossifying fibroma. The differential

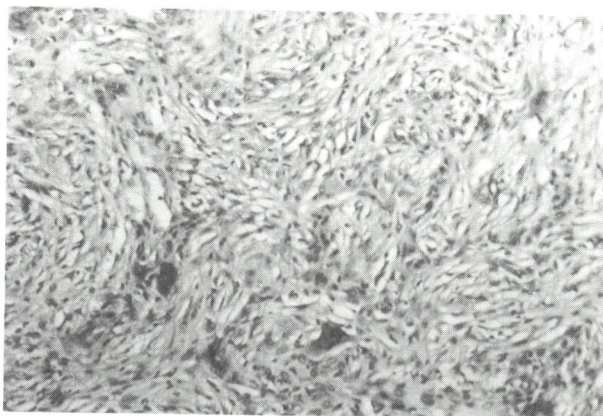

**Figure 22.** Non-ossifying fibroma. Spindle-cell fibroblasts producing some collagen are arranged in a striking storiform pattern. Osteoclast giant cells are scattered throughout. Original magnification × 200.

diagnosis is from giant cell tumour and malignant fibrous histiocytoma. This may be difficult as many giant cell tumours contain areas with fibroblasts and sheets of foamy histiocytes which are often associated with previous pathological fracture, areas of haemorrhage or previous surgery. Malignant fibrous histiocytoma shows more aggressive features both on X-ray and on histological examination (see below).

## Desmoplastic fibroma

In both behaviour and histology, this rare lesion is similar to the fibromatoses in soft tissues. It is slowly progressive and has an infiltrative pattern. However, its effects are local and it does not metastasize. As in fibromatosis, the lesional tissue contains moderate numbers of fibroblasts producing, in some areas, characteristic broad bands of collagen. Mitoses are few. A helpful diagnostic feature is the infiltrative pattern of the margin.

## Malignant fibrous histiocytoma

Malignant fibrous lesions of bone are uncommon and occur in the mature skeleton. Until recently, many poorly differentiated spindle-cell sarcomas were classified under the heading 'fibrosarcoma'. Following the recognition of malignant fibrous histiocytoma in soft tissue (O'Brien and Stout, 1964), this tumour was described as also arising in bone (Capanna et al, 1984; Ros et al, 1984; Huvos et al, 1985; Boland and Huvos, 1986). Initially there was some reluctance among pathologists in accepting this entity in bone; however, it is now generally accepted. The femur and tibia are the common sites, the tumour producing an ill-defined area of bone destruction with a variable amount of periosteal reaction. The tumour is solid and usually grey/white, with yellow/orange areas. The histological features are similar to those seen in malignant fibrous histiocytoma arising in soft tissue. These include a storiform arrangement of spindle cells producing variable amounts of collagen, marked pleomorphism amongst tumour cells but often with sparse mitoses, tumour giant cells and areas including osteoclast giant cells and histiocytic cells, some of which may contain lipid and haemosiderin (Figure 23). Some tumours contain a focal inflammatory infiltrate which is usually lymphocytic. The most useful immunocytochemical markers are $\alpha_1$-antitrypsin and $\alpha_1$-antichymotrypsin. Care has to be taken to demonstrate that cells showing a positive reaction are tumour- rather than non-specific infiltrating histiocytes which may be associated with areas of degeneration and necrosis. However, the absence of positive reaction should not preclude a diagnosis of malignant fibrous histiocytoma provided that other features favour this diagnosis. Again, needle biopsy is usually satisfactory in providing sufficient tissue to make the diagnosis. A number of malignant

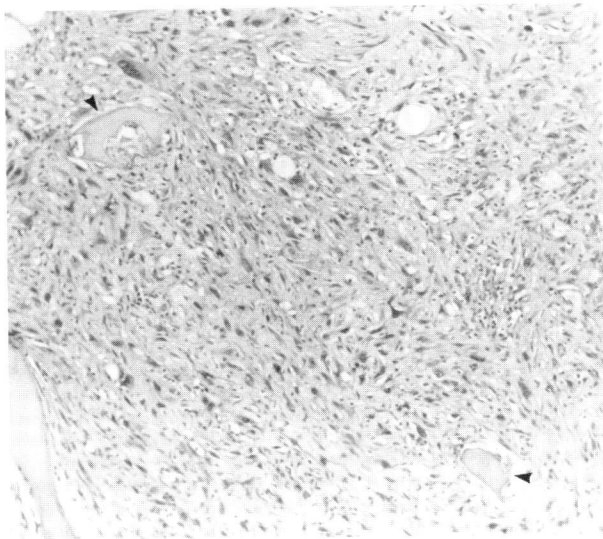

**Figure 23.** Malignant fibrous histiocytoma. Spindle cells arranged in a storiform pattern in a collagenous matrix. The cells are pleomorphic and the tumour has permeated the marrow spaces, stimulating almost total resorption of two of the pre-existing bony trabeculae ( ↑ ). Original magnification × 160.

fibrous histiocytomas in bone are associated with a previous infarct (Mirra et al, 1974) or fracture, or areas of abnormal bone such as Paget's disease. Sanerkin and Woods (1979) describe fibrosarcomas and malignant fibrous histiocytomas arising in relation to enchondromas.

## Fibrosarcoma

Since the recognition of malignant fibrous histiocytoma of bone, the number of tumours diagnosed as fibrosarcoma has decreased, and true fibrosarcoma of bone has become very rare. It is a tumour that affects the mature skeleton. Fibrosarcomas diagnosed in the 10–25 year age group are almost invariably fibroblastic osteosarcoma. The macroscopic appearance and the pattern of growth within bone is very similar to malignant fibrous histiocytoma, but without the yellow areas macroscopically. Histologically, the tumour comprises spindle cells or elongated oval cells classically arranged in a herring-bone pattern of interdigitating fascicles (Figure 24). The tumour cells produce a variable amount of collagen. Some fibrosarcomas are well-differentiated, while others are more pleomorphic. Occasionally a pseudo-sarcomatous metastatic deposit in bone may simulate fibrosarcoma or malignant fibrous histiocytoma. Immunocytochemistry is not usually helpful in these rare cases as epithelial markers such as Cam 5.2 may be negative and connective tissue markers such as vimentin may be positive when this degree of dedifferentiation takes place.

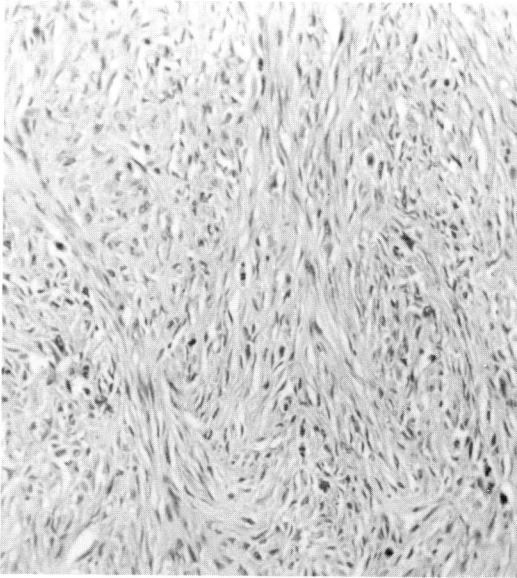

**Figure 24.** Fibrosarcoma. This field shows spindle cells arranged in interdigitating bundles in a collagenous matrix. Original magnification × 200.

## TUMOURS CONTAINING OSTEOCLAST GIANT CELLS (Table 4)

### Giant cell tumour

The definition of giant cell tumour and its variants owes much to the work of Jaffe et al (1940). Giant cell tumour (osteoclastoma), although rare, accounts for 5–10% of primary bone tumours. The tumour occurs in the mature skeleton at the site of a fused epiphysis or apophysis. The

**Table 4.** Tumours containing osteoclast giant cells.

*Benign*
Non-ossifying fibroma
Aneurysmal bone cyst
Benign chondroblastoma
Chondromyxoid fibroma

*Intermediate*
Giant cell tumour
Aggressive osteoblastoma

*Malignant*
Malignant fibrous histiocytoma
Osteoclast rich osteosarcoma
Clear cell chondrosarcoma

*Non-neoplastic*
Brown tumour (hyperparathyroidism)
Pigmented villo-nodular synovitis involving bone

commonest sites are the distal femur, proximal tibia, proximal humerus, proximal femur and distal radius. Typical giant cell tumours are of inter- mediate malignancy, not fitting into truly benign or frankly malignant categories. All giant cell tumours have a very small metastatic potential. The tumour arises towards the end of the bone and classically extends to the undersurface of the articular cartilage of the adjacent joint. The tumour expands the bone but up to a late stage, or modified by pathological fracture, the tumour remains contained within a thin bony shell comprising thinned cortex and woven reactive bone (see Chapter 3). This shell of reactive bone is also a feature of recurrence of giant cell tumour in soft tissue. The endosteal margin is usually well defined. There is no residual bone within the tumour-bearing area. The gross appearance is of soft, rather friable, haemorrhagic tumour tissue which may be reddish-brown or grey. Viable areas have a colour and texture like raw liver. Small blood-filled cystic spaces and bright yellow areas may be seen associated with areas of haemor- rhage and degeneration.

The histological features are a background of mononuclear 'stromal' cells which show both round and spindle forms, containing a variable number of mitotic figures of normal configuration. Distributed throughout this tissue are large numbers of multinucleate giant cells (Figure 25). They are larger

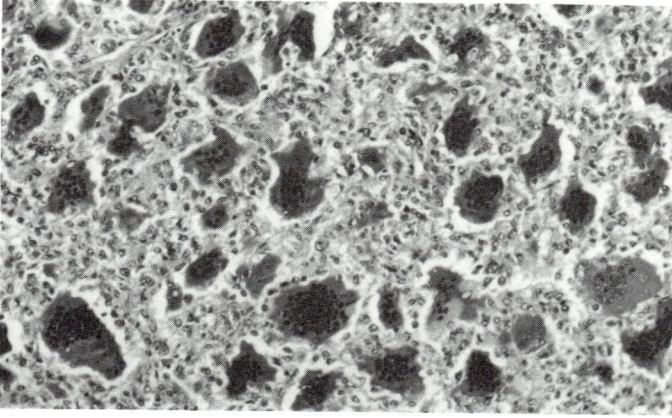

(a)

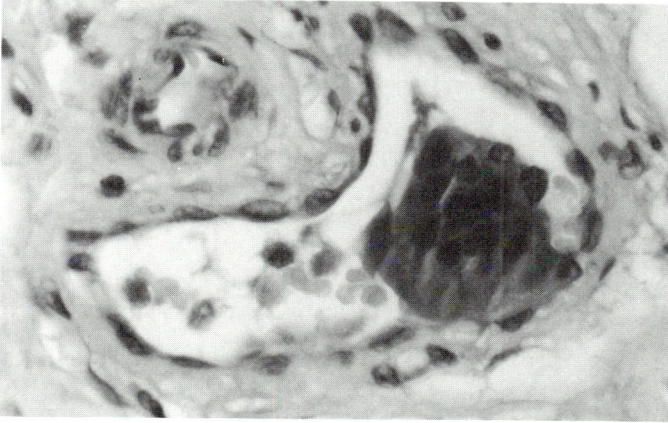

(b)

**Figure 25.** (a) Giant cell tumour. This field shows a typical appearance. Numerous osteoclast giant cells are distributed in a cellular background of mononuclear round and spindle cells. Original magnification × 200. (b) A thin-walled vascular channel cut transversely contains one large osteoclast which is adherent to the endothelial wall at one point. Original magnification × 800.

than normal osteoclasts, but are otherwise indistinguishable from them. Mitoses are never seen in the nuclei of these osteoclast giant cells.

The osteoclast giant cells are identical in giant cell tumour and its variants (Schajowicz, 1961; Johnston, 1977). A feature of all lesions containing these osteoclast giant cells is that they are associated with extensive bone resorption. An obvious explanation is that these large osteoclasts are resorbing the bone. Recent research (Chambers et al, 1985) has shown that giant cells disaggregated from giant cell tumours can resorb bone slices in vitro and that their response to hormones follows a pattern similar to that seen in mammalian-derived normal osteoclasts and normal human fetal osteoclasts. Monoclonal antibodies raised against these tumour-derived osteoclasts react not only with the osteoclasts in giant cell tumour but with osteoclasts in, for example, aneurysmal bone cyst, pigmented villonodular synovitis and human fetal osteoclasts (Horton et al, 1985). This may imply that the osteoclasts in giant cell tumours are non-neoplastic cells (Goldring et al, 1986) which are present in a wide variety of human bone lesions. This has stimulated research to identify the true neoplastic cells in giant cell tumour and to isolate and identify the factors that these tumour cells produce which recruit and activate the osteoclast. A proportion of the 'stromal' cells are mononuclear but mature osteoclasts, while other mononuclear cells show a moderate number of mitotic figures and are the true neoplastic cells. About one-third of giant cell tumours show some production of osteoid within the stroma which is distinct from the reactive shell of bone often seen at the periphery. Alkaline phosphatase is present in occasional tumour cells. Vascular permeation by clumps of tumour cells is a common feature, but the metastatic rate of these tumours is very low (about 1–5%). Another feature of giant cell tumours is the presence of solitary osteoclasts in small vascular spaces (Sladden, 1957). It is possible that these osteoclasts are being recruited into the tumour. It seems likely that the tumour cells are similar to the inactive osteoblasts referred to in the normal cycle of bone turnover as bone-lining cells.

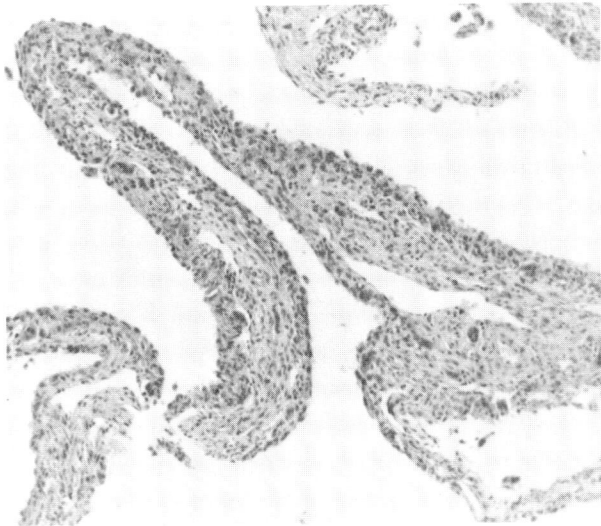

**Figure 26.** Aneurysmal bone cyst. Delicate coiled septae have a smooth margin. They comprise bland spindle cells and numerous osteoclast giant cells. Original magnification × 200.

A grading system has been used by some histologists for giant cell tumour based on the number and size of the osteoclasts and the mitotic activity and degree of pleomorphism seen in the stromal cells (Campanacci et al, 1975; Sanerkin, 1980c). Experience has shown, however, that this grading is of little value in identifying tumours which may recur after surgery or indeed the tiny number which may metastasize. Recurrence after surgery would appear to be more directly related to the thoroughness with which the tumour is removed locally at the time of curettage. Metastasis may occur very occasionally in a tumour which would be classified as grade I, benign and low grade (Eckardt and Grogan, 1986).

The differential diagnosis is from malignant fibrous histiocytoma, osteoclast-rich osteosarcoma, non-ossifying fibroma, benign fibrous histiocytoma and aneurysmal bone cyst. The macroscopic description of the lesion is particularly helpful in distinguishing between aneurysmal bone cyst and giant cell tumour. The X-ray may be acceptable for either lesion, and while haemorrhagic areas are seen in giant cell tumour, solid areas can occur in aneurysmal bone cyst. Also, fragments of giant cell tumour removed by a curette may resemble the septal structures in aneurysmal bone cyst. However, close examination shows a ragged margin on these tissue fragments in giant cell tumour in contrast to the smooth surface of the septae in aneurysmal bone cyst (Figure 26). In addition, the stromal cells in aneurysmal bone cyst are more uniformly spindle shaped, and a larger proportion of cells are alkaline phosphatase positive than is the case in giant cell tumour.

## MALIGNANT ROUND CELL TUMOURS OF BONE

These comprise the following: metastatic neuroblastoma, Ewing's sarcoma, Askin tumour, lymphomas presenting in bone and metastatic small cell carcinoma.

### Ewing's sarcoma

This is a tumour of unknown histogenesis which occurs mainly under the age of 25 years. Often, the diaphysis of a long bone is involved, but these tumours also affect the pelvis and ribs and a similar tumour arises in soft tissue. Because of its malignant nature and its rapid permeation of both marrow spaces in the medulla and vascular spaces in the cortex, it causes much necrosis of pre-existing bone and it is typical of this tumour that much of it may also undergo necrosis, sometimes leaving islands of viable tumour around vessels. Because of this growth pattern, there may be appositional layering of reactive new bone on the pre-existing bony structure, much of which is infarcted. This may cause areas of sclerosis on the X-ray, while in other areas extensive resorption of the pre-existing bone structure may occur corresponding with lytic areas on the X-ray. The periosteal new bone formation pattern too may have the classic 'onion skin layering'; however, a well-defined Codman's triangle may be associated with Ewing's sarcoma.

Occasionally also the bone may appear relatively unaffected radiologically, but a large soft tissue mass may be seen, initially confined under the periosteum, though with an earlier extension into adjacent soft tissue than is usually seen with osteosarcoma.

The cells are small, uniform and round with indistinct cell margins (Figure 27). Mitoses are often relatively few; however, these tumours are uniformly of high-grade malignancy. The classical Ewing's sarcoma contains much intracytoplasmic glycogen, whereas production of reticulin fibres is sparse. Sometimes the reticulin stain may be misleading, especially where there are areas of necrosis and fibrous reaction or where the tumour is in soft tissue outside the bone and is associated with a fibrous stroma. In these situations there may be an impression of reticulin formation, but careful inspection will show that reticulin is sparse and not associated with the actual tumour cells. Some Ewing's sarcomas contain only small amounts of glycogen, and it may be depleted by inappropriate fixation. Glycogen is well preserved in imprint preparations. Because of the necrosis there may be quite a marked inflammatory infiltrate in some areas of the tumour which may raise the alternative diagnosis of osteomyelitis. Ewing's sarcomas may sometimes present with a longer history which is also suggestive of low-grade osteomyelitis. Some problems are associated with biopsy of Ewing's sarcoma. Crush artefact is common in core biopsy of Ewing's sarcoma, as the soft tumour tissue is

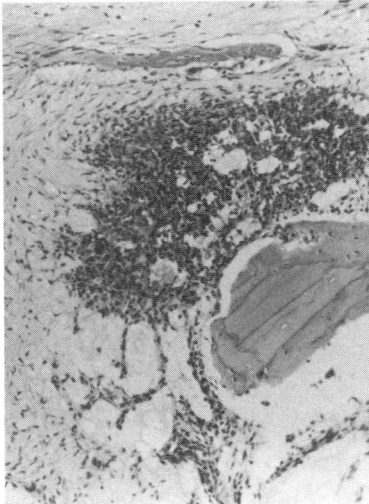
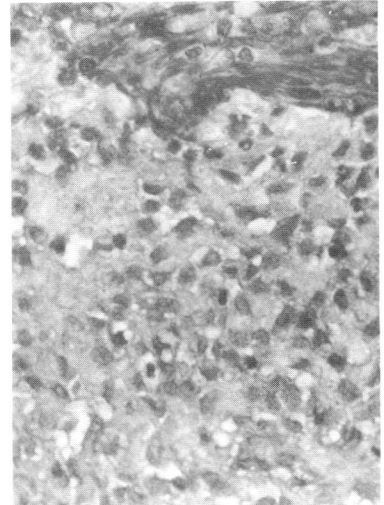

(a)                                                    (b)

**Figure 27.** Ewing's sarcoma. (a) This field shows extensive 'natural' necrosis within a Ewing's sarcoma of femur. Islands of residual viable tumour tissue are surrounded by non-neoplastic reactive fibrous tissue. On the extreme right of the field is a small fragment of infarcted, partly resorbed lamellar bone surrounded by appositional viable reactive bone. Original magnification × 160. (b) Higher magnification of tumour cells from a core biopsy. A sheet of fairly uniform round cells with indistinct cell boundaries is seen. Severe crush artefact has occurred along the top margin of the field. Original magnification × 640.

interspersed with sclerotic bone. Needle biopsy is usually adequate for confirming the diagnosis in Ewing's sarcoma and this tumour makes particularly good imprint preparations on which one can carry out all the special stains necessary to confirm the diagnosis. Below the age of 5 years, it is particularly important to exclude metastatic neuroblastoma. Rosette formation is not a reliable histological marker since it is rarely seen in bone metastasis of neuroblastoma, but has been described in Ewing's sarcoma. Immunocytochemistry is as yet of limited value in the positive diagnosis of Ewing's sarcoma, but the absence of positive reactivity with neuroblastoma markers is helpful in some cases. Vimentin is usually positive in scattered tumour cells.

Chemotherapy given before surgical resection of the tumour usually has a dramatic effect on the tumour, and complete or very extensive necrosis is quite common on examination of the resected tumour site. Occasional tumours which appear to have all the features of a Ewing's sarcoma respond rather poorly to therapy. Recent studies suggest that some extra-skeletal

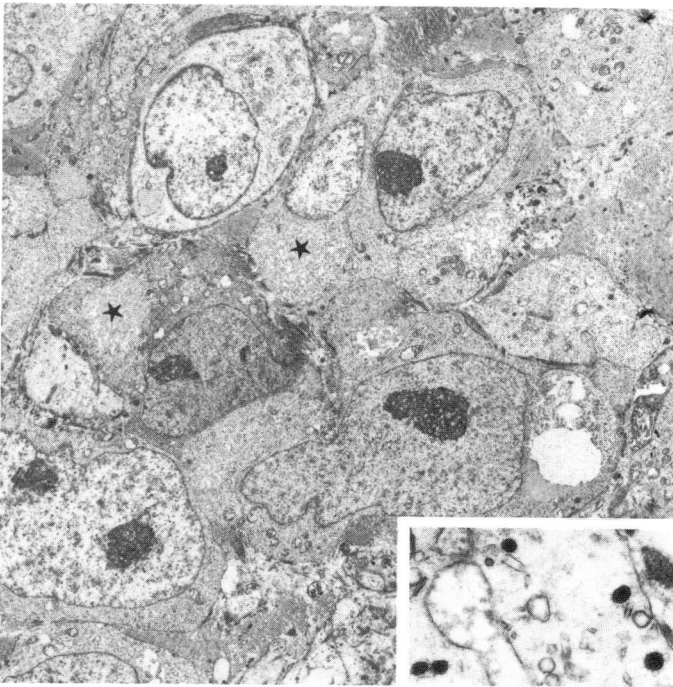

**Figure 28.** Subperiosteal Ewing's sarcoma (same case as Figure 27b). A survey electron micrograph shows a mixture of rounded and somewhat irregular cells with broad cytoplasmic processes. Many cells display glycogen deposits (∗) but they are less prominent than would be expected in a classical Ewing's sarcoma (× 3300). Inset: some of the cytoplasmic processes contained neurosecretory-like granules measuring 110–170 nm in diameter (× 17 300). (Ultrastructural study of this case was provided by Dr Lucienne Papadaki, Department of Histopathology, the Middlesex Hospital Medical School, London.)

'Ewing's' sarcomas are poorly differentiated neuro-ectodermal tumours (Mierau, 1985; Dehner, 1986).

A recent subperiosteal Ewing's sarcoma of the femur showed electron microscopic features of both Ewing's sarcoma and a neural tumour (Figure 28). Askin et al (1979) described a group of malignant small cell tumours of the chest wall in children and adolescents. In these tumours also, electron microscopy suggests a neuro-ectodermal origin. Epithelial markers are used to exclude metastatic carcinoma and common leucocyte antibody is used to exclude lymphoma.

## Other small round cell tumours of bone

The introduction of immunocytochemistry has shown that the vast majority of small round cell tumours occurring in the older age group, formerly regarded as reticulum cell sarcoma, are an assortment of lymphomas presenting in bone. They are rare. Sometimes they are part of a more generalized lymphoma, but a proportion appear to be solitary lesions at the time of presentation involving only one focus in bone (see Chapter 9). The

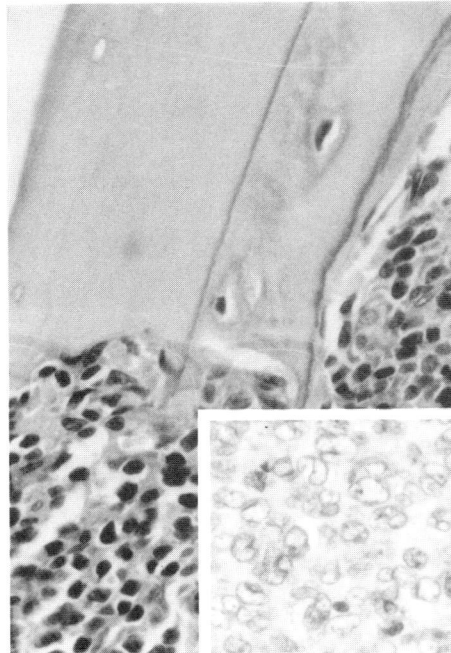

**Figure 29.** B-cell lymphoma presenting in bone. Malignant round tumour cells occupy the marrow spaces and have stimulated extensive erosion of the cancellous bone. An area of infarcted pre-existing bone is seen in the top left area, with a layer of appositional reactive bone on its inner aspect. Original magnification × 200. Inset: higher magnification of tumour cells showing nuclear detail with many cleaved forms. Original magnification × 800.

majority are centroblastic or centroblastic/centrocytic lymphomas with a diffuse growth pattern (Wright and Isaacson, 1983). Occasionally, Hodgkin's disease may present with primary bone symptoms. A study of primary lymphoma in bone (Dosoretz et al, 1982) found that most were of B-cell type and that the presence of cleaved nuclei was associated with a better prognosis.

It is a feature of lymphoma in bone that the tumour at the time of presentation is often widespread in soft tissue beyond the periosteum. However, this does not in most cases preclude conservative surgery, as response to appropriate adjuvant therapy is usually good. Lymphoma permeates the marrow spaces of the bone causing a combination of bone destruction, bone necrosis and reactive new bone formation (Figure 29). The tumour tissue is soft and pale. It is prone to crush artefact. Imprint preparations are useful in establishing a diagnosis. Occasional cells may contain alkaline phosphatase; glycogen is absent. Immunocytochemistry using common leucocyte antigen and markers for B- and T-lymphocytes is also satisfactory on imprints. They are especially useful if there is a need to use further monoclonal antibodies which do not react with fixed tissue. Histological examination shows fairly uniform round tumour cells, larger than the cells of Ewing's sarcoma and with a more open vesicular nucleus. An infiltrate of small lymphocytes is often present. A reticulin stain may show 'packeting' of small clumps of tumour cells by a network of reticulin fibres. Metastatic carcinoma occasionally mimics a primary malignant round cell tumour of bone. Epithelial markers are of value in confirming the true nature of these tumours, the Cam 5.2 being particularly useful in bone as it reacts well in bone decalcified in formic citrate.

## TUMOURS ARISING IN ABNORMAL BONE

These comprise the following: tumours arising in bone infarcts, tumours arising in bone affected by Paget's disease, post-irradiation sarcomas in bone and sarcomas developing in bone affected by fibrous dysplasia.

### Tumours arising in bone infarcts

An association between pre-existing bone infarcts and malignant bone tumours has been described (Mirra et al, 1974). Of four cases described, three were malignant fibrous histiocytomas and one was osteosarcoma. Two arose in Caisson workers. The tumours have no distinguishing pathological features other than their association with a pre-existing infarct. This may be difficult to substantiate histologically as malignant bone tumours frequently cause necrosis in the affected bone. In addition, fibrosarcoma and malignant fibrous histiocytoma have been described arising in relation to enchondromata (Sanerkin and Woods, 1979), possibly in areas of the enchondromata which had become degenerate and infarcted.

## Tumours arising in bone affected by Paget's disease

A variety of sarcomas of high-grade malignancy arise in bone affected by Paget's disease. They include osteosarcoma, malignant fibrous histiocytoma, pleomorphic undifferentiated sarcoma and sarcomas containing numerous osteoclast giant cells. True giant cell tumour may also occur, usually in the skull and jaw. The tumours invariably arise in an area of bone that is affected by Paget's disease: the humerus and femur are most frequently affected. The radiology is most helpful as any malignant tumour may stimulate a local reaction in the affected bone, mimicking histologically the features of Paget's disease. The tumours do not have any histological features to distinguish them other than an association with bone showing the features of Paget's disease (Figure 30).

## Tumours arising in previously irradiated bone

Rarely, sarcomas develop in bone which has been irradiated, usually after an interval of 3 or more years (see Chapter 1). All are of high-grade malignancy. The most common histological types are osteosarcoma, fibrosarcoma and malignant fibrous histiocytoma.

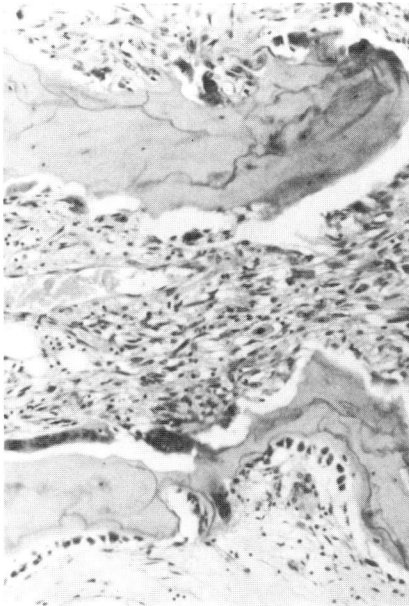

**Figure 30.** Section of bone from humerus showing classic features of Paget's disease with all surfaces covered by osteoblasts or osteoclasts. Evidence of disorderly and rapid turnover is reflected in the mosaic pattern of cement lines within the bone. The marrow spaces are occupied by a high-grade undifferentiated sarcoma. Original magnification × 800.

### Sarcomas arising in bone affected by fibrous dysplasia

Fibrous dysplasia is a developmental abnormality affecting the growing skeleton. Progression of the lesions usually ceases with skeletal maturity. Occasionally a lesion continues to increase in size in young adults—this in itself is not an indication of malignant change. Rarely, malignant change does occur, and in the majority of cases it is associated with prior irradiation. Fibrosarcoma, osteosarcoma and chondrosarcoma have already been described (Campanacci, 1979).

## TUMOURS ARISING IN TISSUE RESTS

These comprise chordoma and adamantinoma.

### Chordoma

This is a tumour of mainly local malignancy which arises from notochordal remnants or rests. The common sites of occurrence are the midline of the upper cervical spine and the sacro-coccygeal region. Rarely, the thoracic and lumbar spine are involved. It is more common in middle age but can occasionally affect adolescents and the elderly. Death is usually due to local extension, but metastases occur in approximately 10% of cases.

Macroscopically the tumour consists of soft, grey, translucent, gelatinous material, very similar in appearance to a myxoid chondrosarcoma. The histological characteristics are of a lobulated tumour with strands and cords of cells arranged like dominoes in a mucoid matrix. The cells contain vacuoles of varying size filled with mucus, referred to as physaliphorus cells (Figure 31). The differential diagnosis is from chondrosarcoma, which may arise in the same sites and have a very similar histological appearance. In the past, attempts have been made to distinguish chordoma from chondro-sarcoma by the use of conventional special stains (Byers, 1981). More recently, the use of immunocytochemistry has enabled a clear-cut distinction to be made, and has confirmed that chordoma is derived from notochor-dal tissue (Salisbury and Isaacson, 1985). Both notochord and chordoma give a positive reaction with the epithelial marker Cam 5.2, while chondro-sarcoma gives a negative reaction.

### Adamantinoma

This is a rare tumour in long bones which owes its name to a histological similarity to the more common adamantinoma of the jaw. The tibia is by far the most common bone affected (90% of all occurrences), and there is an association with pre-existing fibrous dysplasia. The mid-shaft of the tibia is the usual site. The tumour tissue is grey, soft to firm, and usually well demarcated from the adjacent bone. Lobulation and the formation of small cysts may be seen. The histological appearances are of a fibroblastic lesion

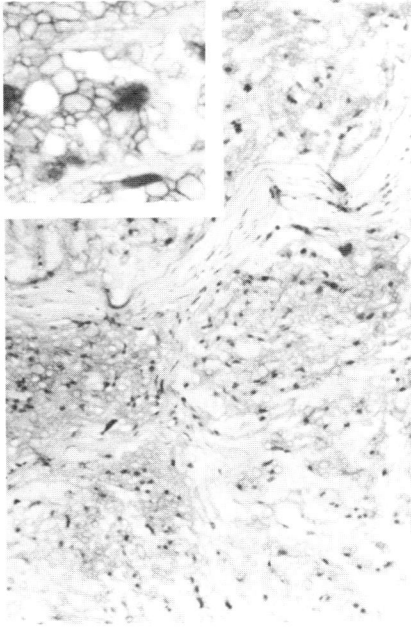

**Figure 31.** Chordoma. A typically lobulated tumour containing cords and strands of cells in a copious matrix. Original magnification × 200. Inset: high power showing vacuolated 'physaliferous' cells. Original magnification × 800.

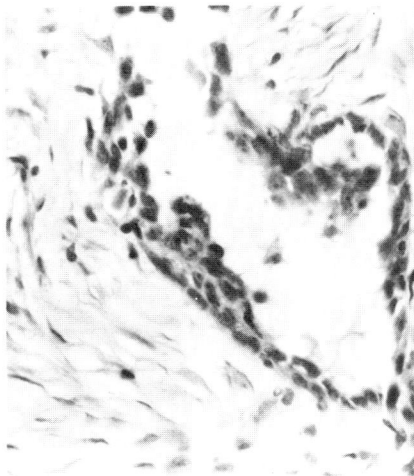

**Figure 32.** Adamantinoma. A spindle-cell background with clefts lined by epithelial cells of rather 'transitional' appearance. Original magnification × 800.

with clefts and spaces lined by epithelial cells that may have a squamous or basal cell appearance (Figure 32). In other areas the epithelial cells are arranged in strands and cords. An electron microscopic study of adamantinoma of the tibia confirmed the epithelial nature of the cells (Rosai, 1969). Other pathologists have noted a similarity of the epithelial cells to proliferating angioblasts, and suggest a vascular origin (Huvos and Marcove, 1975). The main differential, however, is from metastatic carcinoma, particularly if the site and X-ray appearance are atypical. Immunocytochemistry has not proved helpful in this instance: both the epithelial cells in adamantinoma and metastatic carcinoma give a positive reaction with epithelial markers.

## SUMMARY

The introduction of new techniques such as immunocytochemistry has made a significant contribution to the pathology of bone tumours.

The use of alkaline phosphatase on fresh tissue as a marker for malignant osteoblasts has improved the diagnosis in these osteosarcomas where tumour bone formation is scanty. However, in many types of bone tumour accurate diagnosis depends on the ability of technical staff to produce sections of good quality, combined with the experience of the pathologist.

In all cases, close collaboration between the radiologist, surgeon and pathologist is essential.

## REFERENCES

Ahuja SC, Villacin AB & Smith J (1977) Juxtacortical (parosteal) osteogenic sarcoma. Histological grading and prognosis. *Journal of Bone and Joint Surgery* **59A:** 632–647.

Alho A, Connor JF & Mankin HJ (1983) Assessment of malignancy of cartilage tumours using flow cytometry. *Journal of Bone and Joint Surgery* **65:** 779–785.

Askin FB, Rosai J & Sibley RK (1979) Malignant small cell tumor of the thoracopulmonary region in childhood. A distinctive clinicopathological entity of uncertain histogenesis. *Cancer* **43:** 2438–2451.

Bertoni F, Picci P & Bacchini P (1983) Mesenchymal chondrosarcoma of bone and soft tissue. *Cancer* **52:** 533–541.

Bertoni F, Unni KK, McLeod RA & Dahlin DC (1985) Osteoblastoma resembling osteosarcoma. *Cancer* **55:** 416–426.

Boland PJ & Huvos AG (1986) Malignant fibrous histiocytoma of bone. *Clinical Orthopaedics and Related Research* **204:** 130–134.

Byers PD (1968) Solitary benign osteoblastic lesions of bone: osteoid osteoma and benign osteoblastoma. *Cancer* **22:** 43–57.

Byers PD (1981) Chordoma and chondrosarcoma. A study of histological features distinguishing chordoma from chondrosarcoma. *British Journal of Cancer* **43:** 229–232.

Campanacci M (1979) Malignant degeneration in fibrous dysplasia. *Italian Journal of Orthopaedics and Traumatology* **5:** 373–381.

Campanacci M, Giunti A & Olmi R (1975) Giant cell tumours of bone. A study of 209 cases with long term follow up in 130. *Italian Journal of Orthopaedics and Traumatology* **1:** 249–277.

Capanna R, Bertoni F & Bacchini P (1984) Malignant fibrous histiocytoma of bone. The experience at the Rizzoli Institute: report of ninety cases. *Cancer* **54:** 177–187.

Chambers TJ, Fuller K & McSheedy PM (1985) The effects of calcium regulating hormones on bone resorption by isolated human osteoclastoma cells. *Journal of Pathology* **66:** 309–315.

Dahlin DC & Beabout JW (1971) Dedifferentiation of low-grade chondrosarcomas. *Cancer* **28:** 461–466.

Dehner LP (1986) Peripheral and central primitive neuroectodermal tumors: a nosological concept seeking a consensus. *Archives of Pathology and Laboratory Medicine* **110:** 997–1006.

Dosoretz DE, Raymond AK & Murphy GF (1982) Primary lymphoma of bone. The relationship of morphological diversity to clinical behaviour. *Cancer* **50:** 1009–1014.

Eckardt J & Grogan TJ (1986) Giant cell tumour of bone. *Clinical Orthopaedics and Related Research* **204:** 45–58.

Evans HL, Ayala AG & Romsdahl MM (1977) Prognostic factors in chondrosarcoma of bone: a clinicopathological analysis with emphasis on histologic grading. *Cancer* **40:** 818–831.

Goldring SR, Schiller AL & Mankin HJ (1986) Characterisation of cells from human giant cell tumors of bone. *Clinical Orthopaedics and Related Research* **204:** 59–76.

Horton MA, Lewis D & McNulty K (1985) Monoclonal antibodies to osteoclastomas (giant cell bone tumours): definition of osteoclast specific cellular antigens. *Cancer Research* **45:** 5663–5669.

Huvos AG & Marcove R (1975) Adamantinoma of the long bones. A clinicopathological study of fourteen cases with vascular origin suggested. *Journal of Bone and Joint Surgery* **57A:** 148–154.

Huvos AG, Rosen G & Marcove R (1977) Primary osteogenic sarcoma. Pathological aspects in twenty patients after treatment with chemotherapy, en bloc resection and prosthetic replacement. *Archives of Pathology and Laboratory Medicine* **101:** 14–80.

Huvos AG, Rosen G & Dabska M (1983) Mesenchymal chondrosarcoma. A clinicopathological analysis of thirty-five patients with emphasis on treatment. *Cancer* **51:** 1230–1237.

Huvos AG, Heilweil M & Bretsky SS (1985) The pathology of malignant fibrous histiocytoma of bone. A study of 130 patients. *American Journal of Surgical Pathology* **9:** 853–871.

Jackson RP (1978) Recurrent osteoblastoma: a review. *Clinical Orthopaedics and Related Research* **131:** 229–233.

Jaffe HL, Lichtenstein L & Portis RB (1940) Giant cell tumour of bone: its pathological appearance, grading, supposed variants and treatment. *Archives of Pathology* **30:** 993–1031.

Johnston J (1977) Giant cell tumour of bone. The role of the giant cell in orthopaedic pathology. *Orthopaedic Clinics of North America* **8:** 751–770.

Kriekbergs A, Boquist L & Borssen B (1982) Prognostic factors in chondrosarcoma: a comparative study of cellular DNA content and clinicopathological features. *Cancer* **50:** 577–583.

McFarland GB Jr, McKinley LM & Reed RJ (1977) Dedifferentiation of low grade chondrosarcoma. *Clinical Orthopaedics and Related Research* **122:** 157–164.

Merryweather R, Middlemass JH & Sanerkin NG (1980) Malignant transformation of osteoblastoma. *Journal of Bone and Joint Surgery. British volume* **62:** 381–384.

Mierau GW (1985) Extraskeletal Ewing's sarcoma (peripheral neuroepithelioma). *Ultrastructural Pathology* **9:** 91–98.

Mirra JM, Bullough PM & Marcove RC (1974) Malignant fibrous histiocytoma and osteosarcoma in association with bone infarcts. Report of four cases, two in caisson workers. *Journal of Bone and Joint Surgery* **56A:** 932–940.

O'Brien JE & Stout AP (1964) Malignant fibrous xanthoma. *Cancer* **17:** 1445–1455.

Revell PA & Scholtz CL (1979) Aggressive osteoblastoma. *Journal of Pathology* **127:** 195–198.

Ros PR, Viamonte M Jr & Rywlin AM (1984) Malignant fibrous histiocytoma. Mesenchymal tumour of ubiquitous origin. *American Journal of Radiology* **142:** 753–759.

Rosai J (1969) Adamantinoma of the tibia: electron microscopic evidence of its epithelial origin. *American Journal of Clinical Pathology* **51:** 786–792.

Rosen G, Caparros B & Huvos AG (1982) Pre-operative chemotherapy for osteogenic sarcoma. Selection of post-operative adjuvant chemotherapy based upon the response of the primary tumour to pre-operative chemotherapy. *Cancer* **49:** 1221–1230.

Salisbury JR & Isaacson PG (1985) Demonstration of cytokeratins and an epithelial membrane antigen in chordomas and human fetal notochord. *American Journal of Surgical Pathology* **9:** 791–797.

Sanerkin NG (1980a) The diagnosis and grading of chondrosarcoma and fibrosarcoma of bone: a combined cytologic and histologic approach. *Cancer* **45:** 582–594.

Sanerkin NG (1980b) Definitions of osteosarcoma, chondrosarcoma and fibrosarcoma of bone. *Cancer* **46:** 178–185.

Sanerkin NG (1980c) Malignancy, aggressiveness, and recurrence in giant cell tumour of bone. *Cancer* **46:** 1641–1649.

Sanerkin NG & Gallagher P (1979) A review of the behaviour of chondrosarcoma of bone. *Journal of Bone and Joint Surgery. British volume* **61B:** 395–400.

Sanerkin NG & Woods CG (1979) Fibrosarcomata and malignant fibrous histioctyomas arising in relation to enchondromata. *Journal of Bone and Joint Surgery. British volume* **61B:** 366–372.

Schajowicz F (1961) Giant cell tumours of bone (osteoclastoma). A pathological and histo-chemical study. *Journal of Bone and Joint Surgery* **43A:** 1–29.

Schajowicz F & Lemos C (1970) Osteoid osteoma and osteoblastoma. Closely related entities of osteoblastic derivation. *Acta Orthopaedica Scandinavica* **41:** 272–291.

Schajowicz F & Lemos C (1976) Malignant osteoblastoma. *Journal of Bone and Joint Surgery. British volume* **58B:** 202–211.

Sladden RA (1957) Intravascular osteoclasts. *Journal of Bone and Joint Surgery* **39B:** 346–357.

Unni KK, Dahlin DC & Beabout JW (1976a) Parosteal osteogenic sarcoma. *Cancer* **37:** 2644–2675.

Unni KK, Dahlin DC & Beabout JW (1976b) Periosteal osteogenic sarcoma. *Cancer* **37:** 2476–2485.

Unni KK, Dahlin DC & Beabout JW (1976c) Chondrosarcoma: clear cell variant. A report of sixteen cases. *Journal of Bone and Joint Surgery. American volume* **58A:** 676–683.

Wilson JN (1987) Late recurrence following prosthetic replacement for chondrosarcoma (in press).

Wold LE, Unni KK & Beabout JW (1984) Dedifferentiated parosteal osteosarcoma. *Journal of Bone and Joint Surgery* **66A:** 53–59.

Wright DH & Isaacson PG (1983) *Biopsy Pathology of the Lymphoreticular System*, p. 305. London: Chapman & Hall.

# 3

# The place of radiology in diagnosis and management

## D. J. STOKER

Without the assistance of radiology, to the orthopaedic surgeon a bone tumour essentially is a painful swelling. With the availability of a plain radiograph the elements of a coherent differential diagnosis begin to appear. To these must be added other information—clinical, haematological, biochemical, etc., but the imaging modalities remain, short of biopsy, the most important factors in diagnosis and management.

Despite the introduction of new sophisticated imaging techniques, the plain film remains pre-eminent in the primary diagnostic evaluation of any solitary bone lesion. The radiograph is the best imaging method for the demonstration of the pattern of bony destruction, permeation and the zone of transition, basic internal architecture and periosteal reaction. This is not to indicate any conflict between the various imaging methods now available. Indeed, we are fortunate that the newer imaging modalities have extended the capabilities of radiology and not merely replaced one system by another. For the foreseeable future, if one includes a digitalized system, the plain radiograph will remain the main method for radiological diagnosis of musculoskeletal neoplasms. The value of the newer techniques—radionuclide scintigraphy, computed tomography and magnetic resonance imaging—lies more in the staging and management of such tumours, an equally important role. Serious errors in diagnosis most frequently occur when the clinician tries to make the best of films which are inadequate or of poor quality. Constant vigilance is required in control of the radiographic quality to ensure the greatest possible resolution of cortical and trabecular detail, together with the demonstration of soft-tissue shadows. It is a necessary truism to say that the whole of the relevant region must be depicted; so often a misdiagnosis occurs when part of a tumour or even a second lesion lies just off the edge of the radiograph. Equally, not all regions are depicted adequately on standard views, often designed for other purposes; it is important to discuss the radiological investigation of skeletal neoplasms with the interested radiologist at an early stage. Once adequate films are available, diagnosis and further investigation must be achieved through a methodical and analytic approach to each and every film, taking into account all the radiological signs and diagnostic variables.

## THE PLAIN RADIOGRAPH IN DIAGNOSIS

As stated above, a danger exists that the importance of the plain radiograph will be underestimated. Already one sees poor radiographs accepted and used as an excuse to proceed to CT examination, only to provide evidence that good radiography would have shown. Worse, the plain film is sometimes bypassed altogether on the false assumption that new technology is better, whereas the assistance of all appropriate imaging techniques is required in order to gain sufficient information to plan what is best for the patient.

Under certain limited circumstances, the plain radiograph alone is sufficient to establish the diagnosis of a benign and self-limiting tumour or tumour-like lesion. Examples of such lesions, which often do not require intervention, include simple cartilage-capped exostoses, non-ossifying fibromas, sometimes a simple bone cyst (Figure 1), post-traumatic ossi-

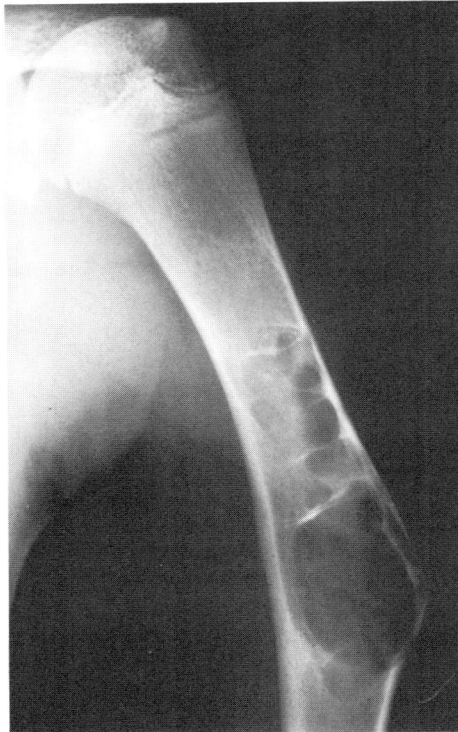

**Figure 1.** Solitary bone cyst of humerus. A well-defined, lucent lesion has expanded the diaphysis of the bone asymmetrically so that the shaft is bowed. The lesion probably arose near the metaphysis but the growth at the proximal metaphysis of the humerus has resulted in displacement of the cyst distally. This is the most common site of origin for a simple cyst. Biopsy is scarcely required for diagnosis, but the lesion could be punctured quite simply and its cystic nature confirmed.

fication, fibrous dysplasia (Figure 2) or a stress fracture. In the majority of symptomatic bone tumours, however, biopsy is essential in order to reach a definitive diagnosis. The radiologist, often from the plain radiograph, can indicate the site most likely to provide adequate representative material for a histological diagnosis. Often, also, a needle or core biopsy performed by the radiologist will prove to be the best means of providing histological material without interfering with future management.

The radiologist does not work in isolation. The diagnosis and management of bone tumours depends on teamwork. The responsibility for the final diagnosis, or indeed, the inability to make a diagnosis, rests with the histopathologist. Both radiologist and histopathologist need to know clinical details, including the age and sex of the patient, the duration of symptoms and whether these included pain. In many cases the radiological diagnosis will be confirmed by the pathologist. In others, the radiologist's differential diagnosis will include the primary diagnosis offered by the pathologist, and this will prove acceptable by the radiologist. Occasionally, the diagnosis

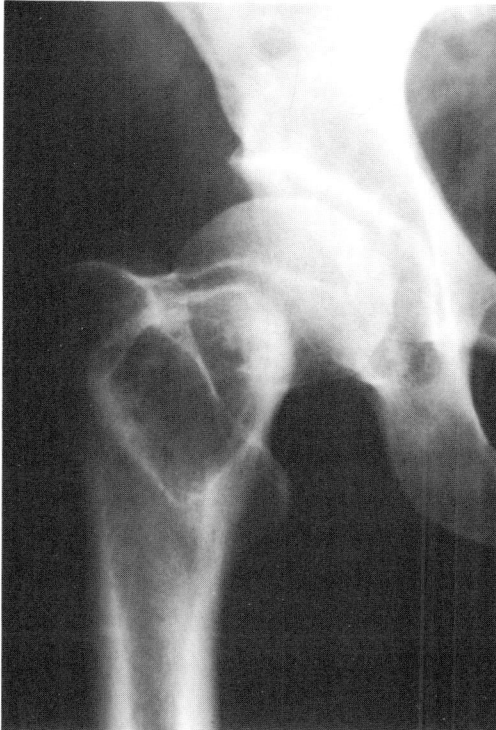

**Figure 2.** Monostotic fibrous dysplasia. Indolent lesions of this type are common in the femoral neck and intertrochanteric region. Note the relatively lucent centre with a thick, sclerotic, rind-like margin. This radiological appearance indicates that the lesion is relatively static, although clear evidence of previous expansion of the bone is shown.

offered by the pathologist will be unacceptable or even bizarre in the light of the radiological features; the radiologist must then challenge its validity. Such diagnostic irreconcilability usually stems from examination of a small or unrepresentative biopsy, which can contain necrotic or reactive tissue; indeed, sometimes only the pseudocapsule of the tumour has been sampled. The radiological information moreover reflects gross pathological anatomy. A frank discussion between the two specialists on the strength of emphasis of various radiological and pathological features will often result in an acceptable diagnosis or at least a course to follow that might result in a working diagnosis for the surgeon.

## GENERAL PRINCIPLES OF RADIOLOGICAL DIAGNOSIS

Orthodox radiology only provides a two-dimensional image of a three-dimensional structure; it can also only differentiate between four types of naturally occurring contrast—water density (most soft tissues), gas, fat and calcium (bone). The relative absence of contrast between muscle and most tumours makes the plain radiograph almost valueless in the diagnosis of a tumour originating in the soft tissues. With bone, the situation is very different. Its well-defined structure and the contrast produced by the presence of fat within the medulla and around the periosteum and muscle bundles enables the form of any destructive process to be depicted and categorized.

### Age of the patient

This is a major consideration in the diagnosis of bone tumours. Many neoplasms show a predominance of incidence confined to perhaps two decades and a range of common and acceptable incidence beyond which it is unwise to make the diagnosis unless the features are unmistakeable.

Carcinomatous metastases are the most common malignancies of bone in patients over the age of 50 years. An atypical metastasis will be encountered in this age group more often than the most radiologically typical primary bone neoplasm. Thus, a sclerotic neoplasm of bone with spiculated periosteal reaction and a soft tissue mass in a man of 70 years is very much more likely to be a metastasis from carcinoma of the prostate gland than a primary osteosarcoma—rare at this age (Figure 3).

The common primary bone neoplasms of childhood—osteosarcoma and Ewing's tumour—are uncommon under the age of 5 years and excessively rare under the age of 2 years. Osteosarcoma is the predominant primary neoplasm of bone in the second decade of life, and Ewing's sarcoma cannot really be diagnosed with any confidence over the age of 30 years. Giant cell tumour of bone is uncommon in children and the older adult; about 85% of these tumours are found between the ages of 18 and 45 years. The likelihood of a neoplasm being a giant cell tumour in a patient with unfused epiphyses at the metaphyseal location of the lesion is very low. In an older patient, the radiological appearance suggestive of a giant cell tumour in a typical subar-

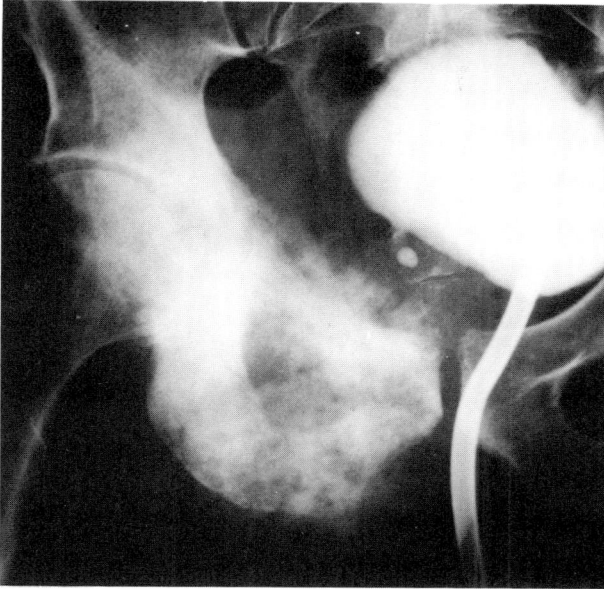

**Figure 3.** Metastasis from carcinoma of the prostate gland. A destructive ischiopubic lesion has produced a large soft tissue extension, much of which is mineralized; the uncalcified element is shown to be displacing the bladder. Although such features constitute the typical appearance of a primary malignancy of bone—an osteosarcoma—in an elderly male patient such a diagnosis would be excessively rare. Metastatic carcinoma is common in this age group, and hence however unusual the appearance, it remains a more likely diagnosis. In this circumstance the calcification is not tumour bone but reactive ossification and/or calcification.

ticular location is more likely to be due to a metastasis (Figure 4). The common primary malignant tumour of the middle-aged or elderly patient is the chondrosarcoma. Although usually less aggressive than osteosarcoma, it is the age of onset that separates these two neoplasms to a great degree.

**Location of the tumour**

Whilst some tumours can arise almost anywhere in the skeleton, certain predilections exist and have to be taken into account.

Primary malignant neoplasms of bone, with the exception of myeloma, are rare in the vertebral column. Thus, any lesion in the axial skeleton in the middle-aged and elderly should suggest a metastasis from carcinoma, or myelomatosis; the presence of similar lesions should therefore be sought in other parts of the skeleton as each of these disorders tends to produce multiple lesions. The most common tumour metastasizing to bone in the first decade of life is neuroblastoma; because the red marrow has not disappeared from the appendicular skeleton, such lesions are often wide-

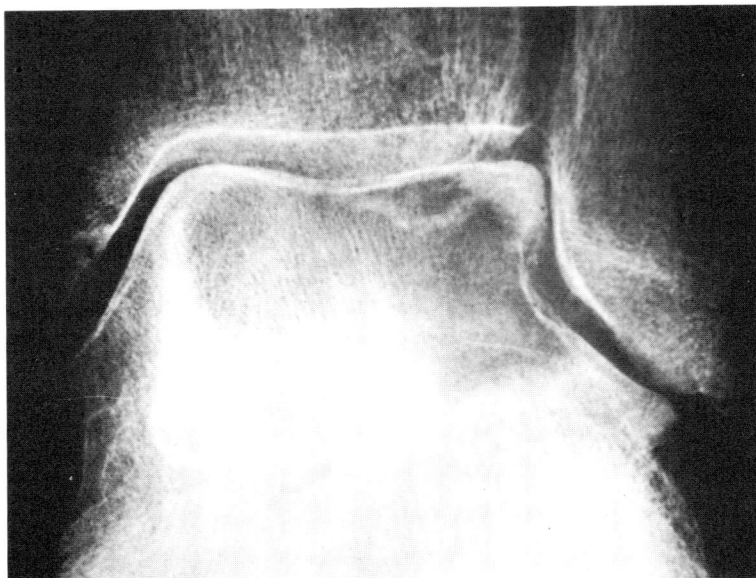

**Figure 4.** Metastasis resembling giant cell tumour. In this middle-aged adult with pain in the ankle, the destructive lesion extending to the subarticular cortex of the talus could be a giant cell tumour radiologically. A lytic metastasis, however, can exactly simulate giant cell tumour in an appropriate age group. Giant cell tumours are relatively uncommon over the age of 45 years, whilst metastases usually affect individuals above this age.

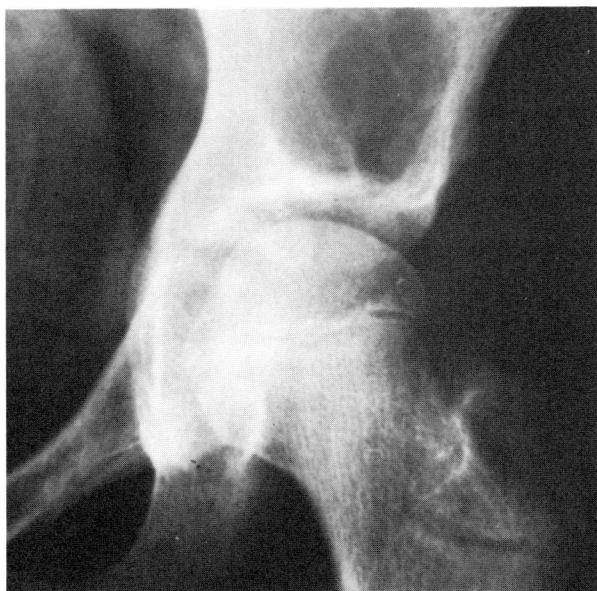

**Figure 5.** Eosinophilic granuloma. A well-defined lytic lesion of the acetabular roof has caused slight expansion of the ilium in this child. Radiologically, the lesion has benign characteristics, although some periosteal reaction has formed. An axial location is typical.

spread. Histioreticuloses such as eosinophilic granuloma and primary histiocytic lymphoma tend also to occur in sites of residual red marrow (Figure 5). In contrast, most primary bone tumours tend to occur in areas of rapid growth, particularly affecting the distal femur, proximal tibia and proximal humerus. Exceptions to this tendency abound, particularly in tumours that present after childhood, and include chordoma with its predilection for involving either end of the spine, chondrosarcoma, predominantly affecting the pelvis and femur (Figure 6), and adamantinoma with a peculiar propensity for involvement of the tibial shaft.

Johnson's metabolic field theory states that 'a tumour of a given cell type usually arises in that metabolic field where the homologous normal cells are most active' (Johnson, 1953). This statement is supported by the fact that many primary tumours of bone arise in the metaphysis. Clear exceptions include malignant round cell tumours which occur most commonly in the diaphyses. It might be argued that these are tumours of red marrow and not bone and it is certainly true that we do not know their cell of origin.

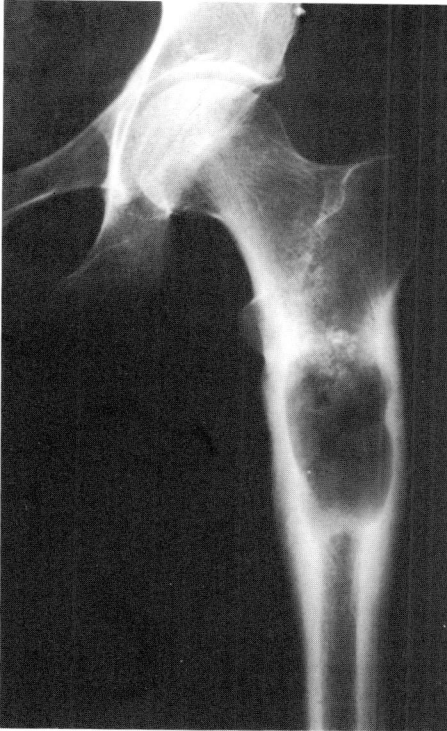

**Figure 6.** Chondrosarcoma of proximal shaft of femur. A lytic lesion is present in the proximal shaft of the femur in this elderly patient. Its relatively slow growth is characterized by scalloping of the cortex and some endosteal sclerosis. A confident radiological diagnosis of chondrosarcoma can be made radiologically on the basis of this appearance; biopsy is, however, required for confirmation before definitive therapy is instituted.

Within the bone, whilst most neoplasms are centred on the medulla, a parosteal osteosarcoma, as its name indicates, is related to the subperiosteal cortex (Figure 7).

Benign bone tumours also are often associated with characteristic sites. A non-ossified fibroma is usually located subcortically in the diametaphysis of

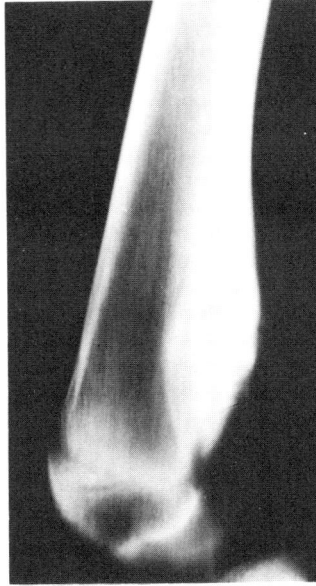

**Figure 7.** Parosteal osteosarcoma. An orthodox tomographic examination in this case shows the typical posterior parosteal location of the tumour. Although the endosteal cortex is thickened, no medullary extension by the tumour is suggested and a good prognosis for surgical excision might be expected. However, CT or MRI examination would be advisable to confirm the limited extension of the tumour.

a long bone in the lower limb (Figure 8; see also Chapter 6, Figure 23). A giant cell tumour almost invariably is subarticular by the time it is clinically and radiologically apparent (Figure 9).

**Rate of growth**

The radiologist, by analysis of the process destroying bone, determines the tumour most likely to possess such characteristics, having regard to the age of the patient and the other radiological features. This is in contradistinction to the histopathologist, who deduces the rate of growth from the cell type and cellular activity of the small area under scrutiny. It is because of these responses to different types of information that the combination of a histological and a radiological opinion provides the most accurate diagnostic assessment in skeletal oncology.

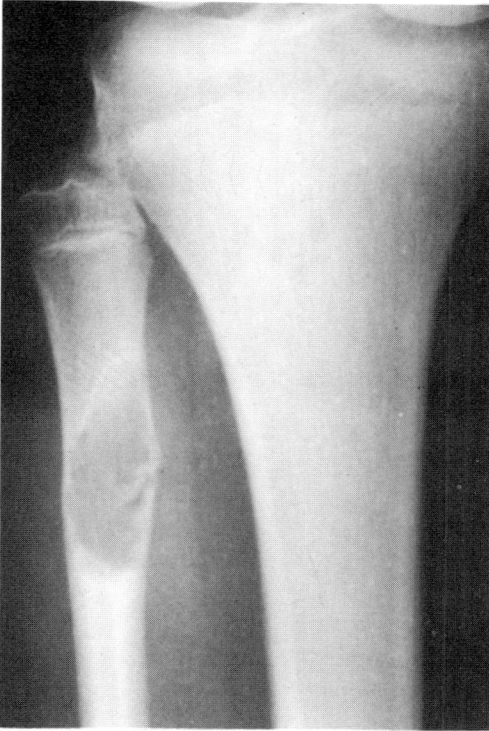

**Figure 8.** Non-ossifying fibroma. A pathological fracture has been sustained through a clearly benign lesion of the proximal part of the shaft of the fibula. Although it has now crossed the shaft, the lesion seems to have had an eccentric origin from the region of the medial cortex.

The determination of the rate of growth of a tumour therefore is a primary responsibility of the radiologist. Much of the clear analysis of radiological observation in this field must be attributed to the work of Lodwick (1971, 1980a, 1980b).

A review of the accuracy of human performance in interpreting the diagnostic radiological features of disease shows that observers can be very accurate in distinguishing between slow- and fast-growing lesions (Lodwick et al, 1980b). It seems unlikely that a computerized program would improve on a simple algorithm in this respect. The prediction of the histological diagnosis is less accurate, indicating that the determination of the rate of growth is merely a necessary first stage in the analysis of a bony lesion. It could be assumed that the experience of the radiological observer must be the most important factor in this second phase of diagnosis.

Most bone tumours arise in the medulla of the skeleton. As a consequence of its large surface area, cancellous bone is destroyed more rapidly than is cortical bone. Unfortunately, however, a lytic region of medullary bone cannot be identified with any certainty, even on a radiograph of good

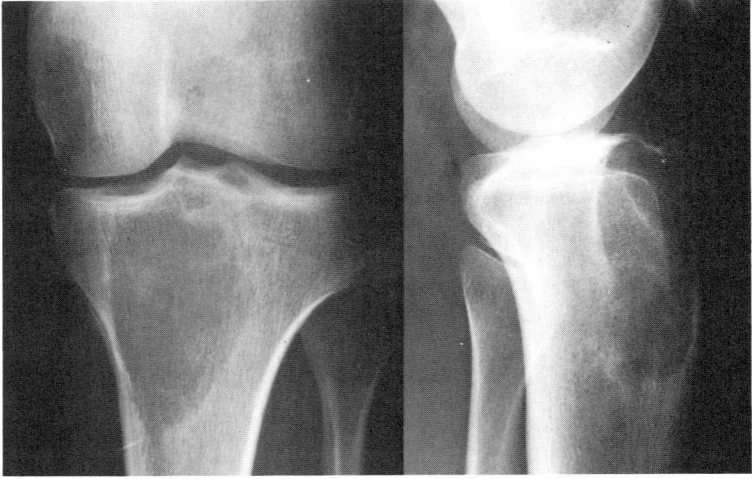

**Figure 9.** Giant cell tumour. A moderately well-defined lytic lesion lies in close relationship to the subchondral cortex of the anterior part of the medial tibial condyle, and this is entirely compatible with the characteristic behaviour of a giant cell tumour at presentation. It should be observed that the tumour also lies in close proximity to the site of the fused apophysis for the tibial tubercle—another acceptable location for giant cell tumour.

quality, until 40–50% of the bone mass has been removed. In contrast, even a small area of erosion of cortical bone will become evident on the plain film.

In most cases the destruction of bone associated with tumours is not a direct effect of the neoplastic cells. It is mediated through resorption by osteoclasts, direct pressure by the tumour mass, by associated hyperaemia or by an alteration in the physiology of the bone (Madewell et al, 1981).

As it enlarges, a neoplasm of bone causes a modification of host bone at its interface with the tumour. This is mediated mainly by the activity of the osteoclasts and osteoblasts of the host bone. The patterns produced reflect the rate of growth of the tumour (Lodwick, 1971), thus:

Grade I—geographical pattern (slow growth)
Grade II—moth-eaten pattern (intermediate growth)
Grade III—permeative pattern (rapid growth)

*Grade I pattern*

This indicates slow erosion of the cortex with sharp margination; destructive change in the medulla will not produce a geographic appearance unless it also produces sclerosis.

Grade I has been divided further into three subtypes, IA, IB and IC.

*Type IA.* This is a geographical lesion with sclerosis of its margin. This exemplifies the typical benign bony lesion such as a solitary bone cyst (Figure 1), quiescent enchondroma, chondromyxoid fibroma (Figure 10), monostotic fibrous dysplasia (Figure 2) and Brodie's abscess.

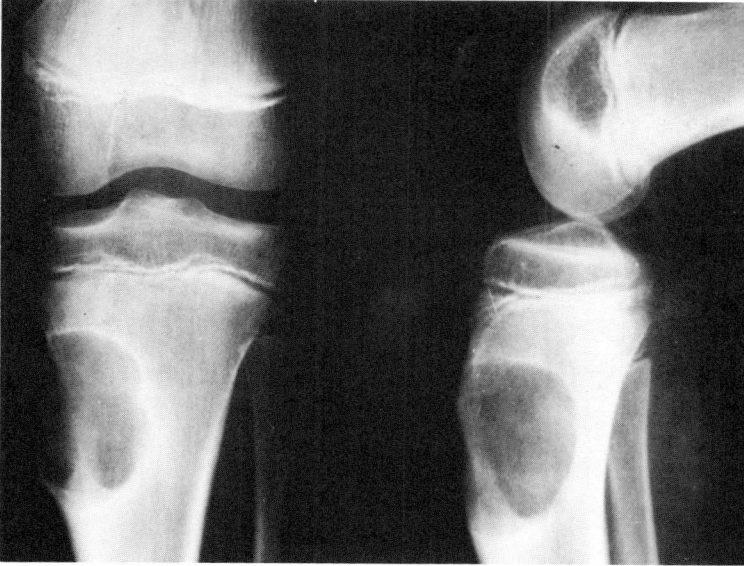

**Figure 10.** Chondromyxoid fibroma. In addition to the characteristic site close to the tibial tubercle, this benign neoplasm shows a cortical defect, a rounded contour and a thin sclerotic endosteal margin—features associated typically with this tumour.

*Type IB*. This is a geographical lesion with no sclerosis of its margin. Type IB lesions often appear 'punched-out' (Figure 11). They do have some medullary sclerotic reaction in that it is the minimal sclerosis of the margin that makes them visible, but this is not an obtrusive feature. However, when the cortex is involved to even a small degree, the lesion becomes visible without the need for cortical sclerosis. This type of radiological appearance is seen in rather more active type IA lesions and especially in benign chondroid neoplasms and more slowly growing giant cell tumours.

*Type IC*. This is a geographical lesion with ill-defined margins. This amounts to a locally infiltrative process, short of a grade II lesion. Neoplasms showing this degree of biological activity include giant cell tumours (Figure 12), active chondromas, chondrosarcomas (Figure 6), certain metastases and low-grade osteosarcomas.

*Grade III pattern*

This is described next. At its least detectable stage radiologically, it involves partial lysis of the cancellous bone of the medulla. Penetration of the entire cortex must be assumed in all moth-eaten and permeated grades (Figure 13). When destruction of the cortex first becomes visible it is ill-defined, but nevertheless such cortical involvement enables the lesion to be identified radiologically. A more reactive medullary lesion, such as a Brodie's abscess,

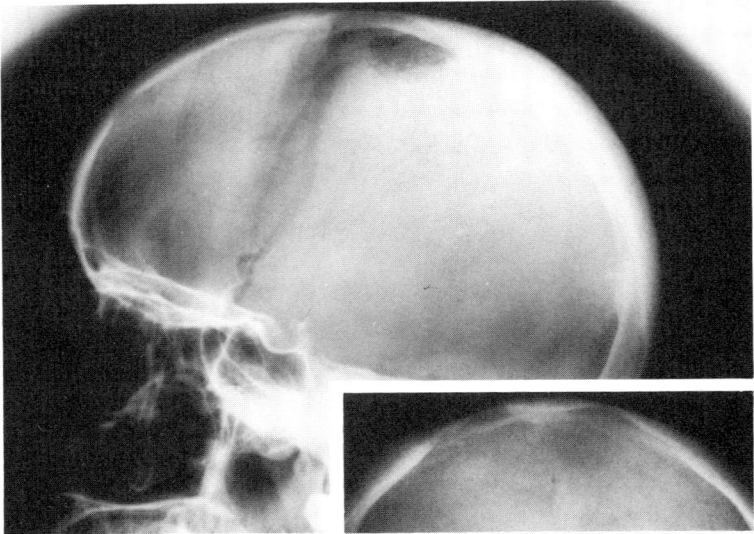

**Figure 11.** Eosinophilic granuloma. A destructive but well-defined lesion is present in the anterior parietal region of the skull of this young patient. In the inset, a projection tangential to the lesion shows the margins to be sharp and bevelled, confirming the benignity of the lesion.

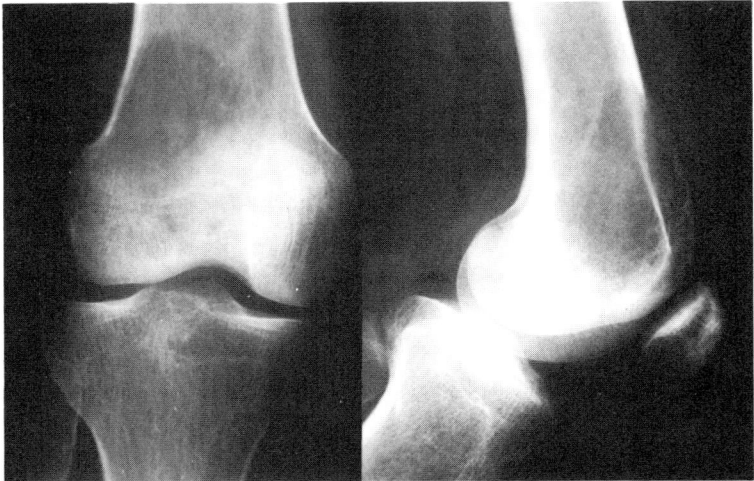

**Figure 12.** Giant cell tumour of bone. This example differs from that illustrated earlier (Figure 9) in that it is located in the femur at and above the level of the patellofemoral articulation. After initial expansion, the anterior femoral cortex is thinned to destruction. Observe that the endosteal margin is ill-defined, suggesting an aggressive tumour. This patient was aged 41 years at presentation. The differential diagnosis includes bone metastasis.

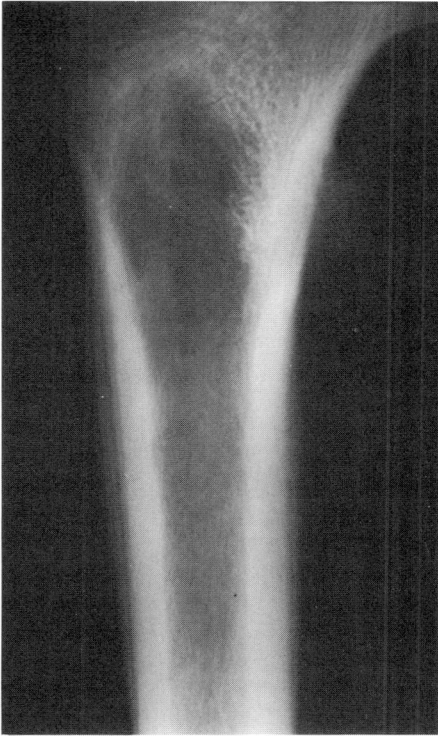

**Figure 13.** Ewing's sarcoma. Ill-defined permeation of the medulla of the proximal femoral shaft is shown together with a multilaminar periosteal reaction. Although this is a finding considered to be classical of Ewing's tumour, such periosteal change is most uncommon in practice.

becomes visible not because of cortical involvement but on account of subtle sclerosis of its medullary margins. This explanation of the difference between geographic and permeating lesions runs counter to that proposed by some authors (Madewell et al, 1981).

*Grade II pattern*

This pattern lies intermediately between the two other grades (Figure 14) and may be difficult to distinguish at times from a coarsely permeating pattern; it probably constitutes the most difficult area of assessment in this classification. It has been suggested that accuracy in grading can be maintained by modifying the categories (Lodwick, 1980b). In this modification, grade III can include moth-eaten and/or permeating patterns but *no* geographical components; grade II can include a similar mixture but with geographical components.

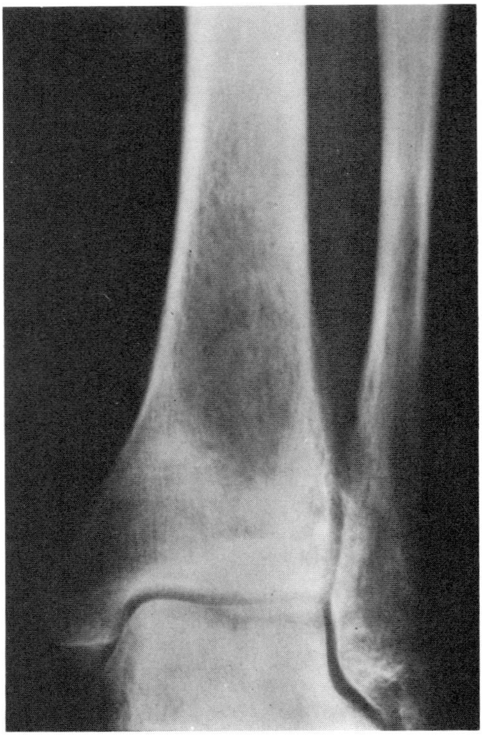

**Figure 14.** Malignant fibrous histiocytoma. This malignant neoplasm, in recent years separated histologically from fibrosarcoma, here shows a moth-eaten appearance. Superimposed on a background of medullary permeation are small, lenticulate lucencies which will probably coalesce as they grow. Such lucencies usually indicate focal erosion of the endosteal cortex. The neoplasm remains poorly defined generally and is highly malignant.

Determination of what constitutes one of these patterns necessitates the introduction of the concept of the zone of transition between normal and abnormal bone. The radiologist has to decide at what point, at the edge of the tumour, the bone is clearly abnormal and where it is entirely normal. An area will remain where it is not possible to say categorically whether the bone is either normal or abnormal—this is the zone of transition. When the zone measures only a few millimetres, the edge is sharp (geographical); when it is indistinct and the zone of transition extends over a centimetre or more, then a more permeating lesion is present. A moth-eaten lesion essentially is a permeating lesion which in addition contains larger, often elliptical or irregular, lytic areas, probably resulting from patchy erosion of the cortex (Figure 14). Usually, the zone of transition is less than a centimetre.

In addition to the pattern of bony destruction, the reaction of the tissues of the host must also be assessed. Slow growth permits the host bone time to surround the tumour with reactive new bone. In the medulla this takes the form of an enveloping endosteal sclerosis, while the cortex (periosteum) responds by producing a shell of new bone of variable thickness. An increase in the rate of growth subsequently will reduce the thickness of this reactive bone.

Sometimes the margin of the lesion varies in its definition. When the variation is relatively minor in degree, especially on serial radiographs, it should be remembered that the radiographic technique can alter the appearance. However, radiographic technical variation cannot make an ill-defined lesion better defined; so if the lesion shows a difference in its borders, it is most probable that the best defined region reflects the true activity of the neoplasm. This must not be accepted if the change is from a relatively slowly growing margin on one side to an overtly aggressive one on another. In this circumstance, the possibility that the lesion has changed its grade of malignancy has to be considered (Figure 15). Such change—'dedifferentiation'—occurs when one part of a neoplasm assumes a different histological appearance, always in the direction of greater malignancy. Thus, a chondrosarcoma may dedifferentiate into a fibrosarcoma or malignant fibrous histiocytoma, or a lower grade of osteosarcoma may

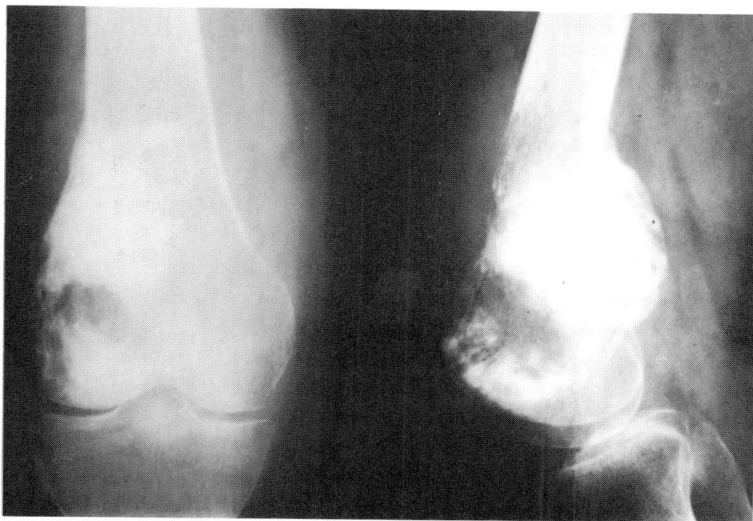

**Figure 15.** Dedifferentiation of parosteal osteosarcoma. The tumour of the distal end of the femur shows a mixed pattern of sclerosis and lysis. The element lying posteriorly is consistent with a parosteal osteosarcoma, but anteriorly a destructive element of greater malignancy is shown. Here the cortex is destroyed and a soft-tissue mass is evident. A biopsy diagnosis of parosteal osteosarcoma had been made earlier at another institution on the basis of the posterior lesion. The radiologist indicated that the lesion had changed, showing appearances reflecting dedifferentiation to a more malignant lesion, and that a further biopsy should be obtained *anteriorly*. The more aggressive element of the tumour proved to be a highly malignant orthodox osteosarcoma.

change to an orthodox and highly malignant variety. Another change that may occur in pre-existing disease is the malignant transformation of benign disorders. Thus, chondrosarcomatous transformation may affect an osteochondroma, and Paget's disease or radiation osteitis may be complicated by sarcomatous change (Figure 16).

The most important diagnostic feature in determining malignancy, or at least local aggressive behaviour, of a neoplasm is the presence of extension into the soft tissues. As the periosteum is not identifiable by any method of imaging, tumour in an extraperiosteal location has to be recognized by implication from whatever radiological signs that are available. Sometimes the periosteum is visualized by the formation of a thin shell of new bone that demonstrates that the tumour is likely to lie within bone (Figure 17). On other occasions, a large, well-defined tumour mass is clearly extraosseous, and this implies malignancy (Figure 18).

Most initial periosteal reactions are non-specific and linear. Multilaminar reactions indicate a periodicity of the tumoral extension. Such an appearance is classically attributed to Ewing's sarcoma (Figure 13). but it is rare even in the presence of that tumour. The formation of parosteal new bone perpendicular to the cortical margin is usually reactive in nature because

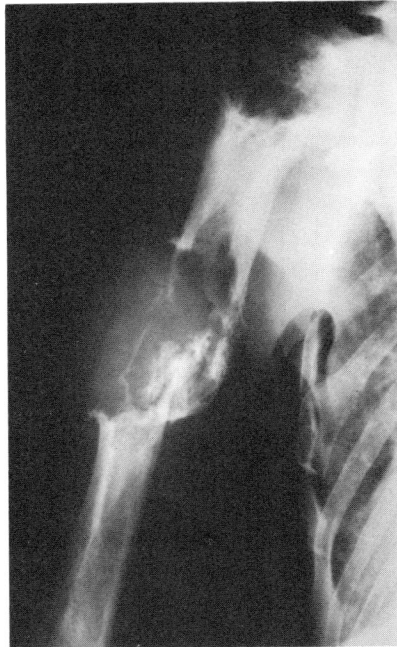

**Figure 16.** Paget's sarcoma. The humerus shows the classical changes of Paget's disease. The diaphyseal lytic lesion cannot be explained except by a complicating neoplasm such as sarcoma, metastasis or possibly giant cell tumour. Observe the associated soft-tissue mass. Histological examination confirmed the presence of an osteosarcoma.

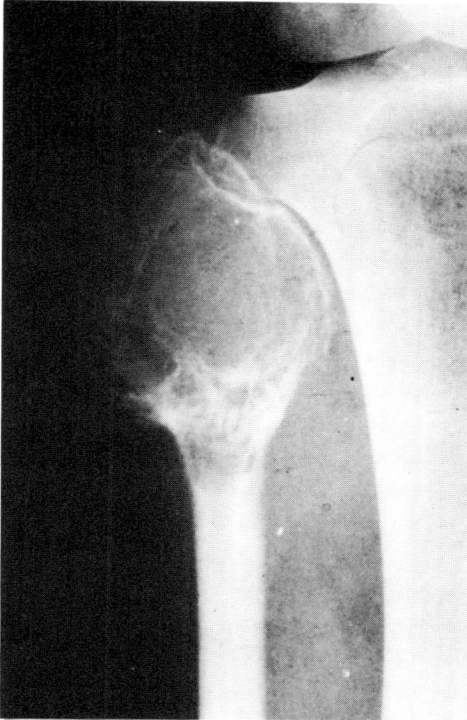

**Figure 17.** Aneurysmal bone cyst. The lytic lesion of the head of the fibula expands the bone, a feature often associated with benign lesions, even if the tumour is locally aggressive. A thin shell of bone covered the lateral aspect of the tumour so that it remained entirely within the periosteum.

such bony spicules follow the lines of the prominent Sharpey's fibres, which bind the periosteum to the cortex until the force elevating it stretches or ruptures them. Although classically associated with osteosarcoma, when the reactive spiculation may be supplemented by the presence of tumoral bone (Figure 18), such a 'sunburst' reaction is by no means confined to that tumour (Figure 3). More delicate perpendicular spicules are to be found in the presence of Ewing's sarcoma, and a sunburst reaction is not uncommon in low-grade chronic cellulitis.

## THE PLAIN RADIOGRAPH IN MANAGEMENT

As already stated, in certain limited circumstances a firm decision on management may be made on the plain film alone. This is usually brought about by the identification of a self-limiting, benign tumour or tumour-like lesion,

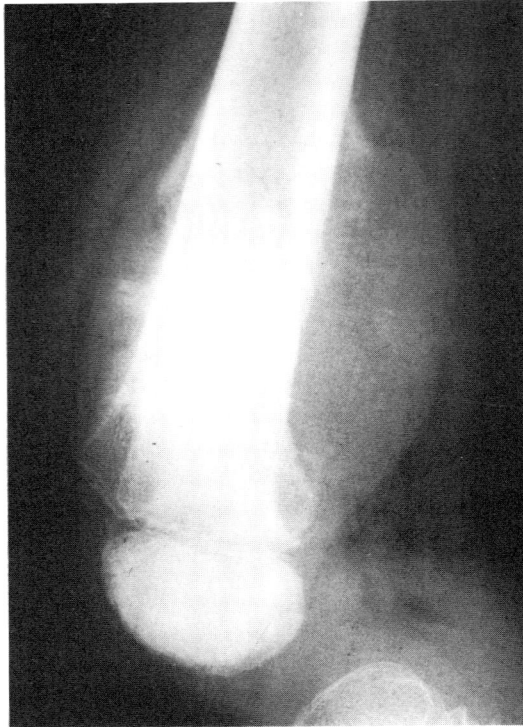

**Figure 18.** Osteosarcoma. In this lateral projection of a typical osteosarcoma of the distal femoral shaft, a large well-defined soft-tissue mass indicates that the tumour is malignant. A smaller mass anteriorly shows ill-defined, perpendicularly orientated bone formation extending from the cortex into the soft-tissue mass. Reactive (Codman) triangles are present.

where the decision is to take no action, or at most to observe the lesion by serial radiographic examinations. In other cases the plain film diagnosis may result in a course of action without further extensive imaging. Such a situation may arise when a solitary bone cyst is diagnosed in a classical site such as the proximal shaft of the humerus, leading to confirmatory cyst puncture and intracystic injection of corticosteroids.

In most cases of intraosseous tumour, however, the radiograph gives only a working differential diagnosis, although this is, quite often, a clearly preferred diagnosis (e.g. Figure 17). Such a diagnosis has to be substantiated, usually by biopsy. Primary neoplasia of bone is rare and, increasingly, cases are likely to be managed in centres where expertise in several specialties is gathered together. The experienced skeletal radiologist can expect to make a specific diagnosis in a high proportion of cases by combining the radiological evidence of the degree of aggressiveness of the lesion with his knowledge of the particular radiographic pattern in the age group under survey.

Subsequently, the radiologist is responsible for defining the anatomical extent of the lesion for the surgeon by complementing the information on the plain film with that of other imaging techniques.

## Relationship to the histological diagnosis

The osteoarticular histopathologist cannot function satisfactorily without radiological information, particularly when biopsy material is under consideration. The radiograph provides the only available information on gross pathological anatomy. Ideally, the histological and radiological opinions will agree. Alternatively, the pathologist's diagnosis is included within the radiologist's short list of likely diagnoses. Of the greatest importance, however, is the situation when the radiologist is unable to accept the histological diagnosis or vice versa. A variety of causes may apply; for example, the radiological appearances may be atypical or the biopsy unrepresentative. In the latter case, certainly, the surgeon must be prevailed upon to agree to a further biopsy procedure after discussing with the radiologist the site most likely to provide representative and diagnostic tissue.

## Staging—defining the extent of the lesion

One of the radiological differences between the extension of a malignant neoplasm and an infection from the bone into the soft tissues is that the malignant tumour is defined better than the infective mass (Figure 18). This results from the fact that we observe such soft tissue masses because of the surrounding fat in the perimuscular tissues. The extent of the inflammatory oedema surrounding an abscess is always greater than that at the periphery of a neoplasm, and hence the fat loses its normal transradiancy at an earlier stage (Figure 19). Differentiation of such changes may be quite subtle and requires good soft-tissue radiography; nevertheless, the observation is extremely valuable. Greater accuracy in staging can be obtained by adding the information obtained from the more recently available imaging modalities—computed tomography (CT) and magnetic resonance imaging (MRI). The objective of staging is the prediction of the degree of risk of local recurrence or distant metastasis and the implication of this on surgical and chemotherapeutic management. In 1980, a system for the staging of musculoskeletal sarcoma was proposed and adopted by the Musculoskeletal Tumor Society (Enneking et al, 1980), subsequently being adopted by the American Joint Committee for Cancer Staging and End Results Reporting (Enneking, 1986) (see Chapter 4). This system depends greatly upon radiological information. Not only does staging specifically relate to the radiographic grade, radionuclide scintigraphy angiography and CT, but many so-called clinical elements of grading, site and distant spread are based primarily on radiological information.

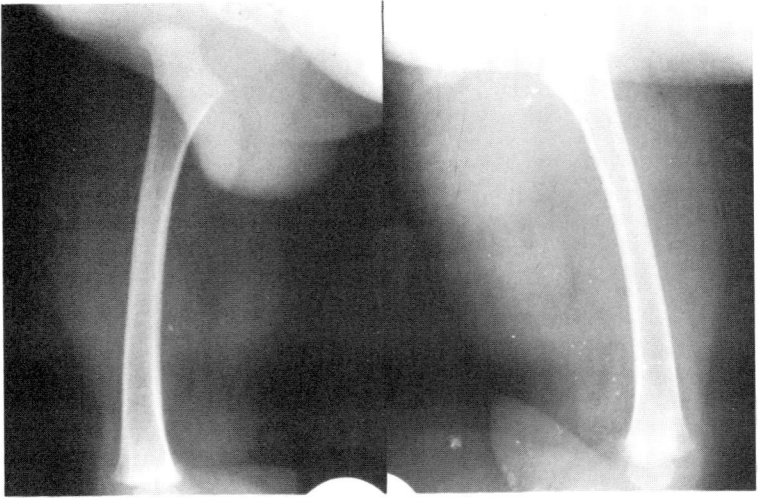

**Figure 19.** Cellulitis of the thigh. The normal limb is shown on the left, the affected thigh on the right. No osseous lesion was found in this infant. The infective process has caused swelling of the thigh with loss of the definition of the muscular bundles as a consequence of inflammatory oedema. Compare this appearance with the margin of the soft tissue extension in Figure 18.

## RADIONUCLIDE BONE SCANNING

This method of imaging is highly sensitive but non-specific, and hence is rarely diagnostic in the field of bone tumours. Probably its most valuable function is in the demonstration or exclusion of multiple lesions. Metastatic cancer is the most common form of malignancy in the skeleton. Lytic metastases may not be visible on a plain film for several months after their demonstration on a bone scan. It is therefore always important to confirm that a lesion in a middle-aged patient is solitary; it may still be a solitary metastasis, but if multiple lesions are evident at scintigraphy, the chances of a primary neoplasm being present diminish markedly. Similarly, certain malignant tumours, notably those of the fibrous series, have a reputation for producing 'skip' lesions in a more proximal location. These are likely to be revealed by a radionuclide bone scan.

In respect of solitary bone tumours, scintigraphy can provide some element of differential diagnosis. Uptake of the phosphorus–technetium complex relates to both the vascular supply and the metabolic activity of the bony lesion. Many highly malignant tumours such as osteosarcoma produce scans with intense activity and irregular outlines (Murray, 1980), often overestimating the extent of the tumoral involvement as the surrounding reactive tissues also take up the radionuclide. The marrow permeation of a Ewing's sarcoma often leads to a lesser activity but may reflect the extent of the involvement by showing activity along the length of the bone far beyond any abnormality detected on the radiograph.

Variation in the uptake of a tumour may reflect its vascular pattern with peripheral uptake in a tumour, such as an aneurysmal bone cyst, which is mainly filled with blood (Gunterberg et al, 1977). Such a deduction is not always possible, however, as it is well known from pathological studies that certain tumours may outstrip their blood supply and undergo central necrosis or haemorrhage. Such complications also will be reflected in reduced central photon activity on a bone scan (Figure 20).

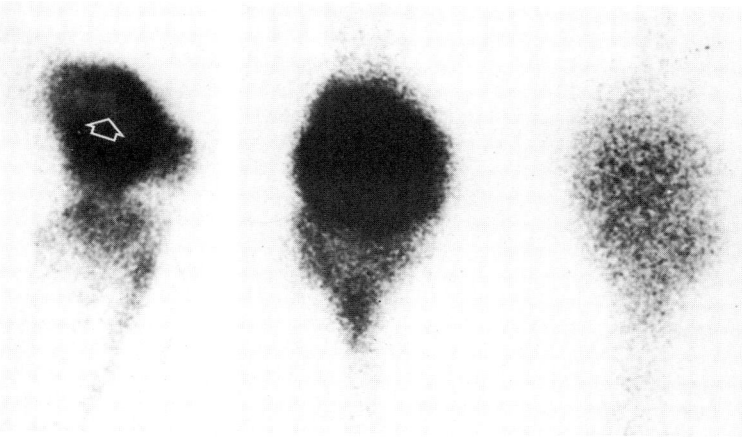

**Figure 20.** Giant cell tumour of distal femur: scintigraphy. A markedly increased uptake of radionuclide has occurred in the location of the tumour. Note the reduction in activity centrally in the lateral projection (arrow). Pathological examination of the tumour revealed massive central haemorrhage and necrosis which probably caused the features evident on the radionuclide scan.

Nevertheless, in terms of staging, radionuclide scans do tend to indicate the extent of the combined neoplastic defect of bone and the surrounding reactive tissue changes and oedema.

## ARTERIOGRAPHY

As it is an invasive procedure, the value of arteriography in the diagnosis and management of bone tumours has always been in dispute. Its value has been stressed in the past (Voegeli and Uehlinger, 1976). In my opinion it has never had an important or necessary place in the diagnosis of such lesions. Its value in the delineation of a soft-tissue extension (Figure 21) has been removed by the introduction of CT and even more so by MRI. In the identification of involvement of major vascular bundles and their relationship to the tumour margin, arteriography has been mainly supplanted by CT scanning following the injection of contrast medium. The depiction of this by axial cuts also has an advantage to the surgeon interested in staging, and

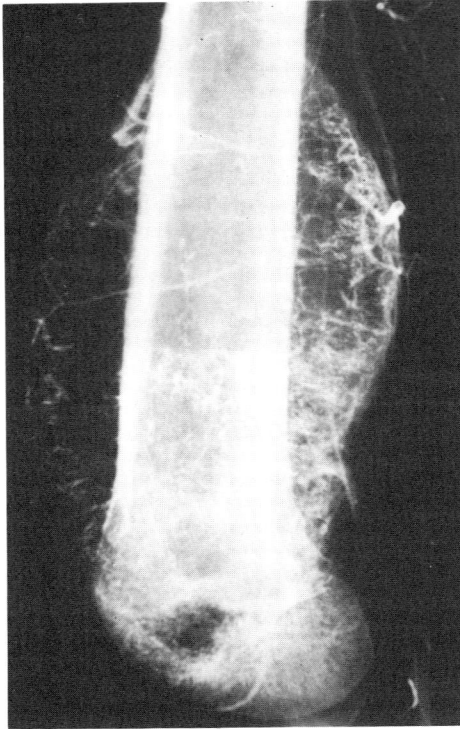

**Figure 21.** Osteosarcoma—arteriography. The extent of the soft tissue mass is shown well by the distribution of normal and neoplastic vessels. The presence of the soft-tissue mass would be clearly visible on a well-exposed radiograph. Nowadays, further evidence in respect of the relationship of the mass to normal structures would usually be provided by CT or MRI.

shows whether the tumour is still within an anatomical compartment. CT itself is in the process of being replaced by MRI for this purpose. None of these methods is, however, infallible, as MRI produces false-positives caused by peritumoral oedema involving the region of the main vessels.

In two areas, arteriography still seems to have a place. Firstly, it remains valuable in the demonstration of tumours of vascular origin, benign or malignant. Secondly, in the embolization of large vascularized tumours that might otherwise be unsuitable for more than palliative therapy, prior diagnostic angiography is essential. Together, these applications relate to only a small percentage of tumours seen by orthopaedic surgeons. Nowadays, angiography can usually be undertaken more quickly and with less risk of complications using digital subtraction arteriography (Figure 22).

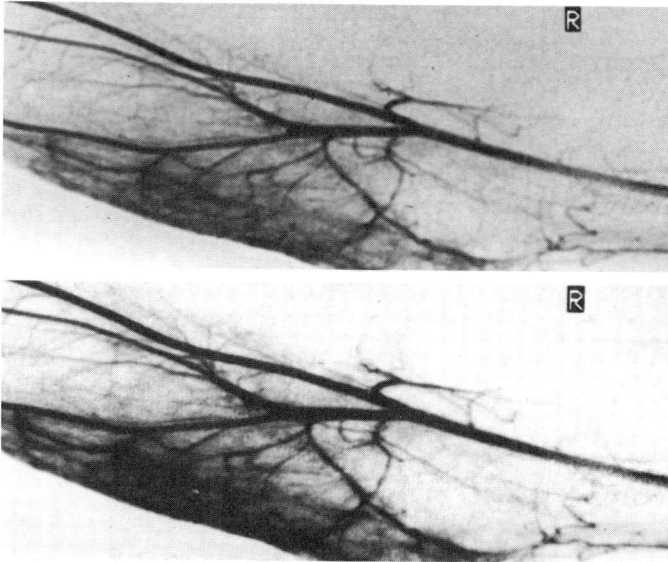

**Figure 22.** Digital subtraction arteriography. This 30-year-old man presented with a recent swelling of his forearm associated with trivial trauma. These angiograms indicate the presence of many atypical vessels consistent with the presence of a benign vascular anomaly. The swelling was considered to be a haematoma and was settled without treatment.

## COMPUTED TOMOGRAPHY

Although it does not play a major part in the primary radiological diagnosis, CT is superior to the plain radiograph in a number of areas of interest. It is of most use in:

1. Determining the intramedullary extension of the tumour on serial transverse axial slices;
2. Determining the presence and extent of extraosseous extension of the neoplasm (Figure 23);
3. Demonstrating the relationship between the tumour and important adjoining structures, in particular the involvement by tumour of major vessels following their demonstration by intravascular injection of contrast medium;
4. Demonstrating certain characteristics of the tumour, such as mineralization of the matrix, which may be important in the diagnosis (Figure 24).
5. Contributing to staging of the disease by demonstrating certain local anatomical relationships and the presence or absence of pulmonary or nodal metastases.

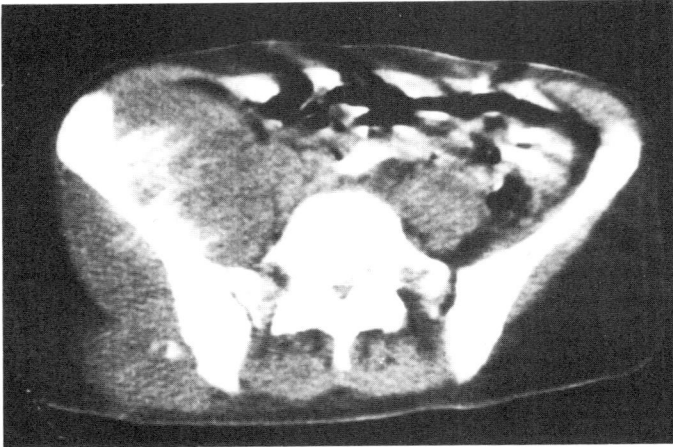

**Figure 23.** CT examination of chondrosarcoma of ilium. A very large mass of tumour lies on both sides of the right iliac wing, the larger part being within the pelvic cavity. Relatively little bony destruction is shown on this CT slice, but radiating spicules extend into the mass from the underlying cortex. Some calcification posterolaterally within the mass indicates the chondroid nature of the tumour in this middle-aged patient.

Some of these attributes are simply sophisticated extensions of linear tomography; others are almost unique to CT or shared in part with MRI.

In terms of superficial lesions, CT will demonstrate that a lesion is completely parosteal or, often in the case of osteochondroma, that the marrow cavity continues into the stem of the lesion. Similarly, it is usually possible to determine if a parosteal lesion originating in soft tissue is involving the cortex itself or simply stimulating periosteal reaction.

CT was the first imaging technique to assess with any degree of accuracy the extent of medullary involvement by a primary neoplasm of bone (Figure 24). It has to be accepted that no imaging technique can be expected to detect a few tumour cells extending along the connective tissue strands of the medullary cavity. Nevertheless, in terms of producing transaxial images every 1.0 centimetre, CT can procure information for the surgeon that enables him to excise the tumour in its entirety, without the necessity of removing normal bone. Measurement of the attenuation value within a representative volume of medulla is more accurate than a visual impression. The measurement in Hounsfield units (Hu) can be compared with the result either of the normal medulla, away from the tumour site, or with the other limb. Similarly, when a tumour is essentially fatty in nature, for example on the plain film, CT can almost always distinguish a benign lipoma with a value equivalent to fat (about $-95$ Hu) from a liposarcoma with a value usually between $-70$ Hu and $+50$ Hu (Figure 25) (Halldorsdottir et al, 1982).

The radiological grading already referred to on examination of the plain radiograph has its counterpart in the CT scan, although this is probably a less reliable and vastly more expensive method of obtaining such information.

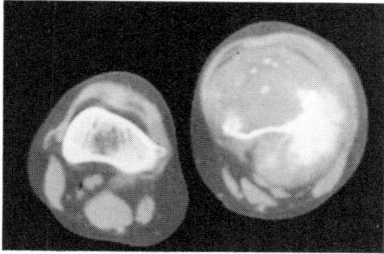

(a)

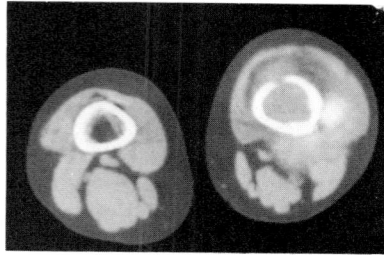

(b)

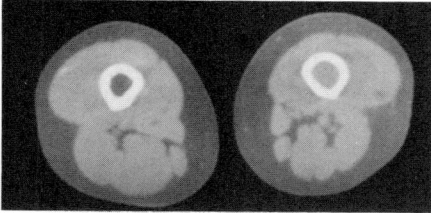

(c)

**Figure 24.** Osteosarcoma. Three CT slices are shown of this neoplasm of the distal end of the femur. (a) shows the soft-tissue extension and tumour bone formation. (b) shows intramedullary tumour soft-tissue extension. (c) shows the extent of intramedullary extension compared with the fat density of the normal marrow in the unaffected limb.

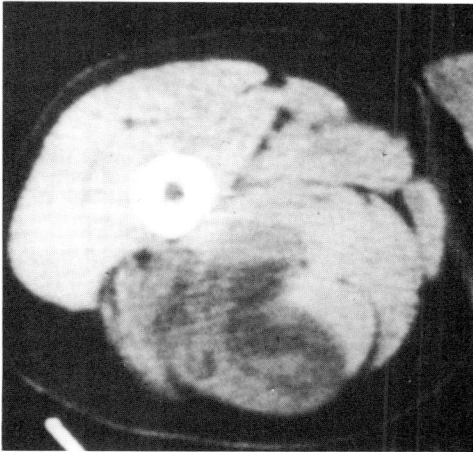

**Figure 25.** Liposarcoma of thigh. This CT scan shows a soft-tissue tumour involving the hamstrings and adductor magnus by infiltration. The tumour shows a non-homogeneous appearance, most of the area being darker than the adjoining muscle. It is, however, not as black as the intermuscular fat, as it is a combination of fat and tumour cells—a malignant fatty tumour.

Thus, CT features signifying geographical and permeating involvement of bone can be shown (Brown et al, 1986). Local recurrences following treatment can be demonstrated, particularly in the medulla and the periosseous soft tissue. CT has less value in this area following the use of metallic prostheses, as artefacts reduce the quality and accuracy of the examination.

As has already been mentioned above, the most sensitive method of detecting metastases, or early involvement of bone by a primary neoplasm, is radionuclide scintigraphy. Radiographic skeletal surveys are much less sensitive and entail greater radiation dose to the patient. A unified approach, logically combining the two imaging modalities, will reduce the number of inappropriate examinations (Mall et al, 1976). In the small but significant number of patients with positive scintigraphic examination and negative radiographs, CT may play an important role. Providing radiographs of good quality are studied to exclude the presence of abnormalities which are clearly non-neoplastic, asymmetry in medullary density may indicate metastatic involvement due to cellular replacement of marrow fat. It has been suggested that a difference of medullary CT number of greater than 20 Hu between limbs is abnormal (Helms et al, 1981).

For many years it has been established that a greater number of pulmonary metastatic nodules can be demonstrated with conventional tomography of the whole lung than with plain radiographic examination of the chest (Neifeld et al, 1977). With the advent of whole-body CT, it has become apparent that this technique is superior to conventional tomography in the demonstration of pulmonary nodules. In 1978, Muhm et al demonstrated that in 35% of their patients more nodules were revealed by CT. In 15.6% of this group, CT revealed nodules where none were shown by whole-lung tomography; in the remainder, CT simply identified more pulmonary nodules in each case. CT has evolved technically since that date, and in a series of 32 patients with osteosarcoma (Vanel et al, 1984), lung tomography demonstrated only half the metastases shown by a third generation CT scanner. It is probable that the main benefit of CT lies in its identification of subpleural nodules, which accounted for about half the metastases. Scintigraphy and tomoscintigraphy are of minimal value in the detection of pulmonary metastases from osteosarcoma in comparison to CT, which remains the diagnostic technique of choice.

## MAGNETIC RESONANCE IMAGING

MRI offers a number of advantages that can be used in the evaluation of musculoskeletal tumours. It involves no ionizing radiation, the resolution of contrast is excellent and continues to improve, and the ability to scan directly in the coronal and sagittal planes suggests advantages for staging and the planning of treatment.

The technique of magnetic resonance depends upon the emanation of radio signals by certain atoms in a magnetic field. Although any atom with an uneven number of protons, and therefore a net spin, would suffice, MRI has concentrated on the hydrogen atom, which is particularly suitable as it is universal in nature and possesses a single proton. The atoms behave as tiny magnets. In a strong magnetic field, at the resonant frequency of the atoms, the nuclei absorb energy and align themselves in a particular direction. When the pulse ceases and the atoms relax and return to their previous random arrangement, like any other spinning magnet, they release energy in the form of an electromagnetic signal at radio frequency. The intensity of the signal in spin-echo imaging depends upon three parameters relating to tissue characteristics and two further instrumental parameters. The tissue characteristics are (a) hydrogen density, (b) the longitudinal magnetic relaxation constant (T1), and (c) the transverse magnetic relaxation constant (T2). Each tissue possesses characteristic values of hydrogen density which are beyond the control of the radiologist. The instrumental variables are the pulse repetition time (TR) and the echo delay time (TE). In general clinical imaging, TR will range from about 300 to 3000 ms, and TE from 30 to 120 ms. A pulse sequence with relatively short TR and TE times is known as a T1-weighted image, whilst a sequence where the TR and TE times are relatively long is known as a T2-weighted image.

The total MR image depends on a number of factors, including proton density, relaxation times (T1 and T2) and flow within vessels. Manipulation of the pulse sequences can alter the relative contribution of each of these elements, although the relative intensities of most musculoskeletal tissues are constant through most combinations of TR and TE in common clinical usage.

Heavily calcified structures, such as cortical bone, contain only a small number of protons. Hence magnetic resonance (MR), which depends upon the presence of protons, produces a poor signal from bone and has little value in the direct evaluation of its structure. As a consequence, MR has no place in the initial diagnosis of a neoplasm of bone. Fortunately, however, fat in the bone marrow and the extraosseous soft tissues produces a high signal intensity with most combinations of TR and TE; hence the cortical bone is identified by default, lying between the marrow and the periosseous fat. Air, ligaments, tendon and fibrocartilage also show a very low signal intensity, while muscle and hyaline cartilage show an intermediate intensity of signal. A significantly different behaviour is shown by fluid-filled structures, oedematous tissue, neoplasia and haematoma. All of these tend to produce elevated values of T1 and T2 and hence show low intensity on T1-weighted sequences and higher intensity on T2-weighted sequences. It should be noted that, just as in CT, a haematoma changes its signal with age. The T1 and T2 constants tend to decrease progressively so that they show high intensity with T2-weighted sequences as well as T1-weighted sequences after a number of days (Swensen et al, 1985).

The intensity of signal obtained in imaging tissues normally found in the musculoskeletal system is summarized in Table 1.

MRI cannot, of itself, differentiate between a malignant and a benign neoplasm. Of more importance is the ability provided for specific demonstration of pathological changes in the bone marrow and the extraosseous tissues. It is into these regions that the spread of neoplasms occurs, and MRI can therefore supply information about the extent and staging of either a

**Table 1.** MR signal intensity in musculoskeletal practice.

*High intensity*
Fat
Bone marrow

*Intermediate intensity*
Muscle
Hyaline cartilage

*Low or very low intensity*
Cortical bone
Ligaments
Tendons
Fibrocartilage
Air

*Variable intensity* (see text)
Fluid collections (joint effusions, subarachnoid space, cysts)
Oedema
Inflammatory tissue
Neoplastic tissue
Haematoma (varies with age)

tumour arising in bone or of metastatic spread to bone. MRI is probably now the most sensitive single method of assessing medullary involvement by tumour (Zimmer et al, 1985). It is also able to demonstrate penetration of cortical bone and involvement of an articular surface; hence it is the most valuable imaging method for staging of musculoskeletal neoplasms (Figure 26).

Early expectations that MRI would be able to identify specific tumour matrix and thus predict the histology have not been realized, except in the case of fluid-filled structures and possibly lipomas. Lipomas can be differentiated from liposarcomas, as with CT (Dooms et al, 1985). The content of a lipoma is normal fat, so that with spin-echo imaging a high-intensity image is shown that is maintained at most pulse sequences. Brightness of this degree is, however, not confined to fat, and difficulty is experienced in distinguishing the signal from a lipoma from that of a soft-tissue haematoma (Sundaram et al, 1987). Fluid-filled structures are indicated when a lesion shows a very long T1 or T2 time. Such structures therefore appear of relatively low intensity on a T1-weighted sequence and brighten considerably when the sequence is more T2 weighted. It may be that future developments of intravenous contrast agents in MRI will improve the ability of the method to recognize various types of tissue.

Both CT and MRI can demonstrate the presence of extraosseous soft-tissue extension (Aisen et al, 1986). When the soft tissue encroachment is bounded by a thin egg-shell of residual bone, and hence may be merely an aggressive benign lesion such as an aneurysmal bone cyst contained by the periosteum, MRI will often not detect the bony rim of the lesion. In this specific circumstance, CT may offer an advantage over both plain radiography and MRI. In other circumstances, the evidence indicates that MRI is superior to CT in differentiating tumour from the adjoining muscle [Figures 26 (c) and (d)] (Aisen et al, 1986; Bohndorf et al, 1986). T2-weighted images

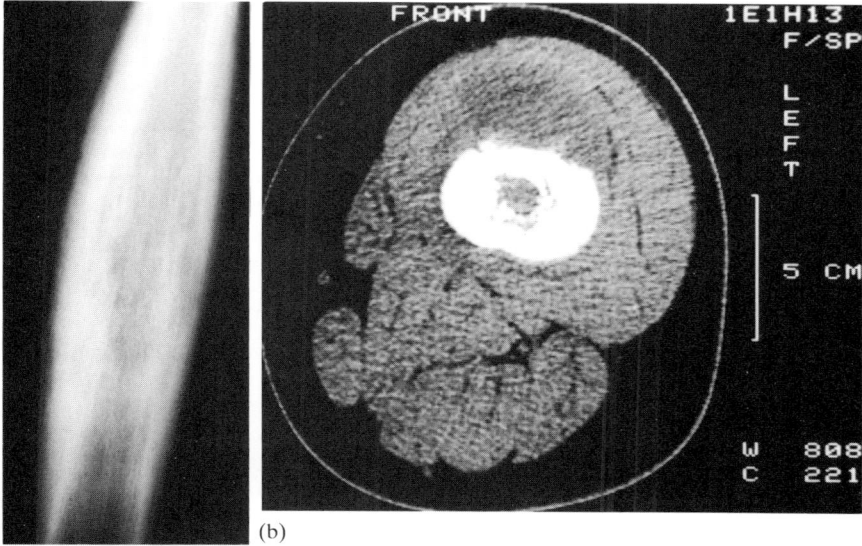

(a)

(b)

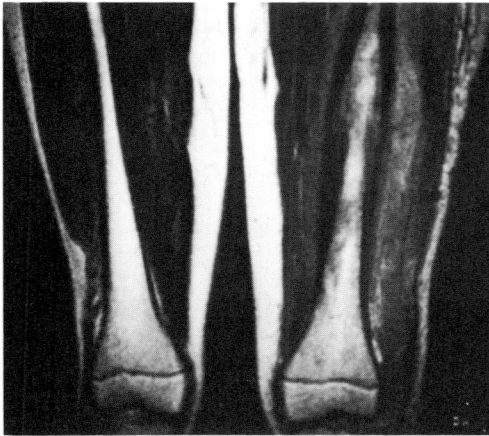

(c)

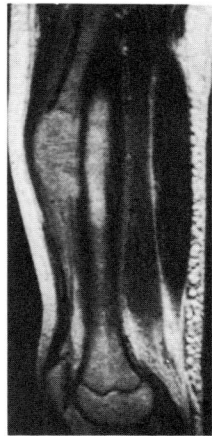

(d)

**Figure 26.** Osteosarcoma (courtesy of Dr K. Bohndorf, Cologne). (a) This expanding and infiltrating lesion of the femoral shaft was reasonably considered at first to be a Ewing's sarcoma. Considerable formation of periosteal new bone is shown. (b) The CT scan shows involvement of the medulla and erosion of the femoral cortex anteriorly. The anteriorly located soft-tissue mass shows a lesser attenuation than the surrounding muscle, but the interface between the normal and abnormal tissue is unclear. (c) Coronal MRI section with T1-weighted image demonstrates the interference with the bright marrow signal seen in the normal right femur. The length of the medullary spread of the tumour is very extensive. (d) This shows sagittal MRI images with variation of the factors, demonstrating both intramedullary and soft-tissue spread. Observe the clear definition of the soft-tissue mass and its relationship to the vastus medialis and rectus femoris muscles.

are most valuable in the definition of extraosseous tumour from peritumoral oedema and surrounding normal tissue. However, it must be stated that, in high-grade malignant tumours, differentiation of neoplastic tissue from peripheral oedema is not always possible (Bohndorf et al, 1986). Improved resolution over CT is particularly evident in coronal and sagittal MRI scans, which are vastly superior to the reformatted images obtained with CT. MRI produces superior images, particularly in the extremities, where the presence of thick cortical bone may result in significant streak artefacts (Richardson et al, 1986). Prosthetic implants or metallic clips may produce local field defects with MRI, but these interfere with the scan to a much lesser degree than do the severe artefacts of CT.

Present evidence suggests that MRI is proving to be more valuable than CT in the preoperative assessment of musculoskeletal neoplasms. It is, moreover, important to reflect that in terms of its potential development and exploitation, MRI technology is at a relatively primitive stage.

MRI is likely to offer considerable advantages in the assessment of response to treatment with radiotherapy and chemotherapy (Figure 27). Successful response to treatment is shown by reduction in tumoral mass and reduction in the intensity of the previous MR signal (Cohen et al, 1984). The precise cause for the latter is not yet clear, but is likely to be multifactorial.

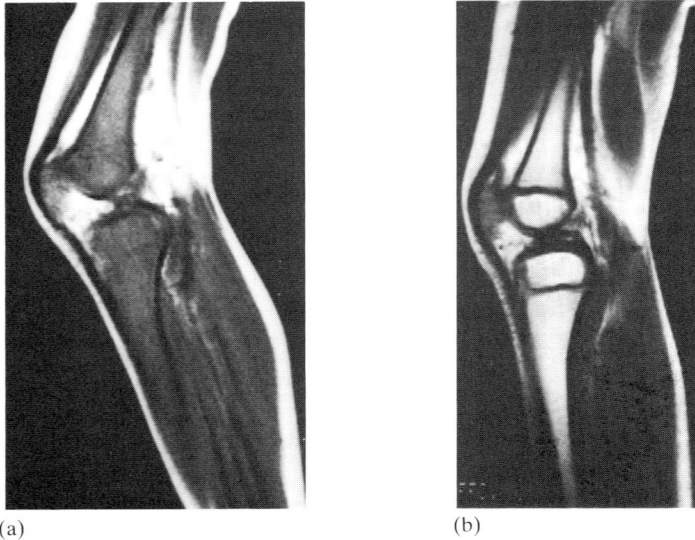

(a)                                                    (b)

**Figure 27.** Leukaemic infiltration of the marrow (courtesy of Dr K. Bohndorf, Cologne). (a) The MRI scan in this child shows the marrow cavity to be grey, much the same as the muscle. This is abnormal. Even in a child one would expect the bright signal of fatty marrow to be evident in the diaphyses. Note the bright signal from the periosseous fat. (b) Following successful therapy, tumour tissue has been replaced by haemopoietic marrow and fat. The signal is now bright and uniform.

## CONCLUSION

In the diagnosis of skeletal neoplasms and tumour-like disorders, radiology plays a major part, prior to biopsy. Even when a histological opinion is available, it should be compatible with the radiological appearances, as the radiological picture reflects gross anatomy, while histological diagnosis is often required from an unrepresentative specimen. In radiological diagnosis the plain film retains an unchallenged place in the demonstration of the pattern of bony destruction, leading to an assessment of the rate of growth of the tumour. The radiograph hence remains, and will do for the foreseeable future, to be the main method for radiological diagnosis. In staging also, the determination of the biological aggressiveness of a neoplasm is a combination of the radiological grade, as exemplified by Lodwick's classification of probabilities and the histological assessment.

Radionuclide scintigraphy is a highly sensitive, but non-specific, investigation. Its main value in this field lies in confirmation of the metabolic activity of the primary lesion and the identification of early or multiple lesions.

Arteriography has limited use in diagnosis, except in the demonstration of tumours of vascular origin. Its employment for the demonstration of soft-tissue extension has now been superseded by CT and MRI.

Both CT and MRI have their greatest value in the demonstration of the extent of the lesion and therefore are pre-eminent in the fields of surgical management and staging. MRI is proving to be better than CT in the demonstration of the extent of spread of a tumour, both within the marrow cavity and into the extraosseous soft tissues. CT retains its superiority in the demonstration of the thinned cortex, mineralization of the tumoral matrix and the identification of pulmonary metastases. While the technical advances of CT are now almost complete, the applications and technical possibilities of MRI undoubtedly will be extended in future years; the use of contrast agents in this new method of imaging has scarcely been explored at the present time.

## REFERENCES

Aisen AM, Martel W, Braunstein EM et al (1986) MRI and CT evaluation of primary bone and soft-tissue tumors. *American Journal of Roentgenology* **146:** 749–756.

Bohndorf K, Reiser M, Lochner B, Feaux de Lacroix W & Steinbrich W (1986) Magnetic resonance imaging of primary tumours and tumour-like lesions of bone. *Skeletal Radiology* **15:** 511–517.

Brown KT, Kattapuram SV & Rosenthal DL (1986) Computed tomographic analysis of bone tumors: patterns of cortical destruction and soft tissue extension. *Skeletal Radiology* **15:** 448–451.

Cohen MD, Klatte EC, Baehner R et al (1984) Magnetic resonance imaging of bone marrow disease in children. *Radiology* **151:** 715–718.

Dooms GC, Hricak H, Sollitto RA & Higgins CB (1985) Lipomatous tumors and tumors with fatty component: MR imaging potential and comparison of MR and CT results. *Radiology* **157:** 479–483.

Enneking WF (1986) A system of staging musculoskeletal neoplasms. *Clinical Orthopaedics and Related Research* **204:** 9–24.

Enneking WF, Spanier SS & Goodman MA (1980) A system for the surgical staging of musculoskeletal sarcoma. *Clinical Orthopaedics and Related Research* **153**: 106–120.

Gunterberg B, Kindblom L-G & Laurin S (1977) Giant-cell tumour of bone and aneurysmal bone cyst—a correlated histiologic and angiographic study. *Skeletal Radiology* **2**: 65–74.

Halldorsdottir A, Ekelund L & Rydholm A (1982) CT diagnosis of lipomatous tumors of the soft tissues. *Archives of Orthopaedic and Traumatic Surgery* **100**: 211–216.

Helms CA, Cann CE, Brunelle FO et al (1981) Detection of bone marrow metastases using quantitative computed tomography. *Radiology* **140**: 745–750.

Johnson LC (1953) A general theory of bone tumours. *Bulletin of the New York Academy of Medicine* **29**: 164–171.

Lodwick GS (1971) *The Bones and Joints*. Chicago: Year Book Medical Publishers.

Lodwick GS, Wilson AJ, Farrell C et al (1980a) Determining growth rates of focal lesions of bone from radiographs. *Radiology* **134**: 577–583.

Lodwick GS, Wilson AJ, Farrell C et al (1980b) Estimating rate of growth in bone lesions: observer performance and error. *Radiology* **134**: 585–590.

Madewell JE, Ragsdale BD & Sweet DG (1981) Radiologic and pathologic analysis of solitary bone lesions. Part I. Internal margins. *Radiologic Clinics of North America* **19**: 715–748.

Mall JC, Bekerman C, Hoffer PB & Gottschalk A (1976) A unified radiological approach to the detection of skeletal metastases. *Radiology* **118**: 323–328.

Muhm JR, Brown LR, Crowe JK et al (1978) Comparison of whole lung tomography and computed tomography for detecting pulmonary nodules. *American Journal of Roentgenology* **131**: 981–984.

Murray IPC (1980) Bone scanning in the child and young adult. Part I. *Skeletal Radiology* **5**: 1–14.

Neifeld JP, Michaelis LL & Doppman JL (1977) Suspected pulmonary metastases: correlation of chest x-ray, whole lung tomograms and operative findings. *Cancer* **39**: 383–387.

Richardson ML, Kilcoyne RF, Gillespy III T, Helms CA & Genant HK (1986) Magnetic resonance of musculoskeletal neoplasms. *Radiologic Clinics of North America* **24**: 259–267.

Sundaram M, McGuire MH & Herbold DR (1987) Magnetic resonance imaging of osteosarcoma. *Skeletal Radiology* **16**: 23–29.

Swensen SJ, Keller PL, Berquist TH, McLeod RA & Stephens DH (1985) Magnetic resonance imaging of hemorrhage. *American Journal of Roentgenology* **145**: 921–927.

Vanel D, Henry-Amar M, Lumbroso J et al (1984) Pulmonary evaluation of patients with osteosarcoma: roles of standard radiography, tomography, CT, scintigraphy and tomoscintigraphy. *American Journal of Roentgenology* **143**: 519–523.

Voegeli E & Uehlinger E (1976) Arteriography in bone tumours. *Skeletal Radiology* **1**: 3–14.

Zimmer WD, Berquist TH, McLeod RA et al (1985) Bone tumors: magnetic resonance imaging versus computed tomography. *Radiology* **155**: 709–718.

# 4

# A system of staging musculoskeletal neoplasms

## WILLIAM F. ENNEKING

The purposes of a staging system for musculoskeletal neoplasms are (1) to incorporate the significant prognostic factors into a system that describes progressive degrees of risk of local recurrence and distant metastases to which a patient is subject, (2) to stratify the states so they have specific implications for surgical management, and (3) to provide guidelines for adjunctive therapies. Over a number of years, staging systems for various classes of malignant tumours have been developed under the auspices of the American Joint Committee (AJC) for Cancer Staging and End Results Reporting. The systems vary among cancers related to the natural course of a particular type of cancer. In 1980, a system for the surgical staging of musculoskeletal sarcoma was proposed, studied and adopted by the Musculoskeletal Tumor Society (Enneking et al, 1980) and subsequently adopted by the AJC.

## THE STAGING SYSTEM

The system is based on the interrelationship of three factors: (1) grade—G, (2) site—T, and (3) metastases—M. Each of these in turn is stratified by components that influence both prognosis and response to treatment. The behavioural changes (latent, active, aggressive, invasive, destructive and metastatic) that form the basis of the staging system together with their clinical, radiographic and staging studies are summarized in Tables 1 (summary), 2 (benign lesion stages) and 3 (malignant lesion stages).

## GRADE

The grade is an assessment of the biological aggressiveness of the lesion. It is neither a purely histological assessment (as in Broders et al (1939), who proposed a 1, 2, 3, 4 grading of malignancies), nor a purely radiographical assessment (as in Lodwick's IA, IB, IC, II and III radiographical classification of probabilities), nor a purely clinical reflection of growth rate, doubling time, size, temperature, tissue pressure or biochemical markers. It is a blending of all of these into patterns. The three stratifications of grade are $G_0$, $G_1$ and $G_2$. Their identifying characteristics are:

## $G_0$ (benign lesions)

*Histological*—benign cytology, clearly differentiated, low to moderate cell-to-matrix ratio.
*Radiographic*—Lodwick IA, IB or IC ranging from clearly marginated to those with capsular broaching and soft-tissue extensions.
*Clinical*—distinct capsule, no satellite lesions, no skip lesions, rare metastases, variable growth rate, predominantly in adolescents and young adults.

**Table 1.** Surgical staging system.

| Benign lesions | | Notation | |
|---|---|---|---|
| Stage 1   Latent | $G_0$ | $T_0$ | $M_0$ |
| Stage 2   Active | $G_0$ | $T_{0-1}$ | $M_0$ |
| Stage 3   Aggressive | $G_0$ | $T_{1-2}$ | $M_{0-1}$ |
| *Malignant lesions* | | Notation | |
| Stage I   Low grade | | | |
| Intracompartmental: | $G_1$ | $T_1$ | $M_0$ |
| Extracompartmental: | $G_1$ | $T_2$ | $M_0$ |
| Stage II   High grade | | | |
| Intracompartmental: | $G_2$ | $T_1$ | $M_0$ |
| Extracompartmental: | $G_2$ | $T_2$ | $M_0$ |
| Stage III   Metastatic | | | |
| Either grade: Intracompartmental Distant metastasis | $G_{1-2}$ | $T_1$ | $M_1$ |
| Either grade: Extracompartmental Distant metastasis | $G_{1-2}$ | $T_2$ | $M_1$ |

**Table 2.** Stages of benign musculoskeletal lesions.

| | Stage 1 | Stage 2 | Stage 3 |
|---|---|---|---|
| Grade | $G_0$ | $G_0$ | $G_0$ |
| Site | $T_0$ | $T_{0-1}$ | $T_{1-2}$ |
| Metastases | $M_0$ | $M_0$ | $M_{0-1}$ |
| Clinical course | Latent, static, self-healing | Active, progressing, expands bone or fascia | Aggressive, invasive, breaches bone or fascia |
| Radiographic grade | $I_A$ | $I_B$ | $I_C$ |
| Isotope scan | Background uptake | Increased uptake in lesion | Increased uptake beyond lesion |
| Angiogram | No neovascular reaction | Modest neovascular reaction | Moderate neovascular reaction |
| CT | Crisp, intact margin—well-defined capsule, homogeneous | Intact margin 'expansile'—thin capsule, homogeneous | Indistinct broached margin—extra-capsular and/or extra-compartmental extension, non-homogeneous |

**Table 3.** Stages of malignant musculoskeletal lesions.

|  | $I_A$ | $I_B$ | $II_A$ | $II_B$ | $III_A$ | $III_B$ |
|---|---|---|---|---|---|---|
| Grade | $G_1$ | $G_1$ | $G_2$ | $G_2$ | $G_{1-2}$ | $G_{1-2}$ |
| Site | $T_1$ | $T_2$ | $T_1$ | $T_2$ | $T_1$ | $T_2$ |
| Metastases | $M_0$ | $M_0$ | $M_0$ | $M_0$ | $M_1$ | $M_1$ |
| Clinical course | Symptomatic indolent growth | Symptomatic mass, indolent growth | Symptomatic rapid growth | Symptomatic rapid growth, fixed mass, pathological fracture | Systemic symptoms, palpable nodes, pulmonary symptoms | |
| Isotope scan | Increased uptake | Increased uptake | Increased uptake beyond radiographic limits | Increased uptake beyond radiographic limits | Pulmonary lesions, no increased uptake | |
| Radiographic grade | II | II | III | III | III | |
| Angiogram | Modest neovascular reactive involvement of neurovascular bundle | Modest neovascular reactive involvement of neurovascular bundle | Marked neovascular reaction, no involvement of neurovascular bundle | Marked neovascular reactive involvement of neurovascular bundle | Hypervascular lymph nodes | |
| CT | Irregular or broached well, capsule but intracompartmental | Extracompartmental extension or location | Broached (pseudo) capsule, intra-compartmental | Broached (pseudo) capsule, extra-compartmental | Pulmonary lesions or enlarged nodes | |

### $G_1$ (low-grade malignant lesions)

*Histological*—Broder's grade 1 and some grade 2, few mitoses, moderate differentiation, distinct matrix.
*Radiographic*—Lodwick II with indolent invasive features.
*Clinical*—indolent growth, extracapsular satellite lesions in the reactive zone, no skip lesions, only occasional distant metastases.

### $G_2$ (high-grade malignant lesions)

*Histological*—Broder's grades 2, 3 and 4, frequent mitoses, poorly differentiated, sparse and immature matrix. High-grade cytological features: anaplasia, pleomorphism, hyperchromatic nuclei.
*Radiographic*—Lodwick III: destructive, invasive.
*Clinical*—rapid growth, symptomatic, both satellite and skip lesions, occasional regional and frequent distant metastases.

The behaviour of $G_0$ benign lesions may be latent, active or aggressive. Their histological features are often poor indicators of their behaviour, and within this spectrum $G_0$ lesions are often better predicted by their radiographic, staging and clinical features (Table 2). The histological characteristics of $G_1$ low-grade sarcomas make their distinction from $G_2$ high-grade lesions on histological grounds predictably accurate, and their radiographic staging and clinical features are supportive and confirmatory of the histological distinction. However, it may be difficult to distinguish $G_0$ from $G_1$ lesions on purely histological features, and, in many instances, the radiographic and particularly the staging studies may be of more value than the histological findings (Table 3).

A promising new method of assessing grade is the determination of the nuclear DNA concentration (ploidy) by flow cytometry. Individual cell nuclei are stained with a specific fluorescent DNA dye and the concentration is assessed rapidly by fluorometric assay of the cells as they pass through a focused laser beam. Normal cells are euploid, and so are most $G_0$ lesions. $G_1$ lesions have both abnormal numbers of cells in tetraploidy and also may show abnormal (aneuploid) cells quite distinctive for high-grade neoplasms. These correlations between ploidy and prognosis have been shown to be valid for other types of neoplasia, particularly myelomas and lymphomas, and preliminary results suggest that this technique may be quite helpful in connective tissue lesions (Kreicbergs et al, 1982).

In summary, surgical grading into $G_0$, $G_1$ or $G_2$ requires histological, radiographic and clinical correlation to achieve accuracy and reliability. Although certain histogenic types of sarcomas may have a preponderance of their $G_1$ or $G_2$ lesions (Table 4), each lesion must be assessed on its own characteristics before a grade is assigned. For example, most parosteal osteosarcomas are $G_1$, but a few dedifferentiate into $G_2$ lesions and accordingly have a much more ominous prognosis. Conversely, although most classic osteosarcomas are $G_2$, occasionally one will be $G_1$ with a much more favourable prognosis.

**Table 4.** Surgical grade (G).

| Benign lesion ($G_0$) | Low-grade malignant lesion ($G_1$) | High-grade malignant lesion ($G_2$) |
|---|---|---|
| Osteoma | Parosteal osteosarcoma | Classic osteosarcoma |
| Osteoid osteoma | Endosteal osteosarcoma | Radiation sarcoma |
| Osteoblastoma | | |
| Exostosis | Secondary chondrosarcoma | Primary chondrosarcoma |
| Enchondroma | | Dedifferentiated chondrosarcoma |
| Chondroblastoma | | Mesenchymal chondrosarcoma |
| Chondromyxofibroma | | |
| Periosteal chondroma | | |
| Fibroma | Fibrosarcoma, well differentiated | Fibrosarcoma, undifferentiated |
| Fibromatosis | Malignant fibrous histiocytoma, well differentiated | Malignant fibrous histiocytoma |
| Giant cell tumour, bone | Giant cell sarcoma, bone | Undifferentiated spindle cell sarcoma |
| Giant cell tumour tendon sheath | Giant cell sarcoma, tendon | |
| | Epithelioid sarcoma | Synovial sarcoma |
| Neurofibroma | | Neural sarcoma |
| Neurolemmomma | | |
| Lipoma | Myxoid liposarcoma | Pleomorphic liposarcoma |
| Angiolipoma | Haemangiopericytoma | Angiosarcoma |
| Haemangioma | Haemangioendothelioma | |
| | Chordoma | Alveolar cell sarcoma |
| | Adamantinoma | |
| | Leiomyosarcoma | Rhabdomyosarcoma |
| | | Ewing's sarcoma |

## SITE

The anatomical setting of the lesion has a direct relationship to the prognosis and the choice of surgical procedure. The three strata of anatomical settings are $T_0$, $T_1$ and $T_2$. These are determined primarily by clinical and radiographic techniques. Staging studies (isotope scanning, angiography, CT, MRI, ultrasonography, myelography, etc.) can make valuable contributions in assessing these settings preoperatively thus:

$T_0$: The lesion remains confined within the capsule and does not extend beyond the borders of its compartment of origin. While the boundaries of the capsule and/or the compartment of origin may be distorted or deformed, they both remain intact.
$T_1$: The lesion has extracapsular extensions, either by continuity or isolated satellites, into the reactive zone, but both the lesion and the reactive zone about it are contained within an anatomical compartment bounded by the natural barriers to tumour extension: cortical bone, articular cartilage, joint

capsule, the dense fibrous tissue of fascial septa, ligaments or tendon (sheath). To be classified as $T_1$, both the lesion and its (pseudo)capsule must be within the compartment. If the reactive zone extends outside the compartment while the tumour remains within, the lesion is classified as extracompartmental. The anatomical compartments of both bone and soft tissue are shown in Table 5.

Three particular points about compartmentalization require elaboration. The skin and subcutaneous tissue are classified as a compartment, even though there are no longitudinal boundaries. In the transverse dimension, however, the deep fascia forms an effective barrier between the subcutaneous and deeper tissues. The parosseous compartment is a potential compartment between cortical bone and overlying muscle. Lesions on the surface of bone that have not invaded either the underlying cortical bone or the overlying muscle but have pushed them apart are defined as intracompartmental. Lesions within muscular compartments that contain more than one muscle (e.g. the volar compartment of the forearm) are considered intracompartmental despite involving more than one muscle.

$T_2$: Lesions extending beyond compartmental barriers into the loosely bounded fascial planes and spaces that have no longitudinal boundaries are

**Table 5.** Surgical sites (T).

| Intracapsular ($T_0$) | Extracapsular, intracompartmental ($T_1$) | | Extracapsular, extracompartmental ($T_2$) |
|---|---|---|---|
| Intracapsular, intraosseous | Extracapsular, intracortical | → | Extracortical extension |
| Intracapsular, intra-articular | Extracapsular, intra-articular | → | Extra-articular extension |
| Intracapsular, skin-subcutaneous | Extracapsular, skin-subcutaneous | → | Deep extension |
| Intracapsular, parosseous | Extracapsular, parosseous | → | Extension into bone or soft tissue |
| Intracapsular, whether intracompartmental or extracompartmental | Extracapsular, intracompartmental soft tissue | → | Extracompartmental soft tissue |
| | | | Extracapsular by extension or origin |
| | Intracompartmental by origin: | | Extracompartmental by origin: |
| | Ray hand | | Midhand, dorsal or palmar |
| | Ray foot | | Mid or hind foot |
| | Posterior calf | | Popliteal fossae |
| | Anterolateral leg | | Periarticular knee |
| | Anterior thigh | | Femoral triangle |
| | Medial thigh | | Obturator foramen, pelvis |
| | Posterior thigh | | |
| | Buttocks | | Sciatic notch, intrapelvic |
| | Volar forearm | | Antecubital fossae |
| | Dorsal forearm | | Periarticular elbow |
| | Anterior arm | | Axilla |
| | Posterior arm | | |
| | Deltoid | | Periclavicular |
| | Periscapular | | Paraspinal, head neck |

classified as extracompartmental or $T_2$ lesions. Extracompartmental involvement may be either by virtue of extension of a previously intra-compartmental lesion, by arising de novo in the extracompartmental tissues, or by inadvertent transmission by trauma or surgical excision. The various sites that are extracompartmental are shown in Table 5. Almost without exception, lesions (or their reactive zones) that abut or involve major neurovascular bundles are extracompartmental by virtue of the extracom-partmental location of these structures.

## METASTASIS

In most staging systems for carcinomas, metastases are stratified by virtue of being regional (N for nodes) or distant (M) since the prognosis and treatment is significantly different for these two sites of metastasis.

For sarcomas, metastatic involvement of either regional lymph nodes or distant organs has the same ominous prognosis and both are designated by M. There are only two strata of metastasis: $M_0$ and $M_1$. $M_0$ indicates no evidence of regional or distant metastases, while $M_1$ signifies either regional or distant metastases.

These three factors—G, T and M—are combined to form the criteria for the progressive stages of benign and malignant lesions (Table 1). Benign lesions that are designated by the arabic numerals 1, 2 or 3 are synonymous with latent, active or aggressive. The characteristics of stage 1 (latent), stage 2 (active) and stage 3 (aggressive) lesions are shown in Table 2. Stages 1, 2 and 3 correspond closely to the Lodwick classification of radiographic features as IA, IB and IC.

Malignant lesions that are designated by the Roman numerals I, II or III are synonymous with low-grade, high-grade or metastatic. These three states of sarcomas are further stratified into A or B depending on whether the lesion is anatomically intracompartmental (A) or extracompartmental (B). The characteristics of these malignant lesions are shown in Table 3. Their radiographic characteristics correspond closely to stages II and III in the Lodwick classification. Only after each lesion has been studied clinically, radiographically and biopsied to ascertain the histological type and cyto-logical grade can it be staged according to its characteristics. Although particular lesions tend to cluster in particular stages (i.e. > 90% of classic osteosarcomas present as stage IIB), others tend to be more evenly distri-buted (i.e. giant cell tumours of bone present approximately in the following proportions: stage 1—10%, stage 2—75%, stage 3—15%).

Clearly, a particular lesion may undergo transition from one stage to another. Benign lesions that are stage 2 active or even stage 3 aggressive during adolescence frequently undergo involution into stage 1 latent lesions after growth has ceased. On the other hand, certain benign lesions of any stage may undergo transformation into stage I, stage II or even stage III sarcomas. Obviously, high-grade stage II lesions and occasionally low-grade stage I lesions become stage III lesions after presentation by virtue of either regional or distant metastases. Certain factors have been implicated directly or by inference in the upstaging of benign or malignant lesions. Radiation has been held responsible for the transition of giant cell tumour, chondroblastoma and other benign lesions to sarcomas. Repeated inadequate surgical interventions have been implicated in the evolution of low-grade fibrous lesions into high-grade fibrosarcomas and in the dedifferentiation of stage I parosteal osteosarcoma into stage II or III high-grade osteosarcoma.

## APPLICATION TO SURGICAL TREATMENT

The application of the staging system to the surgical treatment of connective tissue tumours requires precise definitions of the procedures as well as the stages. The traditional terms of incisional biopsy, excisional biopsy, resection and amputation are difficult to define in biological, anatomical or physical terms. After a number of physical and surgical criteria were postulated, a method of definition was devised, based on the margin the procedure obtained in relation to the lesion and the barriers to its extension.

The description of the four oncological surgical margins, the plane of dissection that achieves them, and the microscopic appearance of the tissue at the margin of the wound are given in Table 6. The four margins are described in surgical terms (intracapsular, marginal, wide and radical) and they reflect the progressive barriers to tumour extension in their natural evolution, e.g. the (pseudo)capsule, reactive zone, intracompartmental normal tissue and compartmental boundaries. Although marginal, wide and radical margins may all be tumour-free, the residual reactive tissue at a marginal margin often contains extensions or satellites, and the residual normal intracompartmental tissue beyond a wide margin occasionally contains skip lesions. For high-grade sarcomas only, a radical margin with an intact barrier of normal tissue between the margin and the reactive zone consistently and reliably can be called tumour-free.

Determinations of margins may be estimated by inspection of the cut surface of either bone or soft tissue. Tetracycline-labelling may be quite helpful in visually identifying the type of osseous margin as it distinguishes reactive bone from normal bone. Often, specimens will have to be taken for histological study from questionable areas to ascertain whether non-neoplastic tissue at a margin is reactive or normal. The microscopic appearance of wide

Table 6. Surgical margins.

| Type | Plane of dissection | Microscopic appearance |
|------|--------------------|-----------------------|
| Intracapsular | Within lesion | Tumour at margin |
| Marginal | Within reactive zone—extracapsular | Reactive tissue ± microsatellites tumour |
| Wide | Beyond reactive zone through normal tissue within compartment | Normal tissue ± skip lesions |
| Radical | Normal tissue, extracompartmental | Normal tissue |

and radical margins is histologically identical (i.e. normal) and the distinction as to the type of margin obtained is made by identifying whether or not the margin is beyond a compartmental barrier. This is usually done by gross inspection or radiographic examination of the specimen. As shown in Table 7, each of the four margins can be achieved by a local or limb-salvaging procedure or an amputation, making eight possible oncological procedures.

Table 7. Surgical procedures.

| Type | How margin is achieved | |
| | Limb-salvage | Amputation |
| --- | --- | --- |
| Intracapsular | Intracapsular piecemeal excision | Intracapsular amputation |
| Marginal | Marginal en bloc excision | Marginal amputation |
| Wide | Wide en bloc excision | Wide through-bone amputation |
| Radical | Radical en bloc resection | Radical exarticulation |

The four types of limb-salvaging procedures are: (1) intracapsular excision, i.e. debulking, cytoreductive excision, etc., carried out piecemeal within the (pseudo)capsule, (2) marginal (local) excision, i.e. en bloc excisional biopsy, shell-out, etc., performed en bloc extracapsularly within the reactive zone; (3) wide (local) excision, i.e. en bloc excision carried out through normal tissue beyond the reactive zone, but within the compartment of origin, leaving in situ some portion of that compartment; or (4) radical (local) resection, i.e. en bloc excision of the lesion and the entire compartment of origin, leaving no remnant of the compartment of origin.

The terms 'excision' and 'resection' are coupled with 'wide' and 'radical' to emphasize the biological differences between the two procedures. Wide excision and radical resection are correct. By definition, wide resection and radical excision become incompatible terms. This is important conceptually, if not semantically, because in Europe the term 'radical', in terms of margin, is synonymous with tumour-free and can in the above terms be either marginal, wide or radical. Therefore, in the European literature, excision and resection are used interchangeably, with 'radical' taken to mean any local procedure with a tumour-free margin.

The four types of operations are amputations that achieve various margins and whose levels pass (1) within the (pseudo)capsule (intracapsular amputation); (2) through the reactive zone (marginal amputation); (3) through normal tissue proximal to the reactive zone, but with the compartment of involvement, usually a through-bone (wide amputation); and (4) proximal to the involved compartment, usually a disarticulation (radical amputation because it removes the entire compartment at risk).

Using these definitions the staging procedure can be used to correspond with the surgical margins and operative procedures and has an anatomical and biological meaning. This correspondence is shown for benign lesions in Table 8, and for malignant lesions in Table 9.

**Table 8.** Relationship of staging of benign lesions to surgical margins.

| Stage | Grade | Site | Metastasis | Margin for control |
|---|---|---|---|---|
| 1 | $G_0$ | $T_0$ | $M_0$ | Intracapsular |
| 2 | $G_0$ | $T_0$ | $M_0$ | marginal or ?<br>intracapsular plus effective adjuvant |
| 3 | $G_0$ | $T_{1-2}$ | $M_{0-1}$ | Wide or ?<br>marginal plus effective adjuvant |

**Table 9.** Relationship of staging of malignant lesions to surgical margins.

| Stage | Grade | Site | Metastasis | Margin for control |
|---|---|---|---|---|
| $I_A$ | $G_1$ | $T_1$ | $M_0$ | Wide—usually excision |
| $I_B$ | $G_1$ | $T_2$ | $M_0$ | Wide—considered amputation vs joint or neurovascular deficit |
| $II_A$ | $G_2$ | $T_1$ | $M_0$ | Radical—usually resection or wide excision plus effective adjuvant |
| $II_B$ | $G_2$ | $T_2$ | $M_0$ | Radical—consider exarticulation or wide excision or amputation plus effective adjuvant |
| $III_A$ | $G_{1-2}$ | $T_1$ | $M_1$ | Thoracotomy—radical resection or palliative |
| $III_B$ | $G_{1-2}$ | $T_2$ | $M_1$ | Thoracotomy—radical exarticulation or palliative |

In its preliminary trials by the Musculoskeletal Tumor Society, this staging system was shown to be practical, reproducible and of significant prognostic value for sarcomas of both bone and soft tissue origin (Eriksson et al, 1980). Subsequent reports have shown its value in surgical planning and treatment evaluation (Eriksson et al, 1980; Gitelis et al, 1981; Bononi et al, 1983; Gherlinzoni et al, 1983; Sim, 1983). The relationship between stage and prognosis is shown for fibrosarcoma of bone and soft tissues in Figure 1 and for malignant fibrous histiocytoma in Figure 2.

Some misconceptions of the original presentation of the definitions of surgical margins and procedures in 1980 need clarification. The common misconceptions concern methods for description of the margins (and procedures) about superficial lesions, extracompartmental lesions and lesions that are inadvertently entered but subsequently re-excised. A superficial lesion in the skin and/or subcutaneous tissue that has not penetrated the deep fascia is intracompartmental. En bloc removal with a plane of dissection to the deep fascia and through normal tissue well around the lesion obtains an extracompartmental radical margin in depth (on the other side of the deep fascia, a natural barrier), but only a wide margin circumferentially (there are no natural barriers within skin and subcutaneous tissue, so an extracompartmental radical margin in the defined sense is not possible). This ambiguity has been resolved by arbitrarily calling a margin of less than 5 cm about the reactive zone 'wide', and a margin of more than 5 cm 'radical'. The 5 cm dimension was chosen because it is a margin for melanoma. Thus, a superficial IA lesion excised en bloc to the deep fascia

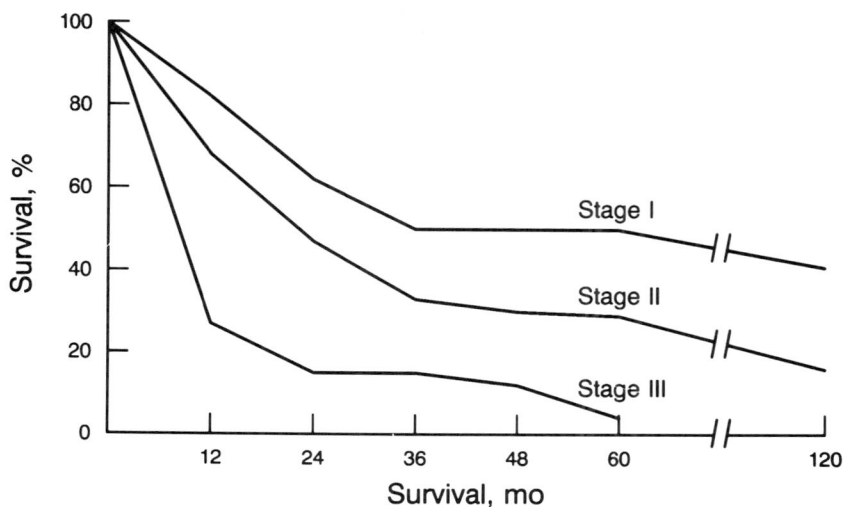

**Figure 1.** Survival related to stage for fibrosarcoma of bone and soft tissue. mo = months.

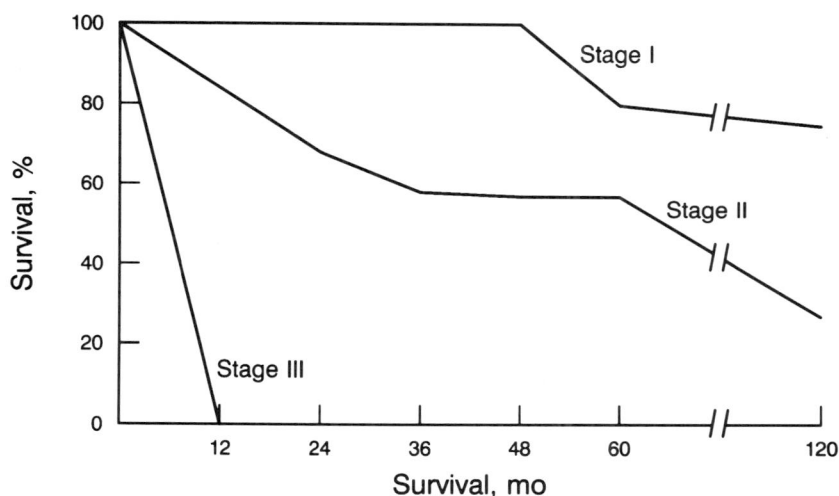

**Figure 2.** Survival related to stage for malignant fibrous histiocytoma of bone and soft tissue. mo = months.

with a surrounding margin of 2 cm has been widely excised, while the same lesion with a 6 cm margin about it has been radically resected. Whether or not these physical dimensions are appropriate for the correspondence of margin and stage remains to be seen.

Extracompartmental 'B' lesions, whether by extension or origin, cannot by definition be radically resected because the extracompartmental spaces and planes have no longitudinal barriers. For such lesions, a local procedure that removes en bloc a lesion with a margin of normal tissue is a wide excision for an en bloc removal. The surgical removal of an extracompartmental lesion that is beyond natural barriers in the transverse plane, but by definition cannot be radical in the longitudinal sense, is arbitrarily defined as a radical resection when the longitudinal margin is at the same level as the origin or insertion of the adjacent muscles. For example, a lesion in the subsartorial canal abutting the femoral neurovascular bundle that was removed en bloc, including the bundle with a plane of dissection beyond the fascial boundaries of the canal (i.e. radical transversely) but with a proximal and distal margin less than the musculotendinous junctions of the sartorius muscle, would have been widely excised. The same procedure with the proximal and distal margins at or beyond the musculotendinous junctions of the sartorius muscle would be a radical resection. If the lesion were removed en bloc by dissection within the canal sacrificing the bundle, the procedure would be a marginal excision. If the lesion were dissected away from the bundle preserving the bundle, the procedure would be designated as either an intracapsular or marginal excision, depending on whether the dissection was within the (pseudo)capsule or extracapsular reactive zone.

If a lesion involves two compartments, i.e. a lesion arising in bone extending into the adjacent soft tissues, then to achieve a radical margin both compartments would have to be removed en bloc. For example, to achieve a radical resection of a lesion of the distal femoral metaphysis extending into the posterior thigh would require removal of the entire femur, hamstrings and sciatic nerve en bloc. From the above it is evident that in certain instances the only practical way of achieving a radical margin is by amputation. This may be particularly true in certain anatomical sites (i.e. popliteal fossae, femoral triangle, axillae, antecubital fossae, flexor canal of the forearm) where radical margin can be obtained by resection, but the virtually functionless salvaged limb hinders rather than aids rehabilitation.

When lesions are entered, the wound is being contaminated and all the tissues exposed are at risk for recurrence. If these at-risk tissues are not removed, the margin is intracapsular. If the tissues are removed, the margin becomes what the subsequent removal achieves in relation to the lesion as if the exposure had not happened. This procedure is said to be a contaminated procedure. For example, if a lesion in the quadriceps were inadvertently entered, exposing the rectus femoris muscle and the lesion subsequently widely excised with a cuff of normal tissue, the procedure would be designated as a contaminated wide excision because some of the exposed more proximal rectus femoris muscle would remain in the wound.

If, under the same circumstance, the entire quadriceps compartment were removed en bloc by extracompartmental dissection, then the procedure would be a (uncontaminated) radical resection. This means that after incisional biopsy, the entire tract at risk must be appropriately excised en bloc with the lesion and tissues to achieve wide or radical margins. It also means that if the (pseudo)capsule is inadvertently entered during attempted excisional biopsy, a great deal more tissue will have to be removed to achieve an uncontaminated wide or radical margin than if such contamination had not occurred. In certain instances contamination may take place in such a way that the only way of achieving an uncontaminated wide or radical margin is by amputation (previously unnecessary to achieve an uncontaminated wide or radical margin), and in other circumstances (e.g. the pelvis) inadvertent contamination may make obtaining an uncontaminated margin of any kind impossible.

It is evident that continuous refinement and classification of these terms, definitions and concepts are needed for them to be of optimal value. A serious consideration of stratification of stage III is also in order. It is becoming clearer that the prognosis of a patient who develops a solitary pulmonary metastasis from a $G_0$ or $G_1$ primary tumour some years following local control is significantly different than multiple metastases from a $G_2$ lesion at the time of presentation or shortly after apparent local control of the primary lesion. It may well be that meaningful stratifications will offer guidelines for the management of these lesions.

The final objective of this staging system—development of guidelines for adjunctive therapy—has yet to be realized. The effectiveness of adjuvant therapy continues to be judged by survival rates of various histogenic types of sarcomas, largely ignoring the influence of the stage, surgical margin or adequacy of the surgical procedure on survival rates. This lamentable state is exemplified by the fact that 10 years after the enthusiastic and widespread adoption of prophylactic chemotherapy, there was serious doubt as to whether the increase in survival rates during this period was the result of adjuvant chemotherapy or improvement in staging techniques with resultant improvements in surgical control of the primary tumour. In the light of this experience it seems clear that data concerning staging, surgical margins and surgical procedures must be gathered to establish what are the significant variables in the assessment of protocols for adjunctive management of musculoskeletal lesions.

## SUMMARY

A system for staging benign and malignant musculoskeletal lesions is presented. This system, first devised at the University of Florida in 1977, was based on data assembled from 1968 to 1976. It was field-tested by the Musculoskeletal Tumor Society and subsequently published (Enneking et al, 1980). In the ensuing 5 years, the system has undergone refinement. It has recently been adapted by the American Joint Committee Task Force on Bone Tumors and proposed by them to the International Union Against Cancer (IUCC) for international usage. Based upon histological grade (G), anatomical site (T) and the presence or absence of metastases (M), it describes the progressive stages, irrespective of histogenesis, that assess the progressive degrees of risk to which the patient is subject. This system is well adapted to current radiological techniques of staging, and serves as a useful guide in the selection of an appropriate definitive surgical procedure. Its usage permits comparative end-result studies on the effect of surgical and non-surgical methods of management.

# REFERENCES

Bononi S, Bacchini P, Bertoni F & Campanacci M (1983) Perosteal chondroma. *Journal of Bone and Joint Surgery* **65A:** 205.

Broders AC, Hargrave R & Meyerding HW (1939) Pathologic features of soft tissue fibrosarcoma. *Surgery, Gynecology and Obstetrics* **69:** 267.

Enneking WF, Spanier SS & Goodman MA (1980) A system for the surgical staging of musculoskeletal sarcoma. *Clinical Orthopaedics and Related Research* **153:** 106.

Eriksson AI, Schiller A & Mankin HJ (1980) The management of chondrosarcoma of bone. *Clinical Orthopaedics and Related Research* **153:** 44.

Gherlinzoni F, Rock M & Picci P (1983) Chondromyxofibroma. *Journal of Bone and Joint Surgery* **65A:** 198.

Gitelis S, Bertoni F, Picci P & Campanacci M (1981) Chondrosarcoma of bone. *Journal of Bone and Joint Surgery* **63A:** 1248.

Kreicbergs A, Boquist L & Larsson SE (1982) Prognostic factors in chondrosarcoma. *Cancer* **50:** 577.

Sim FH (1983) Diagnosis and treatment of bone tumors—a teaching approach. In Sim FH (ed.) *Principles of Surgical Treatment*, pp 164–168. Thorofare, New Jersey: Slack.

# 5

# Limb conservation surgery for osteosarcoma and other primary bone tumours

## HUGH KEMP

Thirty years ago, the prognosis for patients afflicted by osteosarcomas was extremely poor, so poor that Cade (1955) advocated interval amputation for the management of affected patients. The rationale behind this treatment was that if a patient was treated with radiotherapy and survived for 6 months without developing metastases, then, and only then, was it justifiable to treat the previously irradiated primary lesion by amputation. At the present time, because the disease-free interval has been prolonged with the use of cytotoxic drugs, it is possible to take a more rational approach to the surgery of bone tumours.

There are conflicting opinions regarding the contribution that surgery makes to survival. On the one hand it has been suggested that there has been a change in the natural history of the disease with a consequent improvement in the prognosis, while on the other hand it has been suggested that an overall improvement in the surgical technique has in itself improved the prognosis (Taylor et al, 1978a,b; 1985). Both such claims should be treated with considerable caution. Certainly, patients with advanced malignant bone tumours referred from developing countries continue to carry a poor prognosis, so it is possible that earlier diagnosis of indigenous patients is a contributory factor, though the interval from the onset of the symptoms to the initiation of treatment is still, depressingly, on average 6 months. Although early diagnosis of tumours facilitates surgery, it is clear that surgery alone is not solely responsible for the improved prognosis since cytotoxic therapy is used in most cases and it is this treatment which has clearly been shown to improve survival in operable osteosarcoma (Link et al, 1986).

## BONE BIOPSY

Bone biopsy is possibly the most important surgical procedure that is performed in the radical treatment of a patient affected by an osteosarcoma. It is often performed by an inexperienced orthopaedic surgeon in order to establish the diagnosis prior to the referral of a patient to a centre equipped with the facilities to treat the particular problem definitively. In the management of patients with bone tumours there is nothing that is more dishearten-

ing than a local subcutaneous or intramuscular recurrence at a biopsy site
when radical surgery of the primary tumour has apparently been successful
(Cannon and Dyson, 1987).

Several problems are encountered with inexpert biopsy. The biopsy
incision is often incorrectly positioned so that definitive surgery cannot be
performed using an incision that encompasses the original biopsy site
(Figure 1a). The biopsy may be placed correctly in relation to the definitive
surgical incision but may not be sited to avoid muscle contamination. As a
result it may be necessary to excise muscle widely at the time of tumour
resection. Skin and subcutaneous closure is frequently performed using
interrupted sutures which involve a wide margin on either side of the site of
the initial biopsy incision. The greatest difficulties arise when the biopsy is
executed without maintaining the highest standards of sterile techniques,
and infection occurs at the biopsy site which prejudices the subsequent
surgical management. Finally, a biopsy may be so radical that a pathological
fracture occurs as a sequel.

Biopsy of osteosarcomas should therefore be regarded as a major step in
the management of this life-threatening disease. An extensive collective
analysis by members of the Musculo-skeletal Tumour Society (Mankin et al,

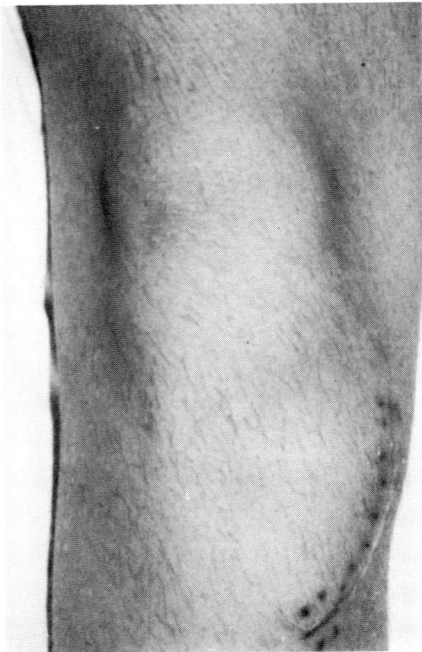

**Figure 1. (a)** Periosteal osteosarcoma occurring on the proximal subcutaneous surface of the
tibia of a young, skeletally immature male. The biopsy is incorrectly positioned and too
extensive.

1982) concerning the misapplication of the principles of biopsy showed that: (a) the incidence of significant problems in patient management due to poor biopsy techniques was 20%, and (b) the incidence of wound healing complications was also 20%. Eight per cent of biopsies produced a significant adverse influence on the prognosis. Five per cent cause or significantly contribute to an otherwise unnecessary amputation and, finally, errors in diagnosis leading to inadequate treatment occur twice as frequently when the biopsy is performed in the referring hospital as when the biopsy is performed at the oncology centre.

In compartmentalizing and staging tumours, too little importance may have been given to the role of the periosteum. Clinical experience suggests that, regardless of the anatomical site of the tumour and despite the cellular morphology of the malignancy, the integrity of the periosteum is a critical factor in determining the prognosis of the particular malignant lesion. If this is true, it is clear that tumour biopsy carries a considerable risk, and that it may convert an intracompartmental lesion to an extracompartmental lesion, with the attendant risks. It may therefore be necessary to revise the approach to bone biopsy in relation to the investigation of such tumours. Bone biopsy should be the ultimate investigation of a skeletal lesion, performed after routine radiographs, isotope scans, computed tomography (CT) scans and magnetic resonance imaging (MRI) scans have been completed. Preferably, the biopsy should be carried out in the centre where the definitive surgery is performed. The biopsy should be carried out by an individual experienced in surgical anatomy and in recognizing, on screening, the relevant area of tumour activity as against reactive bone response. The technique of biopsy is dictated by the nature of the tumour. To reduce soft-tissue contamination it is preferable if possible to perform a needle biopsy, employing a Jamshidi or 'Tru-Cut' needle. When the lesion is sclerotic it is essential to employ a core biopsy that penetrates the full thickness of the affected bone. In performing a biopsy, sterile procedures are essential. If the result of the biopsy is equivocal, the investigations should be collectively evaluated by the histopathologist, the radiologist and the surgeon and, if there is any doubt about the diagnosis, the biopsy should be repeated until a definitive diagnosis has been obtained.

## INDICATIONS AND CONTRAINDICATIONS FOR CONSERVATIVE SURGERY

Patients with osteosarcomas should initially be assessed regarding their suitability for conservative surgery. The investigations include standard radiography, CT scanning of the lesion and chest, and MRI scanning. In our experience arteriography is of little value.

The dicta of suitability for such surgery closely parallel those laid down by Enneking et al (1980). However, at certain sites, such as the knee, the tumours are frequently related to 'bare areas' of bone, and in consequence the mandatory requirement of the removal of 2 centimetres of associated muscle and soft tissues around the tumour cannot always be achieved in performing a wide excision. Evidence on scanning of the involvement of vessels does not preclude tumour resection because affected segments of blood vessels can be excised and grafted. In general, skin and subcutaneous involvement usually precludes conservative surgery as it is only in a rare instance that it is possible to mobilize an adequate myoplastic flap to cover such a defect.

Pulmonary secondaries that are resectable or are slow growing do not exclude conservative surgery to the primary tumour. In these cases the prognosis is poor, but conservative surgery removes the primary tumour and may maintain function.

Only a relatively small number of patients with limb bone sarcomas are not suitable for conservative management by any of the accepted methods when they initially present. The obvious examples are those individuals who present with tumour extensions that are so advanced that there is soft tissue and skin involvement. Some osteosarcomas may fail to respond to cytotoxic therapy, and in the interim between the commencement of cytotoxic therapy and the 'window' when surgery is proposed, they move from the stage of operability to that of inoperability. This is most commonly seen with osteo-sarcomas of certain histological types, namely, osteoclast rich, chondro-blastic or haemangioblastic osteosarcomas.

Atypical tumour spread may also preclude reconstructive surgery. Osteosarcomas with extensive medullary and atypical lymphatic spread are not suitable for conservative limb reconstruction. Patients with pathological fractures in whom spillage has occurred are, in general, probably best treated by amputation. This applies, in particular, to chondrosarcoma. (It may also apply, albeit rarely, to benign tumours such as osteoclastomas which, if clearance surgery is delayed, are capable as a sequel to pathological fracture of extending widely through tissue planes.)

Chondrosarcomas have a very variable natural history. They are most likely to recur after inadequate local resection and, when they do, they tend to show an alteration in cellular pattern towards a higher histological grade such as an increase in binuclear cells. For this reason, even the most benign lesion should be treated with circumspection during excision (Wilson and Scales, 1987). While pathological fractures in any malignant tumour are associated with a worse prognosis, this applies particularly to chondro-sarcomas, not only in terms of local recurrence but also in the likelihood of the development of metastases.

It has previously been accepted that amputation should always be performed through the immediately proximal joint because of the concern that a conservative resection might be complicated by tumour recurrence in the amputation stump. In 1975, Sweetnam suggested that a more con-servative approach could be considered if surgery was associated with chemotherapy. Most oncological surgeons now regard amputation or dis-articulation by the same criteria as they do for wide excision of a tumour. Consequently, if it can be shown that amputation flaps can be cut and the bone divided with adequate tumour resection, then it is permissible to perform an amputation through the shaft of the bone proximal to the tumour.

## VARIATIONS IN TUMOUR BEHAVIOUR

Osteosarcomas are locally invasive tumours. Although initially contained by the periosteum, they ultimately break through, invading the muscle, and eventually involve subcutaneous tissues and skin. Medullary spread is relatively slow to occur and it is exceptional to see extensive medullary spread, though local extension may take place. Enneking and Kagan (1975) drew attention to the occurrence of 'skip lesions' in osteosarcoma, and since then the frequency and importance of such lesions has been debated. Concern regarding this complication has led some surgeons to advocate interval biopsy, that is core biopsies spaced above or below resectable osteosarcoma in order to determine the safe level for wide excision of a resectable tumour. The disadvantage of this technique is that it is obviously possible to take biopsies on either side of a skip lesion if present. The advent of third-generation CT scanners coupled with MRI scanning techniques makes it possible to recognize such lesions and include them in the resection. It would appear that the occurrence of such lesions is less common than was originally thought.

In osteosarcoma, as with other skeletal sarcomas, metastases are blood borne and are usually first detected in the lungs. Such lesions can now sometimes be treated surgically by metastatectomy. A minority of patients exhibit multiple skeletal metastases which may or may not be associated initially with pulmonary lesions, though these nearly always occur relatively soon after disseminated skeletal lesions are observed. Some authors regard these bone lesions as examples of multicentric primary tumours. Usually, only one lesion exhibits the radiological features of a primary lesion, whereas the others have the characteristics of secondary intermedullary deposits (Ross, 1964). This interpretation is supported by the instances where the primary lesion has been excised and multiple skeletal deposits then present at a later stage. Rarely, patients present with lymph node involvement. Such deposits are not necessarily consistent with the lymphatic drainage of the affected area. When they occur the prognosis is poor.

## SURGICAL OPTIONS FOR LIMB CONSERVATION

In general, the majority of appendicular tumours, particularly those related to the shoulder, elbow, hip and knee are very suitable for conservative surgery. The specific tumours treated by such methods include osteo-sarcomas, chondrosarcomas, skeletal malignant fibrous histiocytomas and, more recently, Ewing's sarcomas when the treatment is in combination with chemotherapy and radiotherapy.

In the surgical treatment of osteosarcomas a different discipline is required to the local 'intralesional or marginal excisions' (Enneking, 1980) which may be judiciously employed in the management of benign tumours. Local excision of osteosarcomas is rarely acceptable, though this approach can be performed in certain instances (e.g. parosteal osteosarcomas, which may be excised) provided that a wide margin of normal bone is removed.

Local excision can also be used for certain periosteal osteosarcomas after they have initially been treated by cytotoxic drugs (Figures 1b–d). Occasionally, Ewing's sarcoma can be excised locally, for instance when they arise in the fibula, chest wall or pelvis, provided that they are concurrently treated with such drugs and subsequently with local radiotherapy.

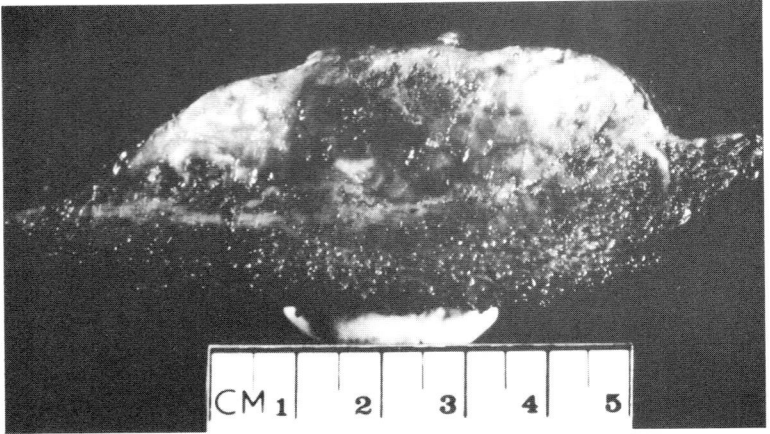

**Figure 1. (b)** Macroscopic specimen of periosteal osteosarcoma after resection.

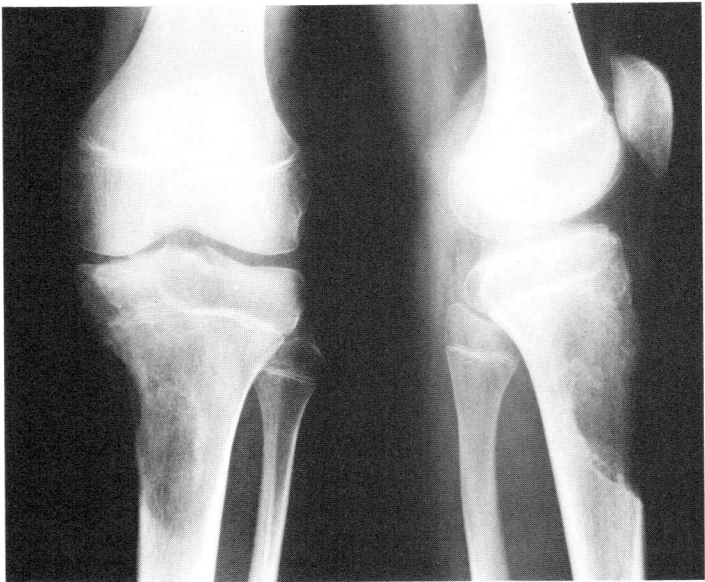

**Figure 1. (c)** Radiograph of resultant defect.

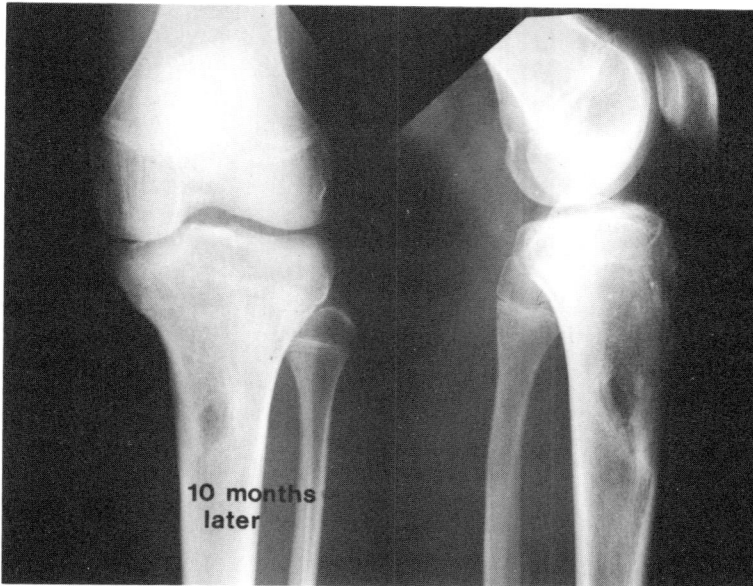

**Figure 1. (d)** Radiograph showing progressive repair of the defect 10 months later.

It is generally agreed that a margin of at least 2 centimetres of normal tissue needs to be removed (Van der Heul and Von Ronnen, 1967). Following a local excision, the creation of an extensive defect in a weight-bearing bone carries a risk of subsequent fracture. For this reason it is extremely tempting to graft the defect that results (Luck et al, 1979; Marcove and Rosen, 1979). In our experience, grafts mask the radiological manifestation of a local recurrence and, for this reason we do not use them. It is our practice to cast brace these patients for between 6 and 12 months, according to the age of the patient, until there has been adequate new bone formation. The criteria for such local surgery are that the lesion needs to be relatively small—in general not more than 5 centimetres in diameter, that the margins are well defined and discrete, and that there is careful histological review subsequently, to ensure that a normal margin of bone has been removed. If the preoperative assessment proves to have underestimated the extent of the tumour, it is mandatory that a further and more radical excision or removal is performed.

There are a number of options available in the conservative surgical management of osteosarcomas following radical removal of the tumour. Allografts to replace part of an affected bone were first advocated by Lexer (1925). Their use in the treatment of tumours has been advocated by Volkov (1970) and in some centres in the USA, notably by Parrish (1973) and Mankin et al (1976). Such procedures have not gained wide acceptance due to the relative morbidity of the grafts which may fracture or be partly absorbed and, in the long term, exhibit degeneration of the articular surfaces. The alternative forms of treatment which are currently widely practised are radical excision coupled with internal fixation and grafting, radical excision and internal prosthetic joint replacement, and tumour excision coupled with a modified Van Nes procedure (1950). The advantage of the former method is that a solid arthrodesis provides a lasting result, even though it may be difficult and protracted to achieve. Possibly, this may also be claimed for a Van Nes procedure or (as it is also called) 'the rotational turniplasty'. However, this operation places a considerable psychological strain on the patient, particularly upon an adolescent. Furthermore, the surgical achievement provides limited benefit to the patient, since replacing the knee joint with a reverse ankle joint can only, at the most, offer 60° of movement from a fixed flexion deformity of between 30° and 40°. Possibly it might be wiser to curb such surgical procedures, limiting the enthusiasm to extending the length of the amputation stump. Having expressed these reservations, it must be acknowledged that this technique has a wide popularity in the management of tumours of the lower limb on the continent and particularly in Germany (Winkelmann, 1983; Winkler et al, 1986).

Merle d'Aubigne and Dejournay (1958) were amongst the first to describe a method for bridging the defect created by tumour excision by the use of sliding inlay grafts. Their techniques were developed by the work of others and, in particular, by Enneking and Shirley (1977), who modified the design of the Kuntschner rod in order to obtain adequate fixation in both the femur and the tibia in continuity. They then filled the attendant defects with free autografts taken from adjacent sites. They reported excellent results in 20 patients treated for tumours about the knee. In 16 surviving patients, 13 were ambulant at 1 year and the remainder within the subsequent 9 months. Others have advanced variants of technique including the use of autografts, autoclaved autografts and allografts in conjunction with prosthetic replacement.

In the UK the main emphasis has been placed on the replacement of defects created by tumour resection with custom-built massive prostheses.

## THE MANUFACTURE AND DESIGN OF PROSTHESES

Major prostheses are preferably designed and custom built for the individual patient. To do this it is necessary to use routine clinical and measurement radiographs of the affected limb. The latter are achieved using a stationary grid and scale. Anteroposterior and lateral views are taken of the affected and contralateral limb (Figures 2a–c). CT scans are essential in determining the point of resection, and MRI scans are now being used to give additional information, in particular, of medullary spread. Obviously, it is an advantage that these are also mensurated. The metals used in the manufacture of prostheses include stainless steel, cobalt chrome molybdenum alloy, titanium (T1–T5) and titanium alloy. Steel is now rarely used. Concave articular surfaces and axle bushes are made of ultra-high molecular weight poly-

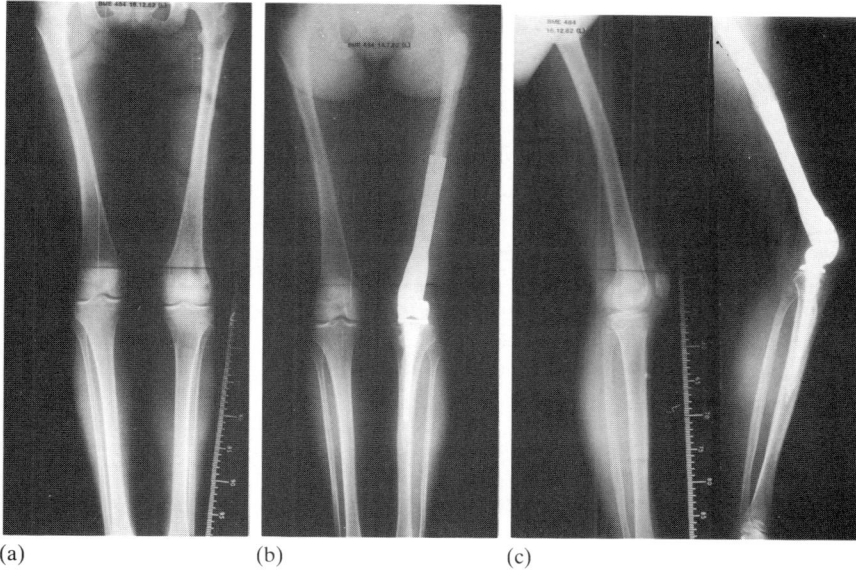

(a)                              (b)                              (c)

**Figure 2. (a)** Measurement films of patient with an osteosarcoma of the left distal femur (anteroposterior view). **(b)** Standing film 8 months later (anteroposterior view). **(c)** Lateral measurement film and standing film 8 months later.

ethylene; the convex articular surface is either metal or ceramic alumina. The intramedullary stem is preferably not less than 14 centimetres in length, though circumstances occasionally dictate the use of a smaller stem. In the adult, the stem is on average between 9 and 12 millimetres in diameter. In cross-section it is normally D-shaped, which prevents rotation in the cement. It conforms to the natural shape of the medullary canal.

The preparation of the medullary cavity is critical; reaming is kept to a minimum because of the damage it can cause to the blood supply. Bone cement should contain appropriate antibiotics and it should always be injected. The nozzle of the syringe should be of adequate length to allow the cement to be inserted as a homogeneous mass, the nozzle being withdrawn as the cement is being extruded. The prosthesis, when inserted, should be held under compression until the cement has set (Scales, 1983). There are now several commercial suppliers of massive prostheses. These prostheses are generally dependent on modular units for their construction and have few of the advantages of custom-built prostheses.

## SURGICAL TECHNIQUES

Although in Britain the main emphasis has been on the replacement of defects created by tumour resection with massive endoprostheses, probably the first such endoprosthetic replacement to be recorded for this purpose was a case reported by Moore and Bohlman (1940) in America. In 1950, at the Royal National Orthopaedic Hospital in the UK, Burrows et al began their programme of tumour replacement (Burrows, 1968). They reported their results on 24 patients in 1975 (Burrows et al, 1975). Since that time, over 860 prostheses have been inserted and, of these, 670 have been for tumour replacements (Tables 1 and 2). The majority of these cases have been treated in two supraregional bone tumour centres in London and Birmingham, namely at the Royal National Orthopaedic Hospital and the Middlesex Hospital (by the author and by Sweetnam), and at the Royal Orthopaedic Hospital, Birmingham (by Sneath).

Although osteosarcomas can occur in any part of the skeleton, they show a propensity for certain sites which bears a close relationship to the regions exhibiting a maximum growth potential. Because of the frequency of bone tumours at certain locations in the appendicular skeleton, relatively standard methods have been developed for their replacement. The common sites for replacements are the distal femur, the proximal femur, the proximal tibia and the proximal humerus. In some instances it has been necessary to replace the whole humerus or whole femur (Figure 3). Rarely, tumours relating to the elbow joint have been prosthetically replaced. Prosthetic replacement of tumours of the distal radius and distal tibia have on occasions been attempted, but these have proved to be totally unsuccessful. If conservative surgery is considered possible at these sites, the lesions are more suitably treated by resection and grafting, using autografts with allografts, or occasionally with xenografts. However, the problems associated with tumours of the distal tibia are considerable and such tumours are in general best treated by amputation.

**Table 1.** Stanmore major prosthesis inserted for tumour, 30 July 1949 to 31 December 1986.

| Prosthesis type | Number inserted |
|---|---|
| Pelvic prosthesis | 11 |
| Total femur | 12 |
| Proximal femur | 160 |
| Mid-shaft of femur | 9 |
| Distal femur | 226 |
| Distal femur and proximal tibia | 4 |
| Proximal tibia | 104 |
| Distal tibia | 2 |
| Total humerus | 13 |
| Proximal humerus | 84 |
| Distal humerus and elbow | 8 |
| Distal radius | 2 |
| Extending prostheses (all sites) | 45 |
| | 680 |

**Table 2.** Bone tumours and destructive lesions treated with a Stanmore major prosthesis up to 31 December 1986.

| Tumour/lesion | Number of cases |
|---|---|
| Osteosarcoma | 253 |
| Parosteal sarcoma | 37 |
| Osteochondroma, enchondroma, chondromyxoid fibroma | 7 |
| Chondrosarcoma | 114 |
| Desmoplastic fibroma | 2 |
| Fibrosarcoma | 23 |
| Osteoclastoma | 98 |
| Malignant fibrous histiocytoma | 29 |
| Massive osteolysis, lipoma | 3 |
| Ewing's sarcoma | 30 |
| Myeloma, lymphoma, liposarcoma, leiomyosarcoma | 9 |
| Other primary bone tumours: | |
|   identified | 7 |
|   unidentified | 3 |
| Metastatic carcinoma | 55 |
| Total | 670* |

* This total is smaller than the number of prostheses inserted (see Table 1) because in 10 patients a temporary prosthesis was used before the permanent one was inserted.

## Proximal humerus

In the management of degenerative lesions of the shoulder, it is usually only necessary to replace the humeral head or the humeral head and the glenoid. This involves the use of an unconstrained prosthesis, such as the Neer's prosthesis, or a constrained joint such as the Stanmore or the Kessel shoulder joint replacement. In using these prostheses it is not necessary to disturb the integrity of the intrinsic musculature forming the rotator cuff, that is the muscles which stabilize the humeral head in relation to the glenoid, nor does it affect the extrinsic musculature which is essentially responsible for active movement of the shoulder joint. In contrast, in treating malignant tumours of the proximal humerus it is almost invariably necessary to excise up to one-third of the proximal humerus. Consequently, even though the humeral deficit is replaced by an internal prosthesis, unless the shoulder musculature can be reconstructed the patient will be left with a hanging shoulder. Such a procedure will allow the patient to use the forearm at the waist level, though it will not allow activities such as lifting. Nevertheless, such a radical clearance may be necessary in the management of Ewing's sarcoma or an osteosarcoma that has extended beyond the periosteum. However, in the majority of patients such a wide clearance is not required and it is possible to perform more conservative surgery in an attempt to reconstitute shoulder function (Ross et al, 1987).

The patient is positioned on the operating table so that the shoulder can be freely moved. The incision resembles in its proximal part the 'sabre' incision originally employed in an anterior approach to the shoulder; it is then continued down the arm along the lateral border of the biceps. This incision

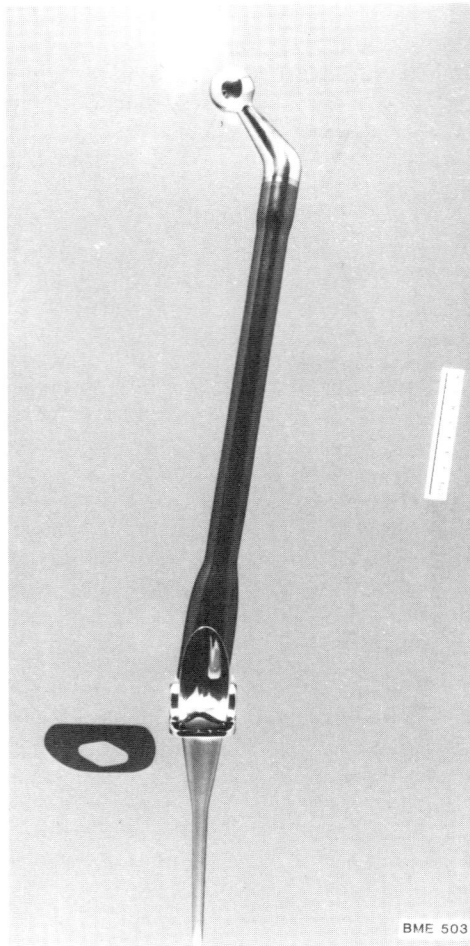

**Figure 3.** Total femoral replacement employed when there has been extensive tumoral invasion of the diaphysis. Tibial plateau plates are used to distribute load bearing.

allows the proximal humerus to be freely exposed. The delto-pectoral groove is identified and the cephalic vein ligated when necessary, the muscles are separated, and the deltoid is then detached from its clavicular and acromial origins. The tip of the coracoid is detached and reflected medially with its associated muscles. This provides direct access to the rotator cuff muscles, namely the subscapularis, supraspinatus, infraspinatus and teres minor. Depending on the extent of the tumour, these muscles are divided approximately at their insertions to leave an adequate clearance of the tumour. The residue of the insertions are then transfixed with stay sutures. If the tumour is extensive in terms of bone involvement, then the pectoralis major, latissimus dorsi and teres major are dealt with in a similar manner after the circumflex nerve and the radial nerve have been clearly identified. The insertion of deltoid should be preserved if this is technically feasible. Occasionally, when a more radical clearance is required it is possible to separate its attachment to the bone though maintaining its continuity with periosteum. When this is not feasible, the insertion of the deltoid is divided and the residual portion of the insertion is tagged with stay sutures. The tendon of biceps brachii is rarely involved in the tumour. If it cannot be lifted out of its sheath, it is divided and its continuity re-established at a later stage. The tumour is then resected and a custom-built prosthesis inserted.

A previously manufactured sleeve of Mersilene EM 54 (Ethicon) is then attached to the prosthesis and its distal tail is tethered to the periosteum of the residual bone (Figures 4a and b). The proximal portion of the sleeve is appropriately shaped at this stage and attached to the residual capsule around the glenoid with interrupted sutures. The posterior, superior and anterior muscles of the rotator cuff are then attached to this Mersilene sleeve, approximating, where possible, to their original insertions. The teres major and latissimus dorsi are attached to the posterior lateral aspect of the sleeve and the pectoralis major is attached to the anterolateral aspect. If the deltoid has been detached, its insertion is carefully replicated on the sleeve and underlying attachments. Finally, the tendon of the long head of the

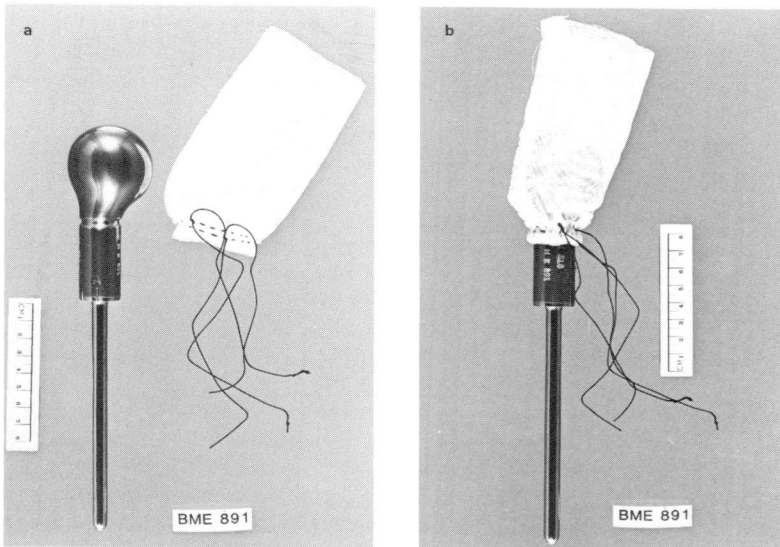

**Figure 4.** (a) Unconstrained prosthesis used in the replacement of the proximal humerus. The Mersilene sleeve acts as an artificial capsule. (b) Sleeve in situ. It facilitates the reconstruction of the rotator cuff and allows the reattachment of the extrinsic musculature of the shoulder.

biceps is reconstituted, or if this is not possible, it is attached to the short head of the biceps after the tip of the coracoid process has been reattached to the body. The divided origin of the deltoid is reattached and the delto-pectoral groove is reconstituted in order to re-establish the anterior axillary fold.

Postoperative management is similar to that employed in treating a patient who has had a Bankart procedure, the arm being held across the chest in a sling and crêpe spica for 3 weeks. The patient is then actively mobilized. Using this method it is possible to obtain some 80° of flexion, 40° of extension and almost full internal and external rotation. Deltoid function does not recover as adequately, and no more than 30° of abduction can be expected in the average case. Occasionally it has been necessary to replace the whole humerus. When this is done a modified Stanmore elbow joint is incorporated in the prosthesis.

*Elbow joint*

Tumours arising in relation to the elbow joint are extremely uncommon. When they occur, they are most suitably treated by wide excision and insertion of a modified constrained elbow joint of the Stanmore type (Figure 5). The tumour is usually most adequately exposed through a posteriorly placed incision.

*Wrist*

Malignant tumours at this site are rare and usually involve the distal radius. In most cases they are more suitably treated by wide excision and arthrodesis of the distal ulna into the carpal bones of the wrist, usually augmented with autologous grafts.

*Proximal femur*

Resecting the proximal femur (see Figure 6) for malignancy can be performed through any of the recognized surgical approaches; however, the posterior or Southern approach appears to be the most versatile. The hip is exposed in the conventional manner, the distal incision being extended along the line of the femur to the level of resection of the bone. If the greater trochanter is not involved in the tumour, the insertions of the gluteus medius and gluteus minimus are elevated from the surface of the greater trochanter with a thin sliver of the underlying bone in order to maintain the continuity of these muscles with the fascia lata. If the insertions of the two abductors have to be divided in order to achieve adequate clearance, the tendons are transfixed with stay sutures and are subsequently stitched into the fascia when the wound is being closed. The remaining muscles can be freely divided through their origins or their insertions and can be left unattached because it has been found that they gain an adequate attachment to the fibrous sheath that subsequently forms around the prosthesis. Earlier attempts to fenestrate the prosthesis, in order to provide more stable attachments, have proved unnecessary.

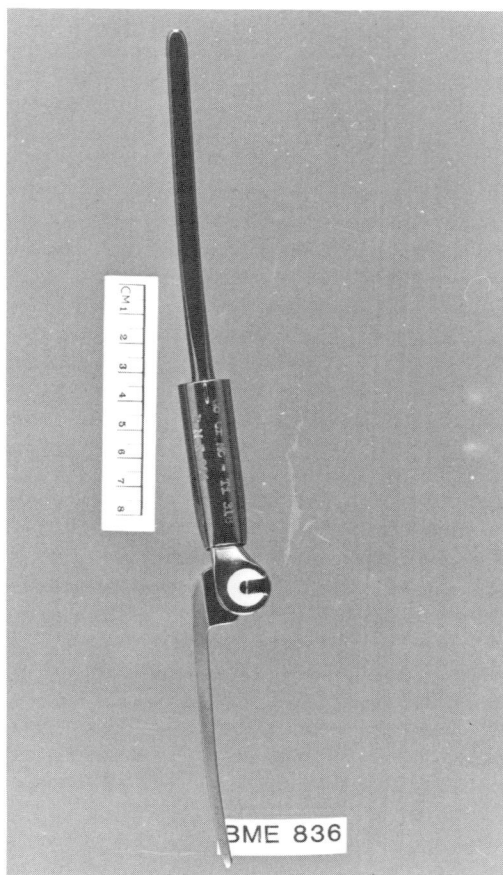

**Figure 5.** A modified constrained Stanmore elbow prosthesis used to replace a distal humeral tumour.

Postoperatively, the patient is nursed on balanced slings with minimal abduction traction for 3 weeks. The patient is then mobilized in a splint of the Erlanger type which prevents adduction and rotation, and this is maintained for 12 weeks to allow fibrous tissue to form around the prosthesis. The reason for this postoperative management is that in the initial series of cases (Wilson and Scales, 1987) there was a high incidence of dislocation in the immediate postoperative period. Using this technique has reduced the frequency of this problem, particularly in the younger patient. Patients who have had massive upper femoral replacement vary considerably in their walking ability. About 40% will exhibit a Trendelenburg gait, the remainder will walk normally, and a minority will even run without a Trendelenburg

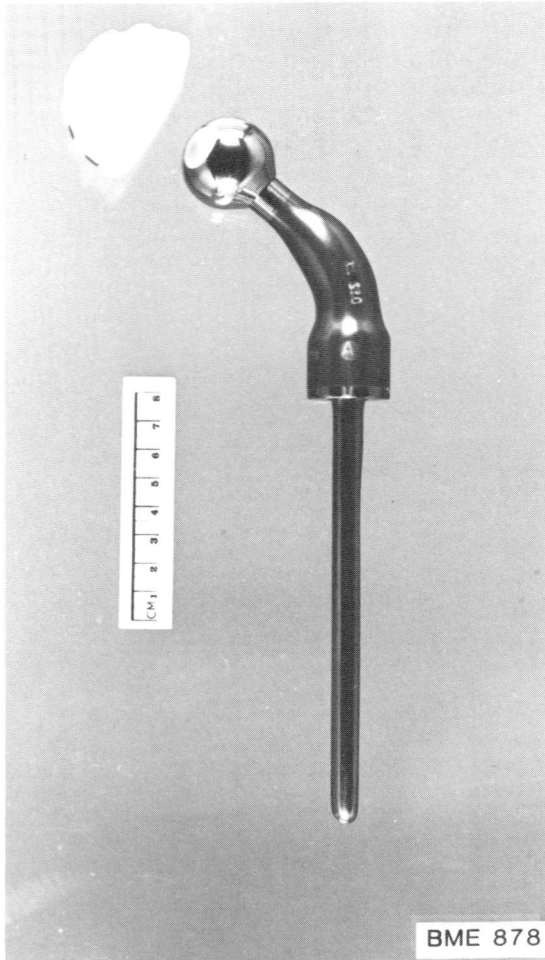

**Figure 6.** A custom-built prosthetic replacement used in replacing tumours of the proximal femur.

gait. Virtually all patients will exhibit a full range of movement. External rotation is increased to between 40° and 60°. The exceptions are those who have received radiotherapy.

*Distal femur*

The distal femur can be approached through either a medial or a lateral parapatellar approach (Bradish et al, 1987). The former approach has certain technical advantages, but the surgical approach is frequently dictated by the site of the initial biopsy. The procedure is normally performed under tourniquet control. The incision extends proximally to the site of election for division of the femur and distally for 5 centimetres below the joint line. The incision is then deepened through the tendon of the quadratus femoris to the midline and curves around the margin of the patella, descending along the medial border of the patellar tendon to its insertion. The quadratus muscles are then reflected on either side of the tumour with an adequate margin of muscle being left in relation to the tumour. The medial and lateral collateral ligaments are similarly divided. The knee joint is progressively flexed and, ultimately, the cruciate ligaments are divided. At this stage, the posterior capsule is exposed and divided along its tibial attachment. The heads of the gastrocnemius and the popliteus are divided, leaving an adequate margin of muscle related to the distal femur. The clearance of the tumour is then extended proximally to the level of the femoral division. Occasionally, after dividing the posterior capsule, the posterior extension of the tumour may make it impossible to identify the neurovascular bundle. In these circumstances the femoral diaphysis is advantageously divided and the dissection extended distally. Surprisingly, tumour extension rarely involves the popliteal nerves, though it may invade the popliteal artery and vein. When this occurs the vessels are resected and grafted with donor grafts taken from the ipsilateral long saphenous vein. We use the Stanmore constrained knee joint with an appropriate custom-built prosthetic extension (Figure 7a). If a medial approach is used, a lateral release of the quadriceps expansion is performed to prevent subsequent patella subluxation, and the medial expansion is then reconstructed to give stability to the quadriceps mechanism. If a lateral approach is used, no attempt is made to repair the lateral expansion. The quadriceps tendon and subsequent tissue layers are approximated with interrupted sutures. The range of movement is shown in Figures 7b and 7c.

*Proximal tibia*

Tumours arising in this region are more suitably approached from a lateral patellar approach, the incision extending from approximately 10 centimetres above the joint line to the preselected point of division of the tibia. The incision is deepened in the manner described (see above) and the femur dissociated from the tibia. The patellar tendon is elevated from the tibial tubercle or it is divided after the distance from the lower pole of the patella to the point of tibial resection has been carefully measured. It is only necessary to identify the lateral popliteal (common peroneal nerve) when the tumour extends laterally and is likely to encompass the nerve. The superior tibio-fibular joint is identified and opened or, if the tumour extends around the area, the fibula is divided below the joint. Muscles of the anterior compartment are elevated from the bone or widely excised in relation to the tumour mass. An attempt should be made to identify and preserve the anterior tibial artery and nerve whenever this is possible, though they can be sacrificed if this is necessary. The posterior aspect of the tibia is then approached and the soleus muscle and the muscles of the posterior

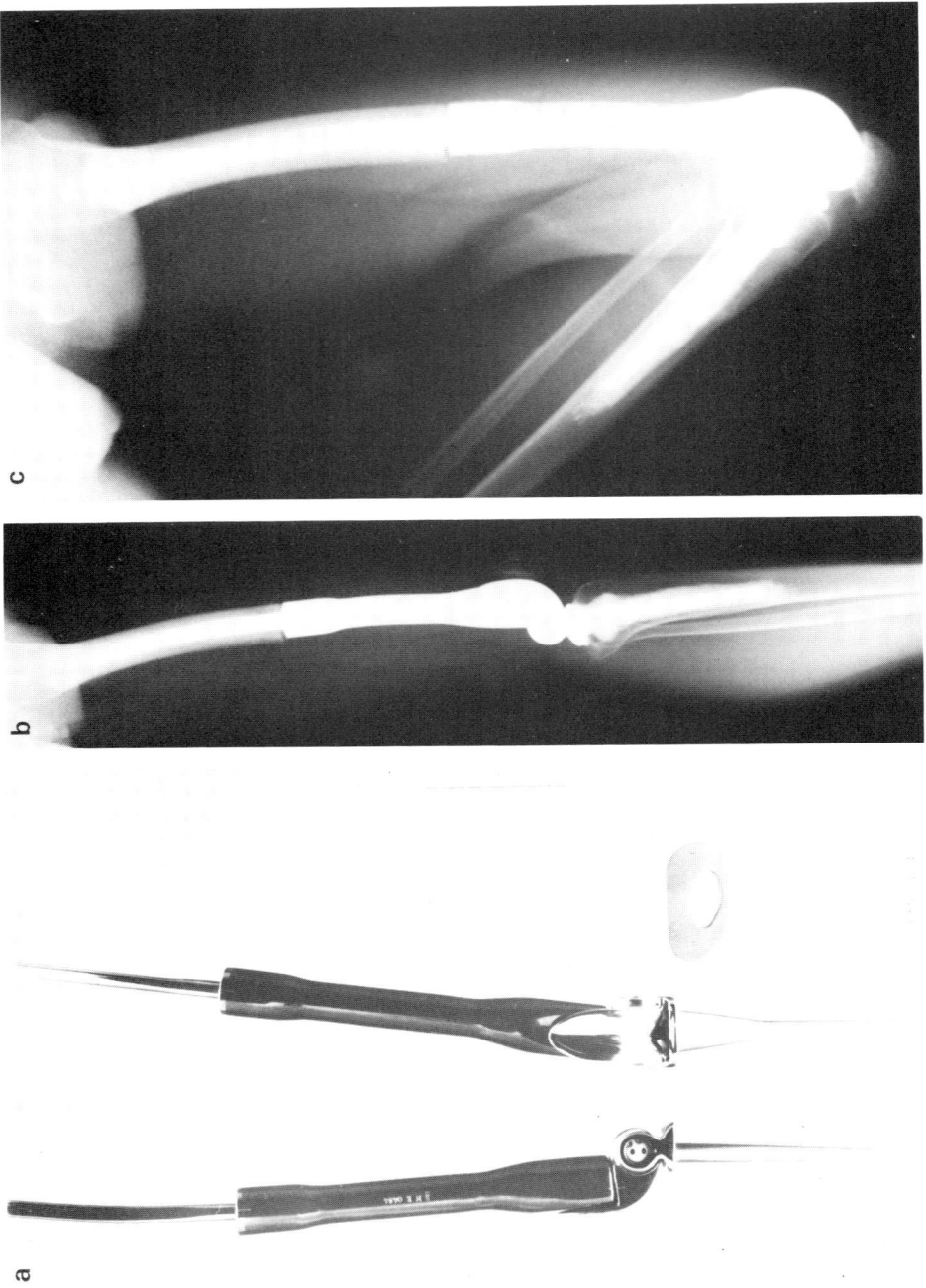

**Figure 7. (a)** Anteroposterior and lateral views of a distal femoral replacement incorporating a constrained joint. **(b)** and **(c)** Lateral radiographs showing range of knee movement after replacement which resulted from a malignant fibrous histiocytoma of the distal femur.

compartment are similarly treated. If the anterior tibial artery can be preserved, it is identified and retracted with the nerve so that the inter-osseous membrane can then be incised. The tibia is then divided at the site of election. The massive tibial replacement is then inserted, followed by a standard component for the femoral side. No attempt is made to reattach the muscles of the anterior or posterior compartments, as their origins incorpo-rate in the fibrous sheath that forms around the tibial prosthesis. However, it is essential to reconstitute the patellar attachment. This is done by attaching the tendon to the tibial prosthesis, employing a ribbon made of polyester tube net (Malmic Lace Ltd). This is threaded through a preconstructed fenestration in the prosthesis so that the two ends of the ribbon can be brought up on either side. The tendon is then drawn down so that the relation of the inferior pole of the patella and the point of transection conform to the initial measurement. The ribbon is then sutured to the tendon. Prior to wound closure the tourniquet is released so that absolute haemostasis can be obtained. In particular, the posterior genicular arterial branches should be identified and ligated. The wound is closed in the manner previously described and is appropriately drained.

Postoperatively, the limb is gently compressed in a crêpe spica until drainage has ceased at approximately 48 hours. At this stage the knee is placed on a constant passive motion (CPM) apparatus. The use of this technique has made a considerable advance in the management of tumours about the knee and also of tumours of the proximal femur. Prior to its usage, the maximum range of knee flexion that could be obtained varied between 80 and 100° (Figures 8a–c). With the employment of CPM apparatus, adhesions of the quadriceps do not occur and the majority of patients achieve virtually full flexion. Patients who have had massive replacements in relation to the knee are often noted to have a knee which is considerably warmer than the opposite side. This is frequently mistaken as an indication of infection, but is due to body heat being conducted through the prosthesis.

*Ankle*

Malignant tumours occur occasionally in the distal tibia. It is feasible to perform an 'en bloc' resection, but grafts between the distal tibia and talus are notoriously slow to incorporate soundly (1–2 years) and, in conse-quence, the patient should be persuaded whenever possible to accept a below-knee amputation as this returns the individual more rapidly to normal ambulation.

**'Growing' prostheses**

In children, the problem of bone replacement is further complicated by the loss of bone growth. This is of particular importance in the lower limb. 'Growing' prostheses have been developed in an attempt to overcome this problem. Developed primarily in the UK by Sneath and Scales (Sneath et al, 1984), the rationale of the prosthesis is to preserve the normal growth potential of the unaffected bone and to replace the resected bone by an

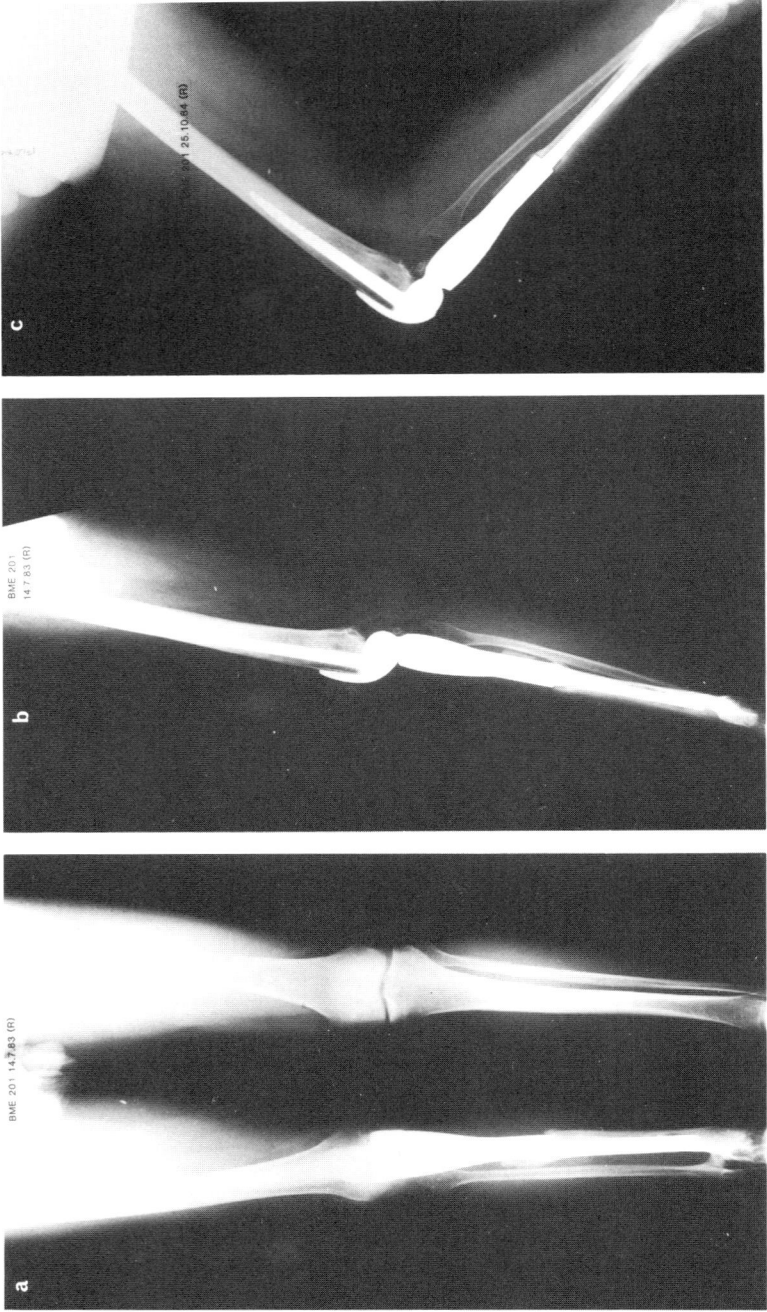

**Figure 8.** (a) Anteroposterior view of tibial replacement performed 10 years earlier. The patient had previously had a fracture of the right ankle. There is heterotopic new bone formation in relation to the prosthesis. (b) and (c) The range of movement in this patient was limited to 80° of flexion. He was treated in a period prior to the use of constant passive motion apparatus.

extendable component. For the unaffected distal femur or proximal tibia with a normal growth plate, the appropriate portion of the constrained knee joint has been modified. A hole is drilled through the epiphysis into the metaphysis. A thread is subsequently tapped into the bone. A threaded high density polyethylene (HDP) tube is then screwed into the metaphysis below the growth plate. Using a template, two grooves are cut into the articular surface of the tibia or femur. The articular surface can then carry a modified knee component supported by a floating table made of titanium alloy that keys into the grooves cut on the epiphyseal articular surface. This is to prevent rotation of the floating table. Below this table there is a piston that fits into the HDP tube. Subsequently, as metaphyseal growth continues, the piston can extend out of the tube without restricting the growth.

The involved bone is replaced with a massive prosthesis (Figures 9a and b). However, this is modified so that it too has a piston action. This piston has a sliding member that prevents rotation from occurring. The piston itself rests within the component on tungsten carbide ball-bearings. In the side of the tube which carries the piston, there is a vent hole to allow the introduction of further tungsten carbide ball-bearings so that, during the growth spurt, it is possible to progressively extend the prosthesis at intervals. Although this prosthesis has many attractions, it has two disadvantages. First, the fibrous sheath that surrounds the replacement prosthesis may be so thick that it prevents the artificial extension of the unit and, second, it is to be expected that a prosthesis designed to fit a child's bone will not necessarily be strong enough to support an adult. It may therefore be necessary to replace these prostheses when growth is complete.

## Pelvic tumours

Pelvic tumours can, on rare occasions, be locally resected, for example a tumour such as a chondrosarcoma with a relatively narrow base arising from the wing of the ilium. Such tumours can be resected without losing stability even when it is necessary to interrupt the continuity of the pelvic ring. Unfortunately, most pelvic tumours require more extensive resection and many patients are treated by hind-quarter amputation. More recently, attempts have been made at more conservative surgery, hemipelvic resection being performed preserving a hanging limb (Enneking and Dunham, 1978; Steel, 1978; Sweetnam, 1983). Alternatively, in selected cases it has been possible to replace the resected portion of the hemipelvis with a custom-built prosthesis. To date, some 12 patients have had such pelvic replacements in the UK.

## Complications of prosthetic replacement

Prosthetic replacement cannot be performed without the risk of complications (Table 3). The major risk is infection. All potential sources of infection, such as decayed teeth, should be treated before the patient begins chemotherapy. When an indwelling subcutaneous (Hickman) line is used to

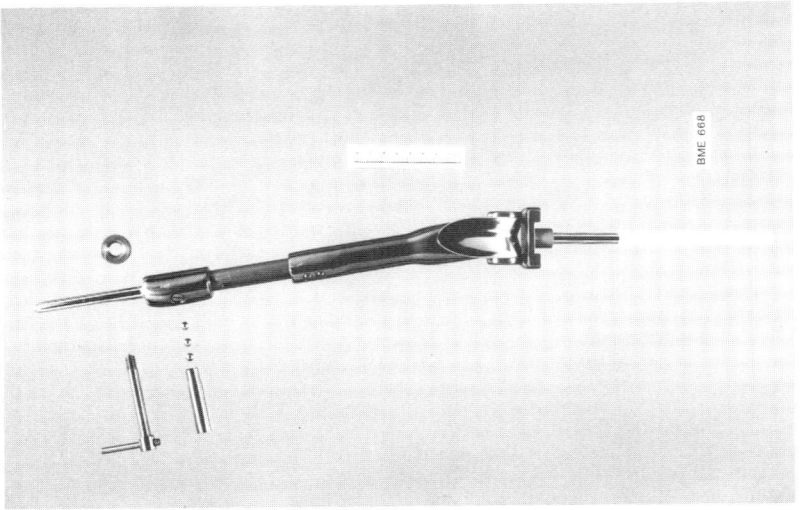

(b)

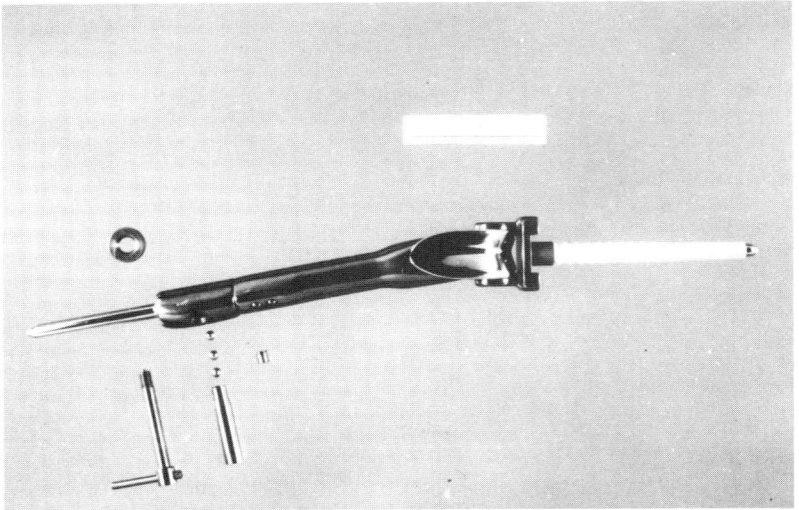

(a)

**Figure 9. (a)** Growing prosthesis in the closed position. **(b)** Growing prosthesis in the extended position. (For details of the prosthesis, see text.)

**Table 3.** Principal prosthesis complications reported by 31 December 1986 in 670 major prostheses inserted for tumour.

| Prosthesis type | Total inserted | Broken prosthesis number | Aseptic loosening number | Deep sepsis number |
|---|---|---|---|---|
| Pelvic | 11 | — | — | 2 |
| Proximal femur | 160 | 4 | 3 | 6 |
| Mid-shaft of femur | 9 | — | 2 | — |
| Distal femur and knee | 226 | 7 | 4 | 6 |
| Proximal tibia and knee | 104 | 1 | 1 | 17 |
| Proximal humerus | 84 | 1 | 4 | 4 |
| Distal humerus and elbow | 8 | — | 2 | — |
| Extending | 45 | 1 | 1 | 2 |
| All other types | 33 | — | — | — |
| Total | 670 | 14 (2.1%) | 17 (2.5%) | 37 (5.5%) |

administer cytotoxic drugs, it should be managed scrupulously. When the lines are flushed and locked with heparin/saline to prevent clotting, precautions should be stringent to prevent the risk of the tubes becoming colonized with such organisms as *Staphylococcus epidermidis*. Surgery should always be performed under full antibiotic cover and the antibiotics should be administered for 24 hours preoperatively and maintained until wound healing has occurred. Ideally, antibiotics should be administered intravenously and serum levels constantly monitored. It is preferable to refrain from using the Hickman catheter for the administration of antibiotics and for blood transfusion in the immediate perioperative period. Surgery should be performed under conditions of maximum sterility, preferably in a laminar air flow theatre. Finally, wound closure in patients on chemotherapy should be with interrupted sutures because of the poor tissue healing potential. Despite these precautions, infection rates are still high at 5.5%. Of these, a small proportion have been of late onset. Only rarely has it been necessary to amputate an affected limb. Loosening of the prosthesis has occurred in 2.5% of cases; however, it has been possible to re-operate on these patients successfully.

In some patients prostheses have broken. This was not an uncommon occurrence before the standards which were laid down for the manufacture of prostheses meant that materials of adequate tensile strength were employed. Breakage has been a relatively rare occurrence over the past 20 years. When it has occurred it has been possible to replace the prostheses in all but one instance. The cause of breakage, in the majority of cases, has been the result of excessive force such as a road traffic accident.

## Axial skeleton

Malignant tumours of the axial skeleton are relatively rare. When they do occur, there is no alternative to radical excision if this is surgically feasible. Unfortunately, because of the problems associated with the surgical approach, they are rarely removed with an adequate tissue margin, and, in consequence, the local recurrence rate is relatively high and the prognosis is extremely poor.

The surgery of tumours of the axial skeleton is essentially a debulking procedure in that the tumour is virtually never removed with an adequate margin of normal tissue. However, it is a justifiable procedure if it is accepted that chemotherapy is more effective when the primary tumour has been largely removed. This concept applies in particular to Ewing's sarcoma where debulking, coupled with subsequent chemotherapy and radiotherapy, is now an established form of therapy.

## SUMMARY

The past 10 years have seen a considerable change of approach in the management of malignant bone tumours. The earlier attempts to replace tumours with allografts appear to have been disappointing and no comprehensive series of results has been published to date. The Van Nes procedure will undoubtedly continue to be used by its advocates, though these patients require continuous emotional and psychological support. They may well come ultimately to revision or amputation, a procedure which, if it has been performed at the start, might have been less traumatic to the individual. The sliding inlay grafts pioneered by Merle d'Aubigne and Djournay can be used at the knee, which is the site of most frequent tumour occurrence. Its success rate is high and the loss of joint movement is a relatively small price to pay for preservation of a limb. However, incorporation and consolidation of sliding allografts in the immunologically suppressed patient takes time and the procedure is only justifiable if cytotoxic therapy improves the long-term prognosis. Massive joint replacement is justifiable even in a patient whose prognosis is poor because of secondaries. The limb is preserved and the patient is rapidly restored to near normal function. Paradoxically, it remains to be shown that this mode of treatment is the best option in a patient whose prognosis is good because such patients may have a normal life-span. Risks are inherent in prosthetic replacement, namely infection, loosening and breakage. There is no doubt that, in reviewing the results over the years and as surgical methods and biomedical engineering techniques improve, so the complication rates decrease; nevertheless failures will occur. In the case of patients for whom the prognosis is good, there are now a substantial number who have had near normal function for 20 years or more. The debate on the best surgical method of management will undoubtedly continue.

## REFERENCES

Bradish CF, Kemp HBS, Scales JT & Wilson JN (1987) Distal femoral replacement—the long term results using the custom made Stanmore hinged total knee replacement. *Journal of Bone and Joint Surgery* **69**B: 276–284.
Burrows HJ (1968) Major prosthetic replacement of bone: lessons learnt in seventeen years. *Journal of Bone and Joint Surgery* **50**B: 225–226.

Burrows HJ, Wilson JN & Scales JT (1975) Excision of tumour of humerus and femur, with restoration by internal prostheses. *Journal of Bone and Joint Surgery* **57**B: 148–159.

Cade S (1955) Osteogenic sarcoma: a study based on 133 patients. *Journal of the Royal College of Surgeons of Edinburgh* **1**: 79–111.

Cannon SR & Dyson PHP (1987) The relationship of the location of open biopsy of malignant bone tumours to local recurrence after resection and prosthetic replacement. *Journal of Bone and Joint Surgery* **69B**: 492.

Enneking WF (1986) A system of staging musculoskeletal neoplasms. *Clinical Orthopaedics* **204**: 9–24.

Enneking WF & Dunham WK (1978) Resection and reconstruction of primary neoplasms involving the innominate bone. *Journal of Bone and Joint Surgery* **60**A: 731–746.

Enneking WF & Kagan A (1975) 'Skip' metastases in osteosarcoma. *Cancer* **36**: 2192–2205.

Enneking WF & Shirley PD (1977) Resection arthrodesis for malignant lesions about the knee. *Journal of Bone and Joint Surgery* **59**A: 223–236.

Enneking WF, Spanier SS & Goodman MA (1980) A system for the surgical staging of musculoskeletal sarcoma. *Clinical Orthopaedics* **153**: 106–120.

Lexer E (1925) Joint transplantations and arthroplasty. *Surgery, Gynaecology and Obstetrics* **40**: 782–809.

Link MP, Goorin A, Miser AW et al (1986) The effect of adjuvant chemotherapy on relapse-free survival in patients with osteosarcoma of the extremity. *New England Journal of Medicine* **314**: 1600–1606.

Luck JV Jr, Vernon Luck J & Schwinn CP (1979) Parosteal osteosarcoma: a treatment orientated study. *Clinical Orthopaedics* **153**: 92–105.

Mankin HJ, Fogelson FS, Thrasher AZ & Jaffer F (1976) Massive resection and allograft transplantation in the treatment of malignant bone tumours. *New England Journal of Medicine* **294**: 1247–1255.

Mankin HJ, Lange TH & Spanier SS (1982) The hazards of biopsy in patients with malignant primary bone and soft tissue tumours. *Journal of Bone and Joint Surgery* **64**A: 1121–1127.

Marcove RC & Rosen G (1979) Radical en bloc excision of Ewing's sarcoma. *Clinical Orthopaedics* **153**: 81–85.

Merle d'Aubigne R & Dejournay JP (1958) Diaphyso-epiphyseal reconstruction for bone tumours at the knee. *Journal of Bone and Joint Surgery* **40**B: 385–395.

Moore AT & Bohlmann HR (1943) Metal hip joint: a case report. *Journal of Bone and Joint Surgery* **25**: 688–692.

Parrish FF (1973) Allograft replacement of all or a part of the end of a long bone following excision of a tumour. *Journal of Bone and Joint Surgery* **55**A: 1–22.

Ross FGM (1964) Osteogenic sarcoma. *British Journal of Radiology* **37**: 259–276.

Ross AC, Wilson JN & Scales JT (1987) Endoprosthetic replacement of the proximal humerus. *Journal of Bone and Joint Surgery* **69B**: 656–661.

Scales JT (1983) Bone and joint replacement for the preservation of limbs. *British Journal of Hospital Medicine* **29**: 220–232.

Sneath RS, Scales JT & Wright KWJ (1984) *The Use of 'Growing' Endoprostheses to Induce or Accommodate Lengthening of the Limb in the Child or the Adult*, p 48. Abstracts of the 16th SICOT Congress, London.

Steel HH (1978) Partial or complete resection of the hemipelvis. *Journal of Bone and Joint Surgery* **60**A: 719–730.

Sweetnam RD (1975) Amputation in osteosarcoma. *Journal of Bone and Joint Surgery* **57**B: 265–269.

Sweetnam RD (1983) Limb preservation in the treatment of bone tumours. *Annals of the Royal College of Surgeons of England* **65**: 3–7.

Taylor WF, Irvings JC, Dahlin DC & Prichard DJ (1978a) Osteogenic sarcoma experience at the Mayo Clinic 1963–1974. In Terry WD and Windhorst D (eds) *Immunotherapy of Cancer: Present Status of Trials in Man*, pp 257–269. New York: Raven Press.

Taylor WF, Irvings JC, Dahlin DC, Edmonson JH & Prichard DJ (1978b) Trends and variability in survival from osteosarcoma. *Mayo Clinic Proceedings* **57**: 695–700.

Taylor WF, Irvings JC, Prichard DJ et al (1985) Trends and variability in survival among patients with osteosarcoma, a 7 year update. *Mayo Clinic Proceedings* **60**: 91–104.

Van der Heul RO & Von Ronnen JR (1967) Juxta cortical osteosarcoma. Diagnosis, differential diagnosis, treatment and analysis of eighty cases. *Journal of Bone and Joint Surgery* **49**A: 415–439.
Van Nes CP (1950) Rotation-plasty for congenital defects of the femur. *Journal of Bone and Joint Surgery* **32**B: 12–16.
Volkov M (1970) Allotransplantation of joints. *Journal of Bone and Joint Surgery* **52**B: 49–53.
Wilson JN & Scales JT (1987) *Recent Developments in Orthopaedic Surgery* [Noble J and Galasko CSB (eds)]. Manchester University Press (Festschrift to Sir Harry Platt).
Winkelmann W (1983) Die Umdrehplastik bei malignem proximalen Femurtumoren. *Zeitschrift für Orthopädie* **121**: 547–549.
Winkler K, Beron G, Kotz R et al (1986) Einflub des lokalchirurgischen vorgehens auf die inzidenz von metastasen nach neoadjuvanter chemotherapie des osteosarcoms. *Zeitschrift für Orthopädie* **124**: 22–29.

# 6

---

# Diagnosis and surgical management of benign bone tumours

FRANKLIN H. SIM
HERBERT S. SCHWARTZ
LESTER E. WOLD

Benign bone tumours continue to pose a myriad of diagnostic and thera-peutic problems. They represent 24% of the 8542 primary bone tumours in the Mayo Clinic files (Dahlin and Unni, 1986). Although relatively rare, they encompass a wide variety of lesions, many with differing biological capabilities. These tumours are classified according to the histological and cytological appearance of the cells as well as by the intercellular matrix the cells produce (Dahlin, 1978). The tumours arise from the major cellular constituents of normal bone and may be classified as chondrogenic, osteo-genic or fibrogenic. However, they also arise from vascular, neurogenic or fatty elements, and some are of unknown origin (Table 1). The conditions that simulate bone tumours must also be considered due to the confusion they cause in diagnosis and treatment. A team approach is essential to achieve optimum management.

## EVALUATION

The clinical manifestations of benign bone tumours are often of insidious onset, making early recognition difficult. Patients with benign bone tumours usually present with local symptoms of pain, swelling or a mass. Occasionally a pathological fracture heralds the onset of the problem. A careful, systematic approach to evaluation is essential. This includes a history and physical examination, pertinent laboratory tests and a plain X-ray, which remains the most specific diagnostic modality. Most of these tumours are detected on plain X-rays, obviating the need for further diag-nostic studies (McLeod et al, 1978; Levine, 1981; Lukens et al, 1982; Hudson et al, 1985). However, small lesions such as osteoid osteoma may require a bone scan and tomography for demonstration (Hudson et al, 1985). Computed tomographic (CT) scanning may also be useful in diag-nosis, particularly for lesions that are located centrally in sites difficult to evaluate radiographically. Careful integration of the clinical and radio-graphic information allows an accurate differential diagnosis. If a benign

---

Table 1. Benign bone tumours of childhood.

| Histological type | Tumours |
| --- | --- |
| Chondrogenic | Osteochondroma<br>Chondroma<br>Chondroblastoma<br>Chondromyxoid fibroma |
| Osteogenic | Osteoid osteoma<br>Osteoblastoma |
| Fibrogenic | Fibroma<br>Desmoplastic fibroma |
| Vascular | Haemangioma<br>Angioglomoid tumour |
| Lymphatic | Lymphangioma |
| Lipogenic | Lipoma |
| Neurogenic | Neurilemmoma |
| Unknown origin | Benign giant cell tumours |
| Conditions simulating primary bone tumours | Fibrous dysplasia<br>Aneurysmal bone cysts<br>Unicameral bone cysts<br>Histiocytosis X |

From Sim et al (1979), with permission.

lesion is suspected, a relatively simple staging work-up may be indicated prior to biopsy. Additional imaging studies may not be necessary; the patient can be observed, as in the case of a typical fibrous cortical defect, or undergo surgery, whichever is indicated. On the other hand, when the plain X-ray suggests a more aggressive lesion, such as a giant cell tumour, additional imaging and evaluation are helpful for accurate staging. CT scanning and magnetic resonance imaging (MRI) are the techniques of choice in determining the precise local extent of the lesion (Zimmer et al, 1984). This information may determine whether the patient should be treated with a joint-preserving curettage or with resection and joint reconstruction.

## BIOPSY

After the clinical and radiographic evaluation, an accurate histological diagnosis is determined by biopsy of the lesion. Reliable histological interpretation usually requires an open biopsy with careful removal of adequate and representative tissue. Despite the benign nature of the lesion, there are numerous pitfalls associated with the biopsy which may adversely affect the functional outcome (Mankin et al, 1982). Much care must be exercised in pre-biopsy planning, keeping in mind the definitive surgical procedural options. In this way, if resection is performed, the biopsy wound can be removed 'en bloc' with the tumour specimen. Transverse incisions on the extremity must be avoided because they make resection of the biopsy wound particularly difficult at the time of subsequent surgery. Great care must be exercised to avoid contamination of the surrounding soft tissues. Such contamination may result in soft-tissue recurrence, a not uncommon event with benign cartilage lesions or giant cell tumours. Meticulous haemostasis is essential to avoid a wound haematoma.

Analysis of frozen sections may give an immediate diagnosis or, if diagnosis must be deferred until the examination of permanent sections, ensure that adequate viable and representative tissue has been sampled. The definitive surgical procedure can be carried out immediately if a diagnosis is given by frozen section. However, many surgical pathologists prefer to wait for permanent sections before rendering a final diagnosis, necessitating a delay in treatment. Although there is no evidence that such a delay affects the final outcome, this should be kept to a minimum if an aggressive lesion is encountered.

## SURGICAL TREATMENT

### General considerations

The goals of treatment of a benign bone tumour are to control the osseous lesion and preserve or restore adequate function. Several treatment options are available. If the lesion is surgically accessible, a decision must be made regarding the extent of surgery necessary to balance the risk of recurrence against the functional deficit resulting from the surgery. Several factors have a bearing on the surgical philosophy used in the treatment of benign tumours: the anatomical site; the natural history of the lesion, including its potential for aggressive local behaviour; and its extent based upon the clinical and radiographic assessment. The problem is greater in children because the lesion, or its treatment, may have a profound influence on the growth potential of the affected bone.

The surgical techniques for the treatment of benign bone tumours vary widely and include biopsy; curettage, with or without bone grafts and cement; excision; resection; and amputation. Chemical or thermal adjuvants also have been advised. Radiation therapy is not recommended for benign tumours, except for aggressive lesions in surgically inaccessible sites, because of the potential for malignant transformation (see Chapter 1).

Recently the classification of the Musculoskeletal Tumor Society has standardized the definition of the surgical procedures (Enneking et al, 1980). The surgical procedures are described in terms of the surgical margins obtained in relation to the tumour and its surrounding reactive zone and in terms of the technique by which these margins are accomplished (Table 2). In an intralesional margin (Figure 1a), such as is achieved with curettage, the plane of dissection violates the pseudocapsule, whereas in a marginal margin (Figure 1b), which is achieved by excision of an osteoid osteoma for example, there is a narrow plane of dissection adjacent to the reactive pseudocapsule. A wide margin (Figure 1c) has a cuff of non-reactive normal tissue peripheral to all its margins, but the entire bone is not removed. A radical margin is obtained by removal of the entire bone.

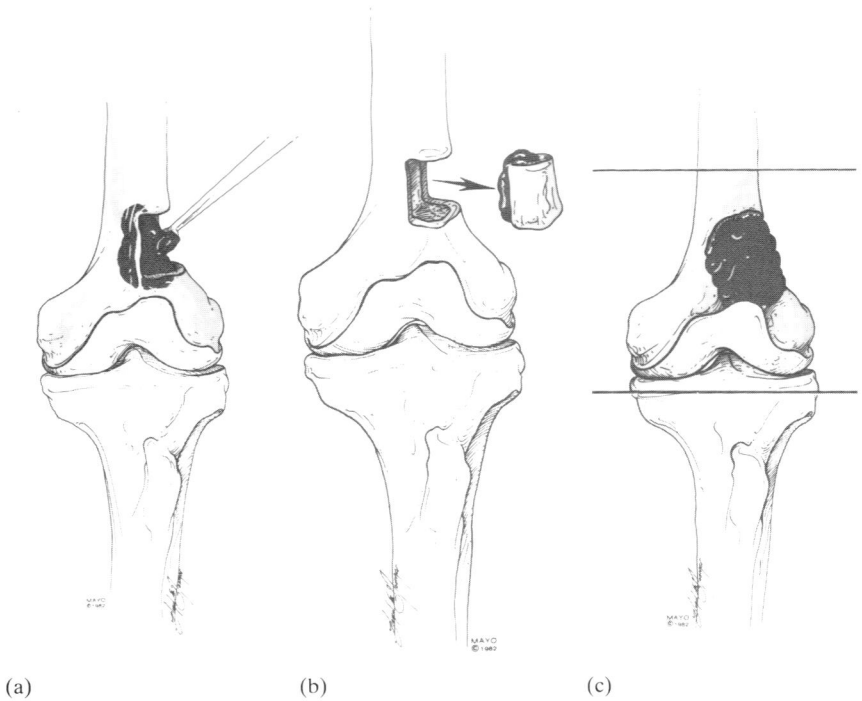

(a)                              (b)                              (c)

**Figure 1.** (a) Intralesional margin. (b) Marginal margin. (c) Wide margin. From Sim (1983), with permission.

**Table 2.** The grading system for surgical procedures in the treatment of bone tumours.

| Grade | Margin | Local treatment | Amputation |
|---|---|---|---|
| 1 | Intralesional | Curettage or debulking | Debulking or amputation |
| 2 | Marginal | Marginal excision | Marginal amputation |
| 3 | Wide | Wide local excision | Wide through-bone amputation |
| 4 | Radical | Radical local resection | Radical disarticulation |

From Enneking et al (1980), with permission. See also Chapter 4.

## Curettage

Most benign tumours may be managed with relatively conservative procedures such as curettage or marginal excision. If curettage is to be successful, adequate technique must be used, because if residual tumour remains,
recurrence is likely. The single most important factor in the success or failure
of curettage is adequate exposure. To achieve this it is necessary to make a
large cortical window and completely exteriorize the tumour cavity. This
may require removal of one-half of the circumference of the end of the bone
(Figure 2). Failure to exteriorize and visualize completely all aspects of the
tumour cavity almost inevitably leads to recurrence of the tumour (Figure
3). We prefer to remove the window in the bone with an osteotome to

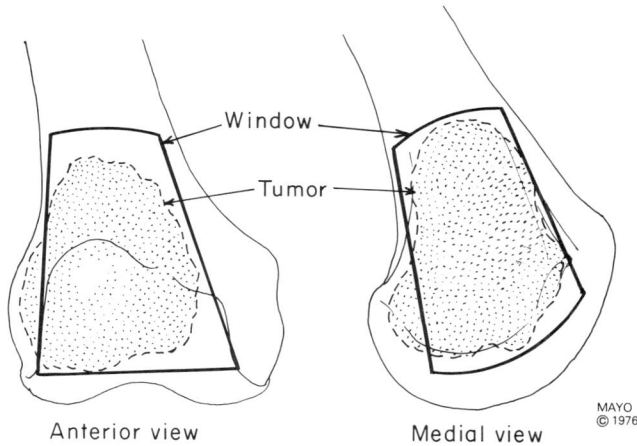

**Figure 2.** Wide exteriorization of lesion of distal femur, demonstrating an adequate excision by
curettage. From Sim (1983), with permission.

connect multiple drill holes rather than with a saw, as the oscillation of the
saw has the potential to spray tumour cells into the surrounding tissue. After
exteriorization, the tumour tissue must be thoroughly excised with a sharp
curette. Care must be taken to avoid contamination of the surrounding soft
tissues, and large spoon curettes are helpful in the initial bulk removal.
Conrad et al (1985) recently advocated suction curettage to help avoid
soft-tissue contamination.

After adequate curettage, a motorized burr is used to extend the margin
into the cortical bone (Figure 4). The cavity is cleansed with pulsatile lavage
with a Waterpik. When all visible tumour has been removed, the tumour
cavity may be cauterized by chemical or thermal agents. We have preferred
local adjuvant treatment with phenol to extend the margin (Figure 3). If this
is used, the soft tissues are packed with Vaseline gauze and moist sponges
and the curetted tumour cavity is filled with phenol for 30–45 seconds. The
phenol, which coagulates protein, is effective in reaching the crevices in the

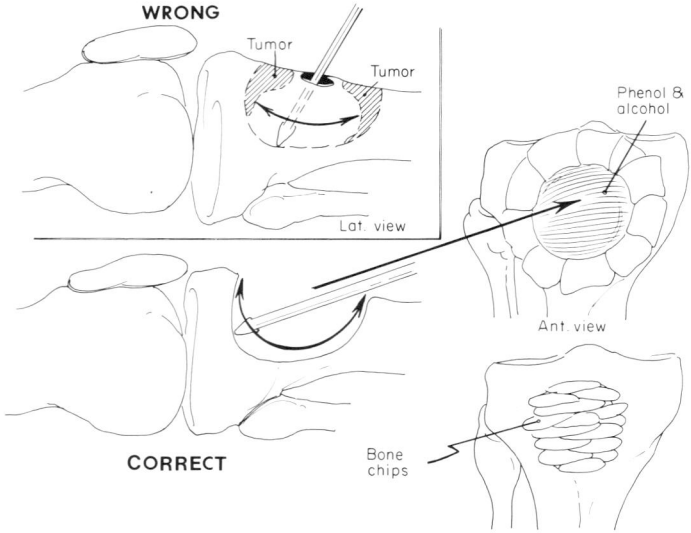

**Figure 3.** Correct and incorrect technique of curettage. From Sim (1983), with permission.

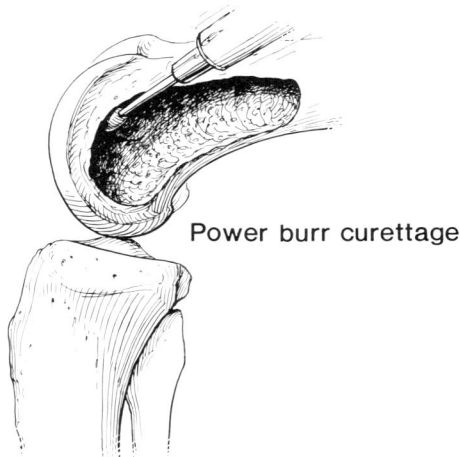

Power burr curettage

**Figure 4.** Motorized burr being used to extend margins of excision into normal bone. Courtesy of Dr Frank J. Frassica.

cortical bone which the tumour has permeated. The phenol is removed and the cavity is rinsed with 95% alcohol. The curetted cavity is then lavaged vigorously with large amounts of isotonic saline. Whether such cauterization is of benefit in decreasing local recurrence has not been definitely established. Johnston (1985) popularized hydrogen peroxide as a chemical adjuvant. Cryosurgery has been used by others (Marcove et al, 1978; Jacobs and Clemency, 1983; Malawer and Zielinski, 1983); however, the high incidence of complications, particularly pathological fractures, has reduced the popularity of this technique.

After tumour excision, it is necessary to restore the integrity of the bone with bone grafts (Figure 5). It is important to fill the cavity completely with abundant bone. Until recently, autologous or allograft bone grafts were used, but more recently methylmethacrylate has proved useful after extensive curettage for some aggressive tumours (Figure 6) (Willert and Enderle,

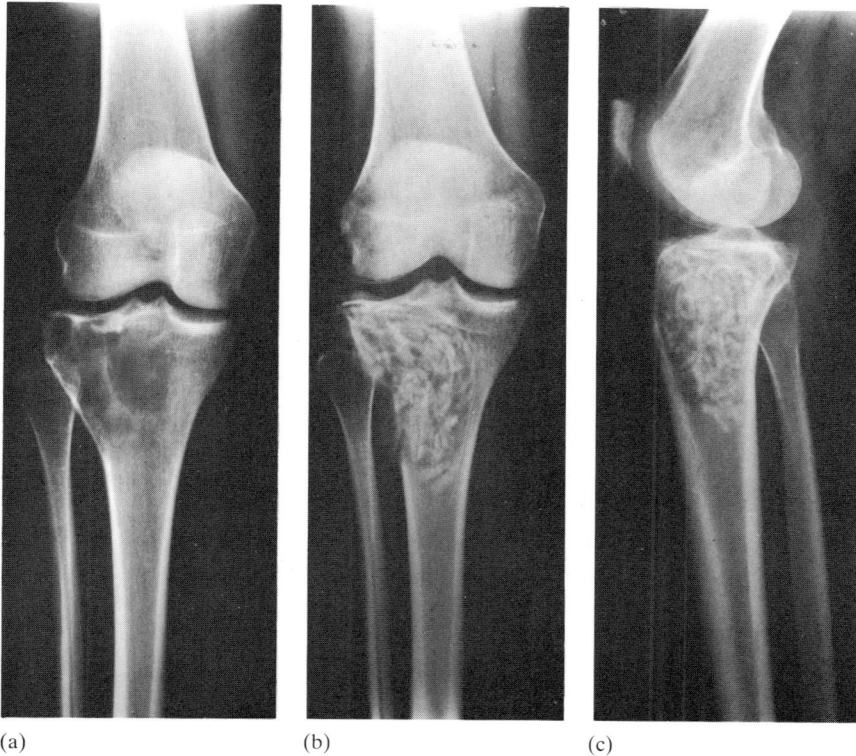

(a)  (b)  (c)

**Figure 5.** (a) Anteroposterior view of proximal tibia showing giant cell tumour. Lesion is eccentrically located and is thinning the cortex and extending to subarticular region. (b) Anteroposterior and (c) lateral view after wide exteriorization of lesion. The lesion has been curetted and cavity chemically cauterized with phenol and alcohol. From Sim et al (1983), with permission.

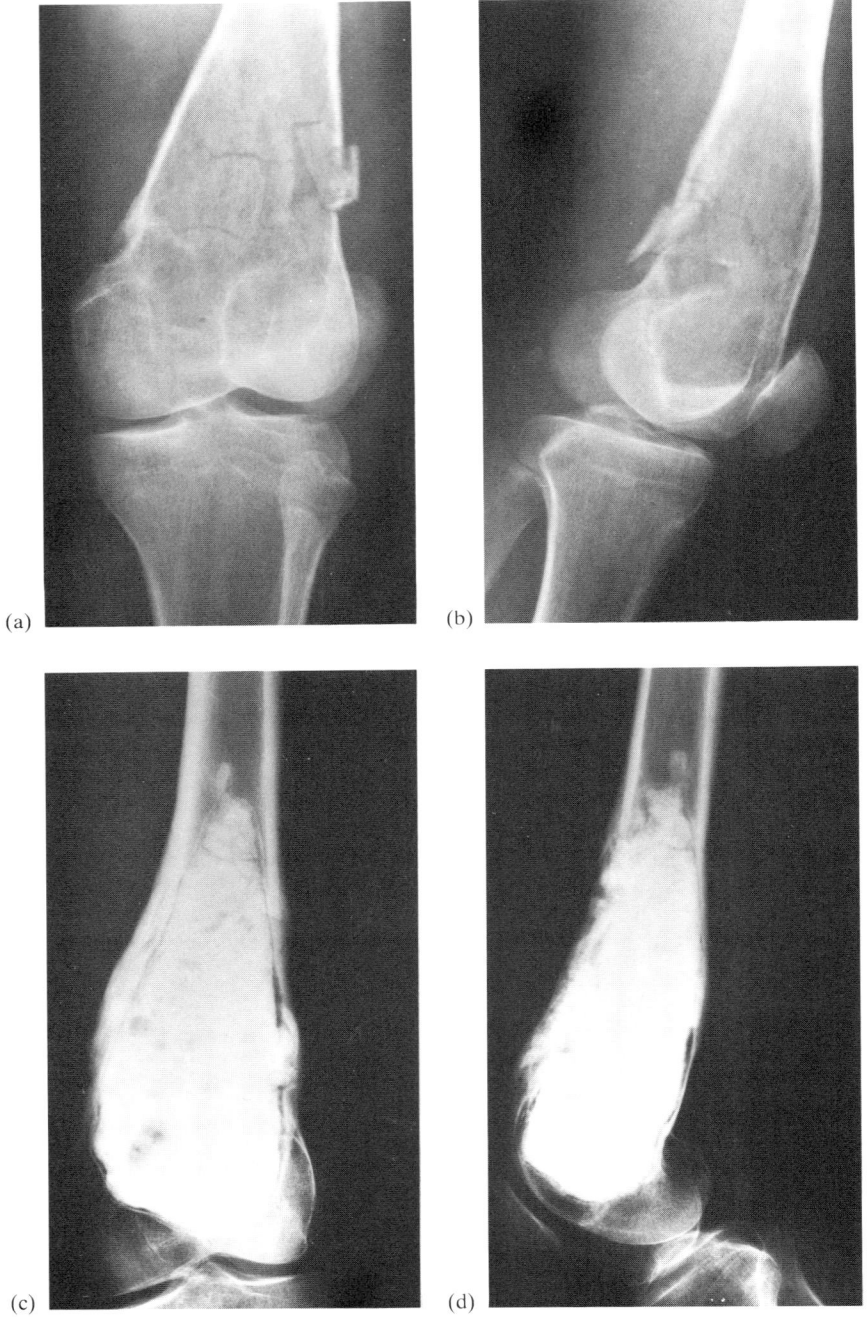

**Figure 6.** (a) Anteroposterior and (b) lateral views of left distal femur showing large giant cell tumour with pathological fracture. (c) Anteroposterior and (d) lateral views 4 years after curettage and cementation.

1983; Persson et al, 1984; Conrad et al, 1985; Johnston, 1985). If bone grafting is carried out, it is extremely important that implantation of tumour at the bone graft donor site is avoided. Separate gloves, gowns, drapes and instruments should be used to minimize the possibility of implantation.

Although it is recognized that autografts are superior to allografts in skeletal reconstruction, allograft chips have advantages in avoiding donor site morbidity (Wilson, 1951). Many of the cavities are large and it is difficult to obtain sufficient autologous bone to fill them completely. However, if allograft bone is available from a limited bone bank using femoral heads, abundant grafts may be used to fill the defects. Our experience with this technique has been successful with healing and blending of the allograft bone with the host bone. One can enhance the incorporation with the addition of host autologous bone. When this technique is used, we usually use a 3 : 1 ratio of allograft to autologous bone.

## Resection

Aggressive or recurrent benign lesions, particularly giant cell tumours that erode through the cortex into the soft tissues or are associated with a pathological fracture, often require 'en bloc' resection with a wide margin to achieve local control (McDonald et al, 1986). However, the major objection to this procedure, when the tumour involves an essential bone or neighbouring joint, is the need for major reconstruction and the subsequent functional loss. Reconstruction after resection presents a complex surgical problem that can be managed by several techniques, depending on the location of the tumour and the functional expectations of the patient (Sim et al, 1987a). The reconstructive techniques include custom prosthetic replacement (Figure 7), osteochondral allograft (Figure 8) (Parrish, 1973; Mankin et al, 1976) and resection arthrodesis (Figure 9) (Marcove, 1980).

In the management of benign tumours it is important to appreciate that the patient will survive his disease after resection. Therefore, the durability and longevity of the reconstructive procedure are of paramount importance. Prosthetic replacement is best reserved for older patients with fewer functional demands, because of the concern for late loosening of the implant. Recent reports have demonstrated the value of osteochondral allografts in joint reconstruction with maintenance of motion and function after resection of benign tumours of the knee, shoulder and wrist (Czitrom et al, 1986). However, if the patient is young and active and expects to place heavy demands on the reconstruction, then a resection arthrodesis is a better choice than either prosthetic or allograft arthroplasty.

## Treatment: considerations related to specific tumours

In the management of patients with benign bone tumours, the choice among the various treatment options discussed will vary with the histological type and biological potential of the tumour, as well as its surgical stage. Moreover, clinical, social and economic factors, as well as the patient's own wishes and expectations, are important to consider. While not comprehen-

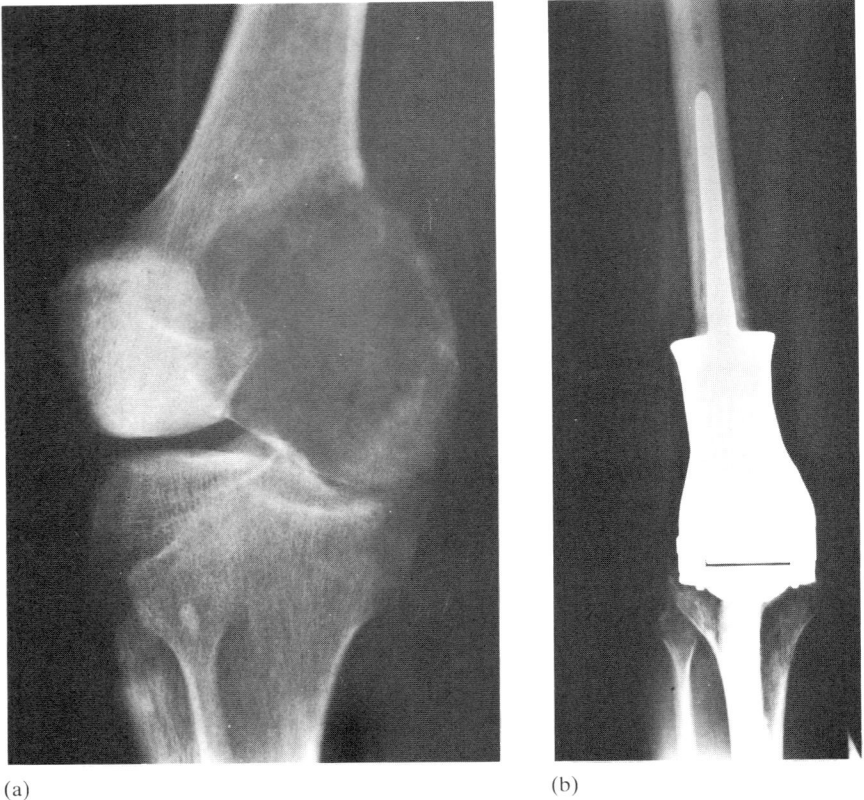

(a)                                                                          (b)

**Figure 7.** (a) An extensive giant cell tumour of distal part of femur with extensive destruction of entire medial femoral condyle. The articular surface was entirely involved and was judged not to be salvageable. (b) Patient was treated with primary wide resection and reconstruction with custom-made prosthesis. From McDonald et al (1986), with permission.

sive, this section outlines some of the major treatment methods for the more frequently encountered benign tumours and lesions simulating tumours.

## Giant cell tumours

These are benign, locally aggressive lesions which acount for approximately 20% of benign tumours (Dahlin and Unni, 1986). A slight predilection for females has been noted. Typically they occur in patients in their third and fourth decades of life, with 85% of the patients aged more than 20 years. Giant cell tumours are usually found in the epiphyseal region of long bones, extending up to the articular surface. They are most commonly located in the region of the distal femur or proximal tibia, which accounts for one-half of the lesions, followed by the distal radius, proximal humerus and sacrum (Larsson et al, 1975).

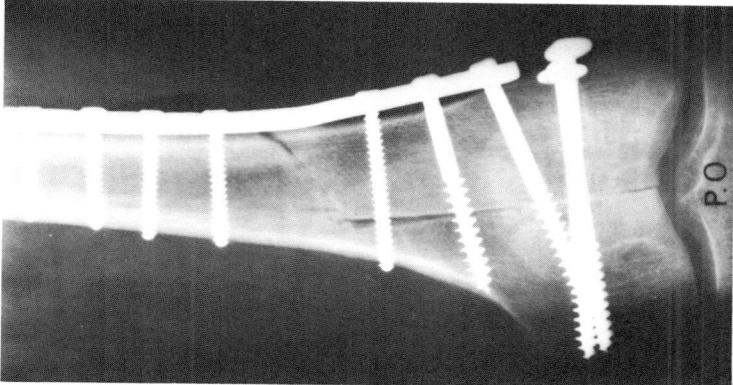

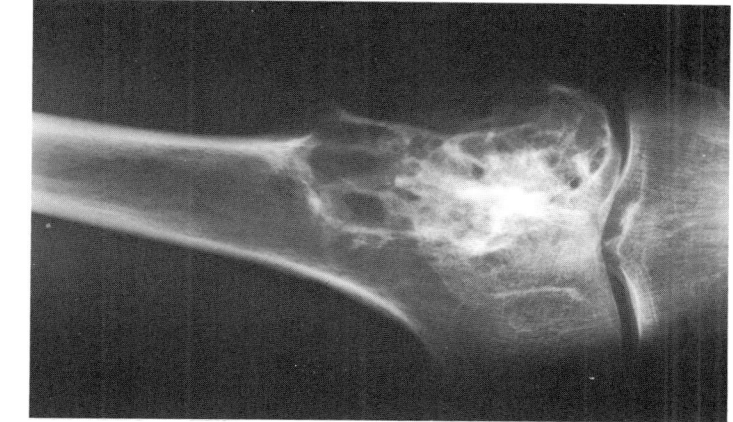

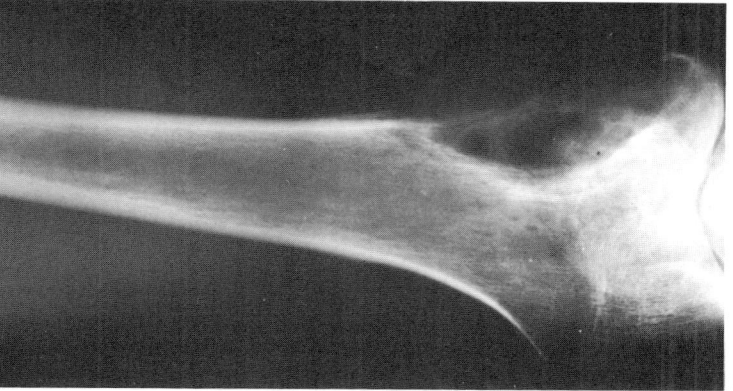

**Figure 8.** (a) Preoperative radiograph of giant cell tumour in distal part of femur. Patient was treated with curettage and bone grafting. (b) Recurrence of lesion with pronounced cortical lysis and involvement of subchondral bone. (c) Because of almost complete destruction of medial condyle, patient was treated with excision and allograft replacement of medial femoral condyle. P.O. = postoperative. From McDonald et al (1986), with permission.

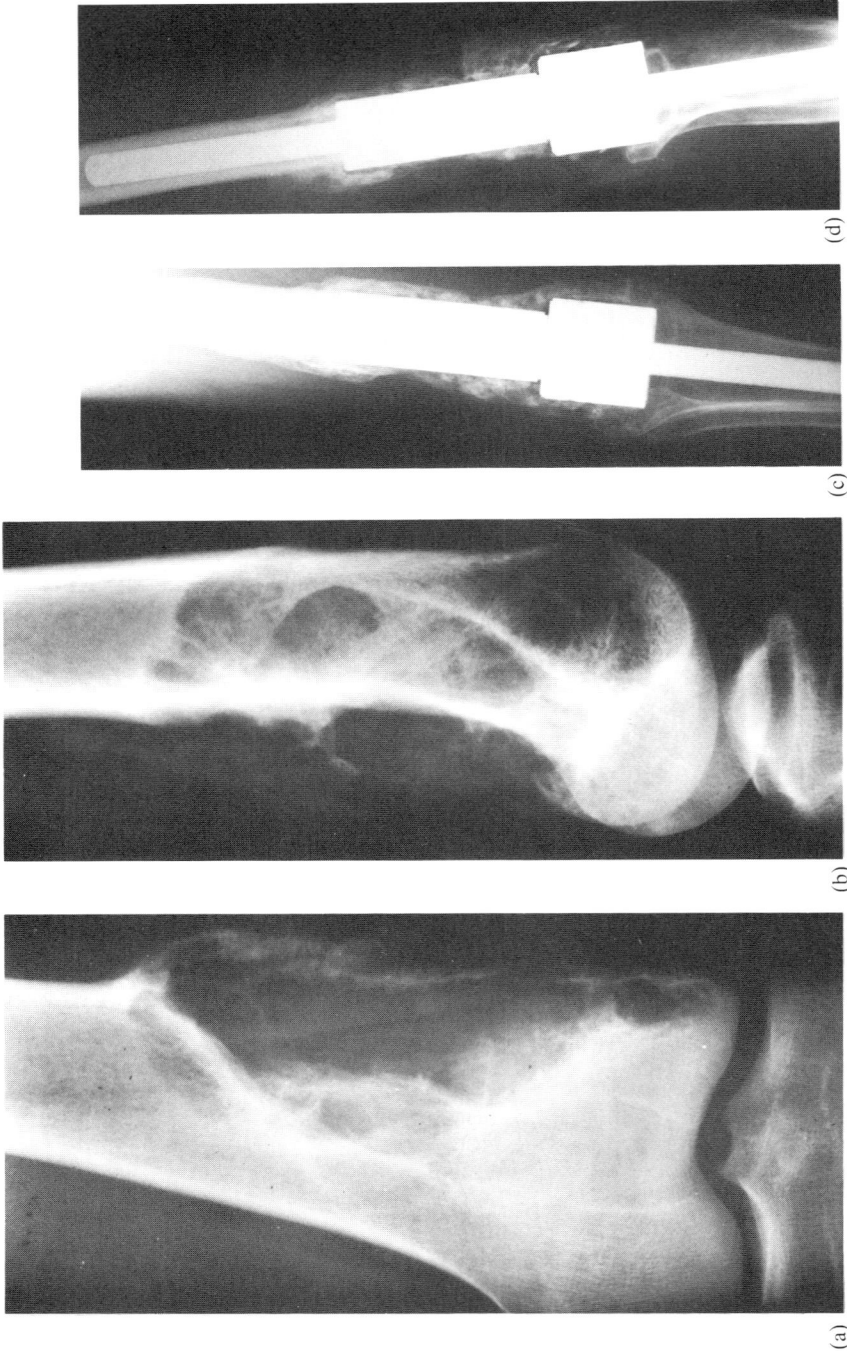

**Figure 9.** (a) Anteroposterior and (b) lateral views of desmoplastic fibroma of distal femur. (c) Anteroposterior and (d) lateral views of distal femur 10 months after resection and reconstruction with titanium prosthetic arthrodesis. Figures (a) and (b) from Sim et al (1984), with permission. (c) and (d) from Sim et al (1987b), with permission.

Radiographically the lesions appear to be very aggressive (Figure 10) (Campanacci et al, 1975). When located at the end of a long bone, they have characteristic features, appearing lytic and centrally located and extending to the subarticular region. Although they may be marginated, more commonly they fade gradually into the surrounding normal bone. As the lesion enlarges, it loses its eccentricity and involves the entire end of the bone. The tumour frequently breaks through the cortex of the bone and extends into the soft tissues. In the spine, they appear as lytic lesions centred in the vertebral body.

Histologically the tumour is composed of proliferating round to oval mononuclear cells which contain an oval-shaped nucleus. Mitotic figures are common. Multinucleated giant cells lie uniformly scattered in the sea of mononuclear cells (Figure 11). The multinucleated cells have nuclei that are similar to the nuclei of the stromal cells. Histological grading of giant cell tumours is controversial. Although Jaffe et al (1940) described three grades of benign giant cell tumours based on the amount of cellular atypia and the number of mitotic figures, attempts to predict clinical behaviour on the basis of histological grading have not been uniformly successful. We have not graded giant cell tumours histologically because of the unreliability of grading systems and the inability to predict tumour behaviour (Dahlin, 1985). The concept of malignant giant cell tumour has further confused the issue. Malignant giant cell tumours are thought to be a separate clinical entity which consists of a sarcoma that is either juxtaposed to zones of typical benign giant cell tumours, or occurs at a site of previously documented benign giant cell tumour (Dahlin and Unni, 1986). Most commonly, sarcoma occurs after treatment of a benign giant cell tumour with radiation therapy. The incidence of malignant tumour ranges from 1 to 15% (McGrath, 1972; Campanacci et al, 1975; Sanerkin, 1980; Duncan et al, 1983). Radiation therapy has been strongly implicated in the malignant conversion of giant cell tumours (Dahlin, 1985).

A further source of confusion is the rare occurrence of metastasis from histologically benign giant cell tumours (Dahlin et al, 1970; Goldenberg et al, 1970; Sung et al, 1982). The usual site of metastasis is the lungs, and the histological appearance of the metastatic lesion is indistinguishable from that of the primary lesion. In the Mayo Clinic series of 411 giant cell tumours, eight developed benign-looking metastases (Rock et al, 1984). Multicentric giant cell tumours rarely occur. Eighteen cases have been reported in the literature, and no apparent clinical or histological differences have been noted between these and the solitary lesions (Sim et al, 1977a; Averill et al, 1980; Peimer et al, 1980).

Treatment of benign giant cell tumour has been one of the more controversial areas in the management of bone tumours. In most lesions the main question is whether to attempt curettage with bone grafts or cement or to carry out a complete resection. Total removal by resection of the tumour with a surrounding margin of normal uninvolved tissue provides the best chance for cure (Dahlin, 1985). However, because most giant cell tumours occur at the end of an essential bone involving a major joint, such as the knee, wrist or shoulder, the resection requires a major reconstructive procedure with

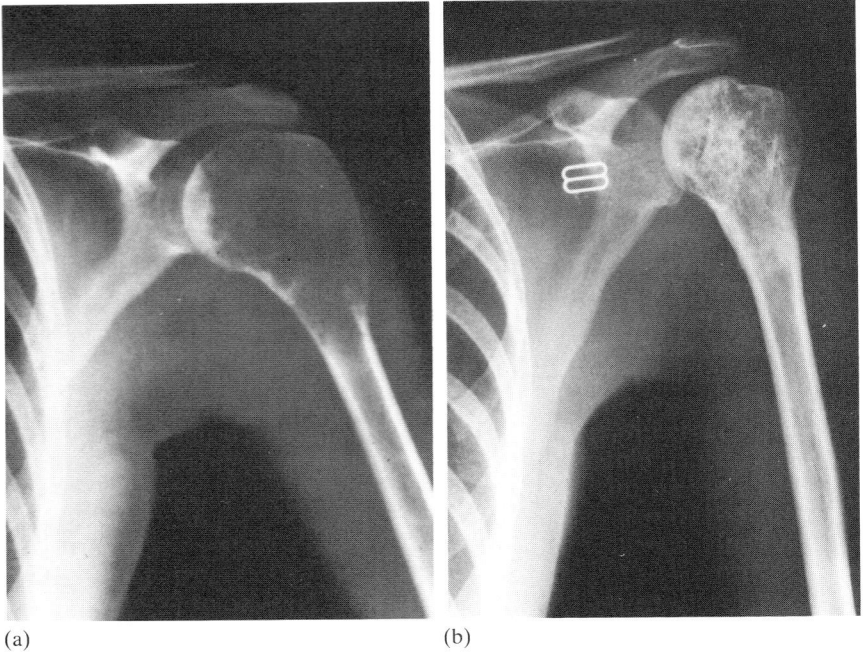

(a)                                                            (b)

**Figure 10.** (a) Anteroposterior x-ray of left proximal humerus showing extensive destruction from giant cell tumour in a 16-year-old boy. (b) There is no evidence of recurrence 4½ years after radical exteriorization, curettage and bone grafting. From Sim et al (1979), with permission.

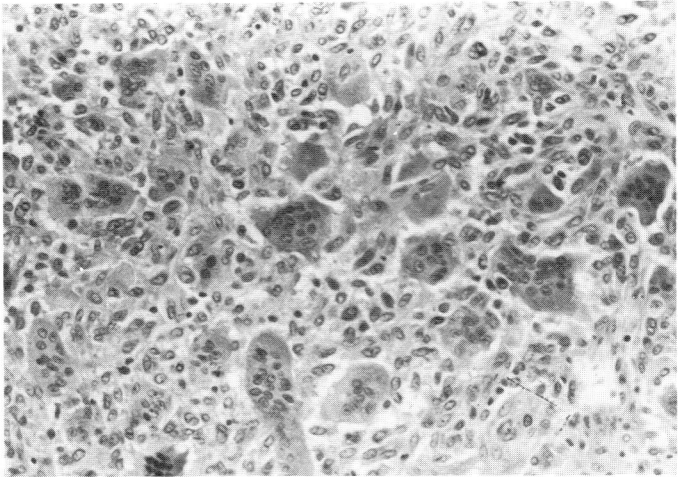

**Figure 11.** Giant cell tumour of bone shows uniform admixture of multinucleated giant cells lying in mononuclear cell stroma. Nuclear cytological features of mononuclear and multi-nucleated giant cells are similar (stained with haematoxylin and eosin).

resulting functional deficit (Figures 7 and 8). On the other hand, curettage with preservation of the joint offers the best functional restoration (Figures 5 and 10). In general, curettage is associated with a recurrence rate approaching 50% (Campanacci et al, 1975; Marsh et al, 1975; Willert and Enderle, 1983; Persson et al, 1984; Conrad et al, 1985; Johnston, 1985; Campanacci et al, 1986; Sim et al, 1987a). In long bones the recurrence rate decreases to 25%. A tumour selected for curettage should be relatively small, radiologically quiescent and entirely intraosseous. The only significant risk encountered from curettage in these selected patients is the risk of recurrence. The risk of metastasis of residual or recurrent tumour and the risk of malignant transformation are essentially negligible and should be ignored as a consideration in the determination of the initial surgical procedure.

On the other hand, if the lesion is large, radiographically aggressive in appearance, has broken through the cortex or articular cartilage, or a pathological fracture is present, then complete resection is indicated. However, because most benign giant cell tumours are somewhere between a small, entirely intraosseous lesion and a large lesion with cortical destruction, treatment requires considerable judgement on the part of the surgeon. The patient's own wishes are an important factor in planning treatment. Some patients are willing to accept a risk of recurrence if there is a chance of avoiding sacrifice of a major joint. On the other hand, other patients prefer an initial resection despite the functional loss in order to avoid the prospects of recurrence.

Recently bone cement has been used in aggressive giant cell tumours after curettage (Figure 6). Originally the technique was used when insufficient bone graft was available, or in lesions for which resection and reconstruction was the only choice. The early results were encouraging and subsequently a number of workers began using methylmethacrylate routinely in giant cell tumours (Vidal et al, 1969; Wouters, 1974; Mándi and Kiss, 1976; Persson and Wouters, 1976; Baddeley and Cullen, 1979; Camargo and Camargo, 1985; Conrad et al, 1985). This technique has several advantages. First, and probably most important, a more aggressive and extensive curettage can be carried out to remove the tumour more effectively without the usual concern for subsequent fracture or collapse of the articular surface. Second, the immobilization time is minimal and function is more quickly resumed. Third, the radiological aspects of tumour recurrence are quickly revealed because the recurrence is adjacent to the cement and involves previously normal bone. Fourth, should there be a recurrence, the original therapeutic options are still available. If the original considerations still apply, one has the option of a conservative procedure, such as curettage and further cementation, or a resection and subsequent reconstruction can be carried out.

Besides the role of cementation in filling the defect and supporting the subchondral bone, an adjuvant effect of the methylmethacrylate on residual tumour has been postulated (Willert and Enderle, 1983; Persson et al, 1984; Conrad et al, 1985). Some have felt that the methylmethacrylate may extend the curettage and kill any residual tumour left in the bone. Possible mechanisms are microvascular disruption, mechanical trauma, chemical toxicity or thermal injury. The most widely accepted explanation is that tumour necrosis after cementation is attributable to thermal injury from the heat of polymerization.

From a clinical standpoint, a decreased recurrence rate has been noted in patients treated by curettage and cementation compared with treatment by curettage and bone grafting (Willert and Enderle, 1983; Persson et al, 1984; Camargo and Camargo, 1985; Taminiau and Wouters, 1985). Although the postulated role of methylmethacrylate remains controversial, most feel that the reason for the decreased recurrence rate is not the cement itself, but the ability to do a better job of excising the tumour. When the surgeon elects to use cement, he can be more aggressive in curettage and excision; thus, the more extensive surgical technique appears to be the key that has resulted in a reduced rate of local recurrence.

From the technical standpoint, after wide exteriorization, aggressive curettage, use of a high-speed burr and Waterpik irrigation, methylmethacrylate is placed into the bony cavity, ensuring that the cement fills every recess. The mechanical stability of the affected area may be improved by additional internal fixation when necessary, such as with a condylar plate. As the cement becomes more firm, pressurization by hand ensures filling of all of the cavity. It is also important to ensure cement containment, keeping the cement out of the soft tissue, tendons and ligaments.

Practically there appears to be some benefit to using methylmethacrylate to replace subchondral cancellous bone. Theoretically there are specific concerns (Ewald et al, 1982; Manley et al, 1982; Radin et al, 1982; Wilkins et al, 1985). Several studies have indicated that methylmethacrylate is an imperfect substitute for subchondral cancellous bone. The cement provides an unhealthy environment for the overlying cartilage by altering the biomechanical transmission of forces, and may lead to articular cartilage degeneration. Over the short term the joint seems to hold up quite well, but there is concern as to how long the joint can tolerate the abnormal biomechanical situation. Willert (1985) reported that 38% of the patients in his series had symptoms of osteoarthritis. Because of the biomechanical situation, potential tissue reaction and the young age involved, several investigators recommend temporary cementation with removal of the cement 2 years later, replacing it with autogenous bone grafts (Willert and Enderle, 1983; Conrad et al, 1985; Taminiau and Wouters, 1985).

Even though the cementation technique may be useful in the management of these difficult problems, it is best to reserve it for selected cases. Our preference is to carry out curettage and bone grafting for less extensive lesions, using resection and reconstruction for the very aggressive lesion with associated soft-tissue extension, loss of articular cartilage or pathological fracture (Dahlin, 1985). Curettage and cementation is used for lesions between these two ends of the spectrum. However, depending on the wishes of the patient, it may be reasonable to try curettage and cementation even in more extensive lesions, when resection and reconstruction is the only other choice. Although the incidence of recurrence is higher in this type of lesion, no bridges have been burned, and one can ultimately resect and reconstruct if necessary.

## Osteoid osteoma

Osteoid osteoma is a well-recognized, peculiar, small, benign bone tumour that accounts for 11% of benign bone tumours (Figure 12) (Dahlin and Unni, 1986). The lesion may occur in any age group, but 90% occur between the ages of 5 and 20 years. Males are more frequently affected than females. Although it may occur in any bone, including unusual locations such as the carpal bones, it most frequently occurs in the femur or tibia. Clinical features are distinctive: there are complaints of unremitting and gradually increasing pain. Night pain is particularly prominent. Referred pain to remote sites and associated muscle atrophy often suggest a neurological cause for the pain (Sim et al, 1977b). Moreover, the lesion may mimic idiopathic scoliosis, suggesting osteoid osteoma when the scoliosis worsens in the supine position. Relief by low-dose aspirin is dramatic. Moreover, prostaglandin inhibitors have also been noted to be effective, and increased concentrations of prostaglandins have been documented around the lesion.

When the clinical history suggests the possibility of an osteoid osteoma, plain X-rays usually confirm the presence of a lesion which is usually less than 1 cm in diameter. When the X-ray is equivocal, tomograms may show the lesion more clearly (Figure 12b); the lesion demonstrates intense uptake on the technetium bone scan. Radiologically, a small radiolucent nidus, often with a central area of calcification surrounded by reactive sclerotic bone, is seen when the cortex is involved. A less sclerotic reaction is seen when lesions are located in the cancellous portion of the bone. For instance, a lesion localized in the intracapsular portion of the femoral head and neck is noteworthy by its lack of surrounding sclerosis. A tumour located in the end of the bone may cause significant regional osteoporosis and synovitis in the neighbouring joint. In the spine the lesion is usually in the neural arch at the apex of the concave side of the curve.

Pathologically, the nidus is grossly somewhat more red than the surrounding cortical bone, from which it is easily distinguished. It is composed of a tightly woven mass of osteoid trabeculae rimmed by osteoblasts (Figure 13). Loose fibrovascular connective tissue is seen between the bony trabeculae. The lesional tissue may be densely sclerotic at times.

Treatment of an osteoid osteoma is by surgical excision. Exact identification of the lesion is important, and this usually means that it must be excised under X-ray control. Intraoperative bone scanning has been helpful in identifying the elusive nidus. A well-planned operative approach is essential. Proper identification of the nidus must be made before and after en bloc removal, with the use of X-rays of the excised blocks of bone and with serial blocks of the specimen by the pathologist. The use of tetracycline labelling also has been useful as a method for identifying the nidus under ultraviolet light. Depending on the size of the defect after excision, bone grafting may be necessary. In instances in which the tumour is curetted and not completely excised, the patient will continue to have pain and will probably require a second surgical procedure (Marsh et al, 1975). This

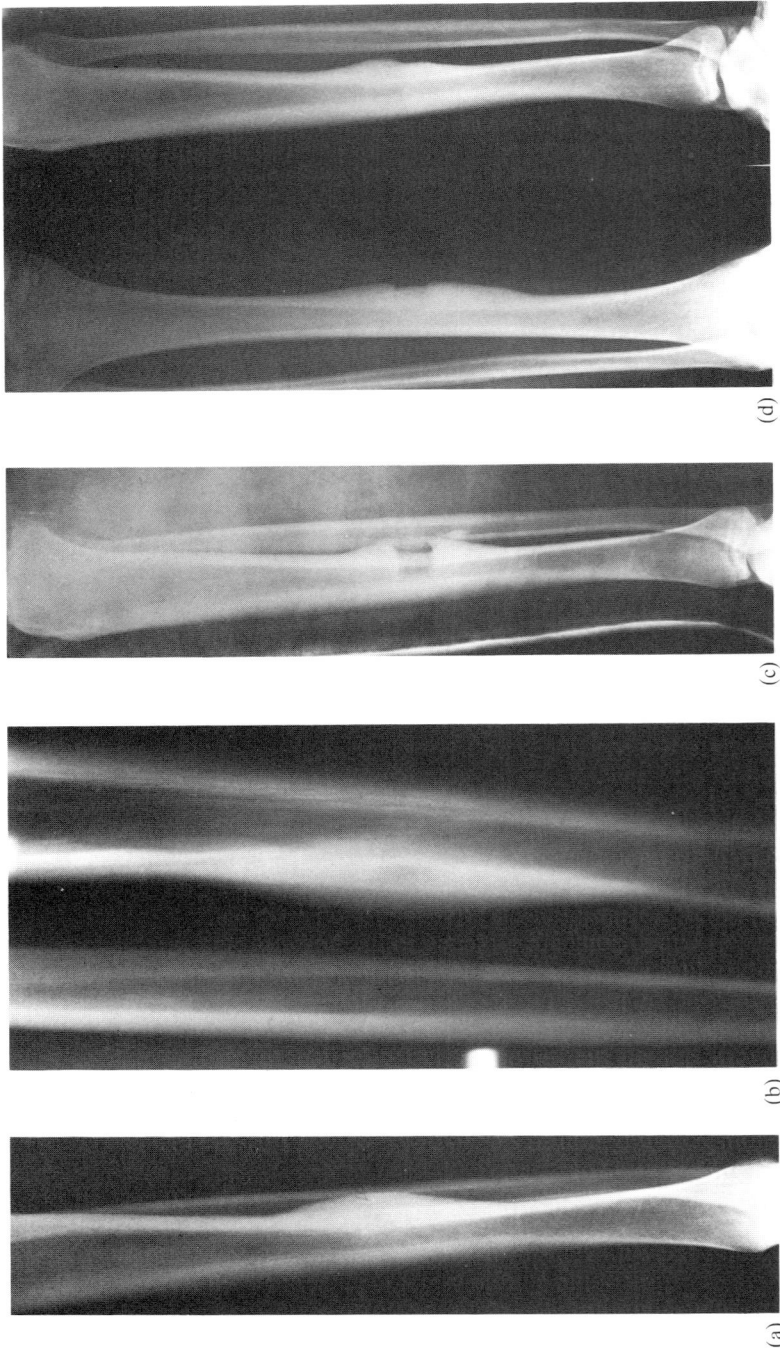

**Figure 12.** (a) Lateral view of right tibia showing typical osteoid osteoma with lucent central nidus and surrounding active cortical sclerosis. (b) Anteroposterior tomogram localizing radiolucent nidus. (c) Lateral view of tibia after excision of lesion. (d) Anteroposterior and lateral views of tibia demonstrating healing of bone grafts. From Sim et al (1983), with permission.

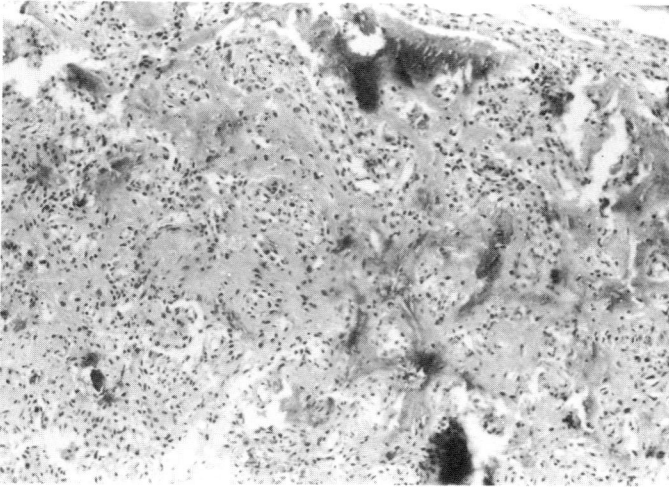

**Figure 13.** Osteoid osteoma shows abundant irregular osteoid within the nidus. Between the osteoid the lesional tissue is relatively hypocellular and cytologically lacks pleomorphism or anaplastic features (stained with haematoxylin and eosin).

emphasizes the importance of adequate excision of the lesion. Curettage is to be discouraged because of the risk of leaving the nidus behind and the difficulty in making a pathological diagnosis of the specimen.

*Benign osteoblastoma*

This is a relatively rare tumour that tends to occur in young people, with 70% found in individuals aged less than 20 years (Dahlin and Unni, 1986). It occurs more commonly in males than in females. Although histologically the lesion appears similar to osteoid osteoma, it is a progressively growing lesion of larger size. Although any bone may be involved, these lesions have a predilection for the vertebral column. In addition, the pain pattern is generally not that associated with osteoid osteoma. Scoliosis and muscle spasm, as well as neurological deficits, are often seen in lesions located in the spine (Marsh et al, 1975).

Pathologically, these lesions are situated in cancellous bone and appear fairly well circumscribed. The microscopic appearance is variable. Trabeculae of osteoid lie within a loose fibrovascular connective tissue and generally show prominent osteoblastic rimming of the trabeculae (Figure 14). Numerous giant cells may be present. At times, worrying osteoblastic activity with mitotic figures may be seen. There may also be areas that are histologically similar to aneurysmal bone cysts.

The X-ray appearance is quite varied and is often not distinctive. When localized to a long bone, the lesions are usually in the diaphyseal area. A central rarified area may be present and may reach a large size. Surrounding

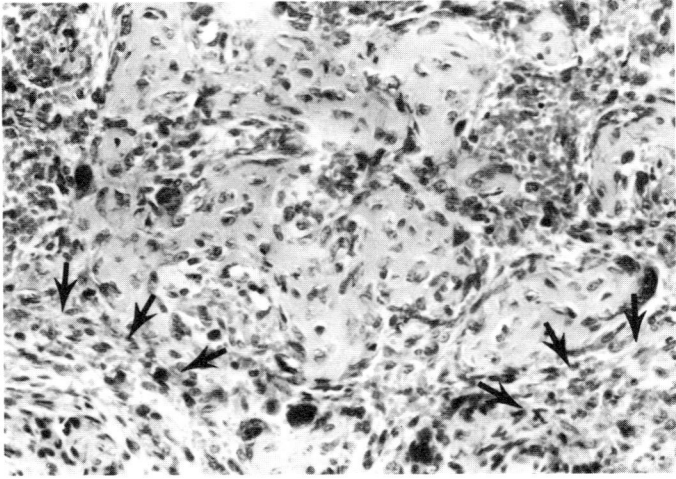

**Figure 14.** As with osteoid osteoma, osteoblastomas display abundant irregular osteoid. Prominent osteoblastic rimming of bone may be apparent and stroma is loose and highly vascular ( ↑ ) (stained with haematoxylin and eosin).

sclerotic bone may be apparent. Spine lesions are usually expansile and may be mineralized.

The benign nature of osteoblastoma necessitates a conservative surgical approach. Usually adequate curettage and bone grafting achieve effective local control, or the lesion may be amenable to simple excision and grafting. The removal does not usually require a wide margin of intact bone around the lesion. If the lesion involves the spine, complete removal by local excision or curettage is carried out with preservation of the spinal cord and emerging nerve roots. Bone grafting to stabilize the vertebral column is often necessary.

*Osteochondroma*

Osteochondroma is the most common benign lesion of bone and accounts for 40% of all benign tumours (Dahlin and Unni, 1986). The true incidence is probably higher because occult asymptomatic lesions are frequently encountered radiographically. The lesion is more common in males and approximately 60% of patients are aged less than 20 years when the lesion is excised. The tumour usually develops in the metaphyseal region of long bones and enlarges by progressive endochondral ossification of a growing cartilage cap. The cap is attached to a bony stalk (pedunculated) or to a broad base (sessile). The osteocartilaginous exostosis is frequently multiple and may be familial. When multiple, there may be a dysplastic appearance of the involved bone, but each tumour has the same characteristics as a solitary lesion. Patients with multiple lesions have a higher risk of sarcomatous change (10% compared with 1% of solitary lesions) (Dahlin and Unni, 1986).

On radiological examination the bony stalk is seen projecting from the surface of the bone, usually away from the adjacent joint (Figure 15a). The cortical bone of the tumour is continuous with that of the underlying bone, as is the medullary cavity. Calcification is frequently seen in the cartilage cap. Grossly, most osteochondromas have a smooth cartilage cap, about 2–3 mm thick (Figure 15b). If the cap is irregular, or greater than 2 cm, careful histological examination is necessary to rule out the possibility of sarcomatous change. Microscopically the cartilage cap is characterized by mature chondrocytes arranged in a single-file pattern that mimics the appearance of normal epiphyseal cartilage. There is an associated region of endochondral ossification with fatty or haematopoietic marrow between the trabeculae.

Treatment of osteochondromas is individualized depending on the clinical circumstances (Jaffe, 1943; Harsha, 1954; Morton, 1964a; Solomon, 1964). Most osteochondromas, either solitary or multiple, are simply observed. Removal is indicated if the lesion is large enough to cause symptoms from mechanical irritation or if it is growing rapidly. At times, removal may be indicated for cosmetic reasons. When excision is carried out, the lesion must be removed at the base of the exostosis in order to remove the entire cartilage cap. Bone grafting is used in large osteochondromas if the bone is weakened when the lesion is removed. Because patients with multiple osteochondromas have a higher chance of developing sarcomatous change, they require careful follow-up.

*Chondroma*

Chondromas account for approximately 10% of all benign tumours (Dahlin and Unni, 1986). These lesions are found at any age and within virtually any bone. When located within the bone, they are referred to as enchondromas; less frequently they are located in the region of the periosteum where they are referred to as periosteal chondromas. Enchondromas are more commonly found in the small bones of the hands and feet, particularly in the phalanges.

Enchondromas are usually asymptomatic and often are discovered on radiographs performed for an unrelated condition. In fact, if the lesion is painful and there is no evidence of a pathological fracture, then the possibility of malignancy must be considered. On radiographs, the lesion appears as a well-marginated zone of lysis that contains evidence of calcification (Figure 16). Lesions in the hands and feet are not usually malignant (Takigawa, 1971). However, a large lesion in a long bone associated with scalloping of the endosteal surface or lytic areas in a mineralized lesion are radiographic features which should arouse suspicion of malignancy.

Histologically, enchondromas appear as lobules of typical benign hyaline cartilage of variable cellularity. The chondrocytes lie in lacunae and have small inconspicuous nuclei. The degree of cellularity and cytological atypia is somewhat dependent upon the site of the lesion. Tumours of small bones or in a periosteal location can show considerably greater cellularity and nuclear atypia, yet still behave in a benign manner.

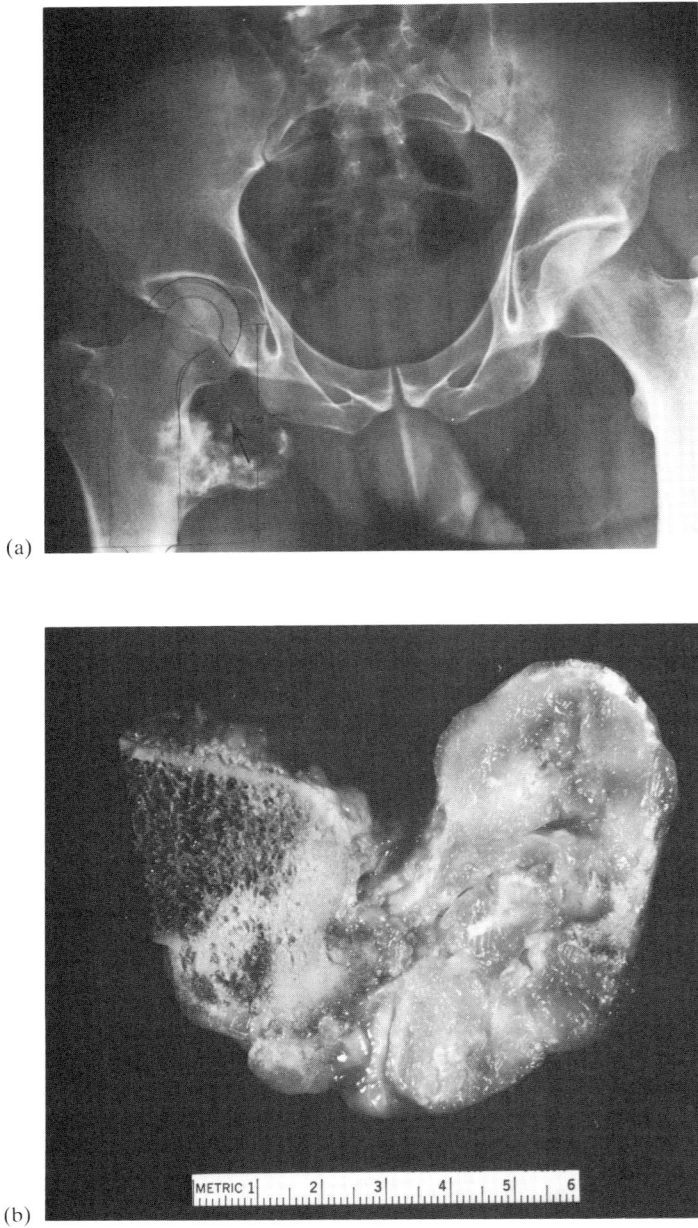

**Figure 15.** (a) Anteroposterior view of pelvis and proximal femur (measurement film) showing large osteochondroma in lesser trochanteric region. Thick, irregular cartilage cap ( ↑ ) suggested the possibility of secondary malignancy. (b) Excised specimen with underlying margin of normal bone. From Sim et al (1983), with permission.

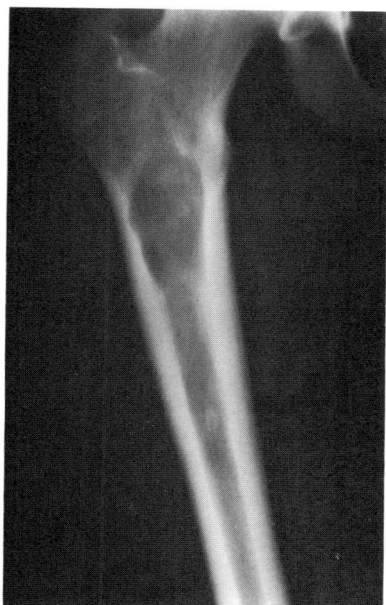

**Figure 16.** Anteroposterior x-ray showing benign enchondroma in right proximal femur in an 11-year-old patient. From Sim et al (1979), with permission.

The periosteal chondroma (Figure 17) is seen on X-ray as a well-demarcated, saucer-shaped erosion of the underlying bone, with extension into the surrounding soft tissues (deSantos and Spjut, 1981). There is no involvement of the underlying medullary bone. Periosteal chondromas have greater cellularity and the cells may be more abnormal than the typical chondroma. At times this may cause confusion with chondrosarcoma (Lichtenstein and Hall, 1952).

Rarely will the patient have evidence of multiple chondromas (Figure 18). When there is widespread involvement and an element of dysplasia, the condition is referred to as Ollier's disease. In addition, multiple chondromas may be associated with angiomas of soft tissue, a condition referred to as Maffucci's syndrome (Lewis and Ketcham, 1973).

A benign-appearing asymptomatic enchondroma that is not structurally weakening the bone warrants observation. On the other hand, if the lesion is symptomatic, curettage and bone grafting are usually curative. When the lesion is associated with a pathological fracture, it is best to do the curettage after the fracture has healed and the continuity of bone has been restored. Periosteal chondromas should be excised en bloc (Lichtenstein and Hall, 1952). In multiple familial enchondromatosis the treatment depends on the clinical features of the individual lesions.

(a)

(b)

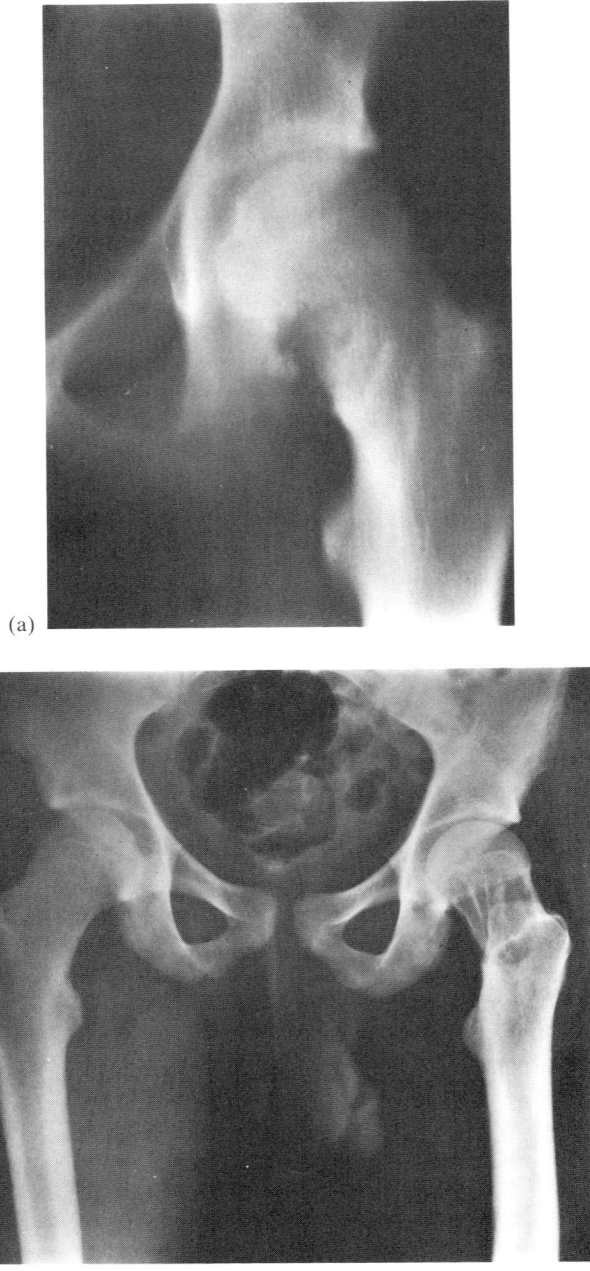

**Figure 17.** (a) Anteroposterior tomogram of right hip showing periosteal chondroma in femoral neck. Cortical irregularity and mineralization suggest the possibility of malignancy. (b) Anteroposterior view of hip after excision and bone grafting. From Sim et al (1983), with permission.

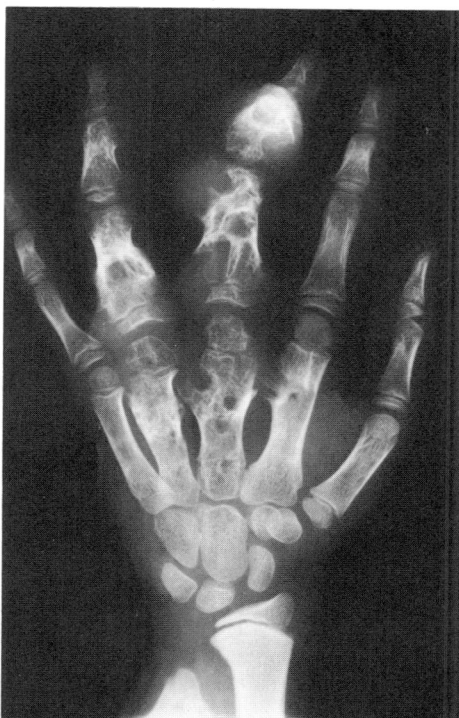

**Figure 18.** Anteroposterior X-ray showing multiple chondromatosis in left hand. From Sim et al (1979), with permission.

## Chondroblastoma

This is a rare benign cartilage tumour that accounts for 1% of benign bone tumours (Sirsat and Doctor, 1970; Dahlin and Ivins, 1972; Huvos and Marcove, 1973; Dahlin and Unni, 1986). There is a 2:1 male predominance and the tumour affects patients aged less than 20 years in 70% of the cases. Chondroblastoma is usually found in the epiphysis of a long bone but can occur in a wide variety of bones. However, 70% occur in the femur, tibia and humerus (Huvos and Marcove, 1973).

Radiographically, most of the lesions appear as a lucent defect involving the epiphyseal area, either solely or with metaphyseal extension (Figure 19). In 25–50% of cases one can appreciate a fluffy, amorphous calcification or ossification. Although most of the lesions are less than 4 cm in diameter, their size can vary considerably. They are usually oval or spherical in shape and eccentrically situated. Approximately one-half of the tumours exhibit cortical involvement, with scalloping or ballooning of the cortical margins similar to aneurysmal bone cysts. Ninety per cent of these tumours appear well marginated, two-thirds have a sclerotic rim, and a periosteal reaction is seen in approximately 10%.

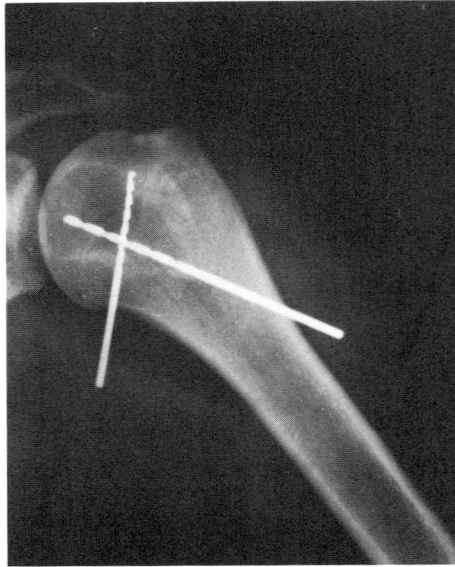

**Figure 19.** Interoperative x-ray showing localization of typical chondroblastoma in proximal humerus marked by two drill bits. From Sim et al (1983), with permission.

Microscopically, the lesions are histologically similar to a benign giant cell tumour but they produce a chondroid matrix. Scattered within a sheet-like proliferation of mononuclear cells are multinucleated giant cells and fibro-chondroid islands. Calcification may be seen in the chondroid islands as well as in a lace-like chicken-wire pattern surrounding the mononuclear cells of the tumour. Secondary cystic changes, similar to aneurysmal bone cysts, are seen in 15–20% of cases (Dahlin and Unni, 1986). Although chondroblastomas generally behave in a benign fashion, there are rare documented cases of pulmonary metastasis from typical benign chondroblastoma. Malignant transformation has been documented in six cases; however, the majority occurred after radiation treatment and are considered post-radiation sarcomas (Sirsat and Doctor, 1970; Dahlin and Ivins, 1972, Huvos and Marcove, 1973; Persson and Wouters, 1976).

Recognition of this entity is important because of its relatively non-aggressive nature and greater curability compared to giant cell tumours. Curettage and bone grafting have been successful in controlling the tumours after the first operative intervention in 90% or more of cases (Schajowicz and Gallardo, 1970; Dahlin and Ivins, 1972; Huvos and Marcove, 1973). Recurrence is more common in the presence of inadequate surgical excision and superimposed aneurysmal bone cyst-like tendencies.

Occasionally the location of the lesion is such that it can be completely excised with a surrounding shell of normal bone without significantly compromising the function of the neighbouring joint. On occasion, massive soft-tissue recurrence or compromise of the articular surface necessitates resection and replacement with an allograft, prosthesis or arthrodesis. Radiation treatment should be reserved for cases not amenable to surgical excision.

## Aneurysmal bone cysts

Aneurysmal bone cysts are thought to be reactive, non-neoplastic processes rather than true benign bone tumours (Dahlin and Unni, 1986). Even though other lesions may have areas that histologically resemble aneurysmal bone cysts, they are now recognized as a separate and distinct entity (Tillman et al, 1968). It is important to differentiate aneurysmal bone cysts from various benign conditions that have aneurysmal bone cyst-like areas, such as giant cell tumour, chondroblastoma, chondromyxoid fibroma and fibrous dysplasia. Moreover, aneurysmal bone cyst may occasionally be confused with telangiectatic osteosarcoma because the rapid growth pattern and histological appearance may be similar.

Little is known of its pathogenesis. Dahlin and Unni (1986) consider that it arises de novo (Dahlin and Unni, 1986). Increased vascular pressure from alteration of the vascular dynamics has been postulated as a cause. Another theory is local release of a fibrinolytic material that destroys the bone and results in a cystic lesion.

Seventy-five per cent of the lesions occur in patients aged less than 20 years. These lesions tend to occur in the metaphyseal region of a long bone or in the vertebrae. The radiographic appearance is characteristic—an eccentric, well-outlined area of rarefaction with a classic ballooned or aneurysmal cystic expansion (Figure 20a). Typically, a surrounding rim of sclerosis from periosteal new bone formation occurs. The lesion may be very aggressive and may result in cortical destruction, soft-tissue extension and the formation of Codman's triangles. This appearance often suggests malignancy. Approximately 20% of aneurysmal bone cysts occur in the spinal region where a lytic expansion of the dorsal elements is typical. These lesions often involve multiple adjacent vertebrae.

Microscopically, aneurysmal bone cysts contain numerous cavernous spaces, usually filled with non-clotted blood. There may be a surrounding thin layer of subperiosteal new bone formation. These tumours are loosely arranged. The septa are thin and may contain bony trabeculae referred to as fiberosteoid. Although mitotic activity may be brisk, the spindled stroma cells lack atypia, which should avoid confusion with malignancy. Benign giant cells may be frequent and may cause confusion with a giant cell tumour.

Aneurysmal bone cysts are amenable to various types of treatment (Sim, 1984). Excision is preferred when the lesion is located in an expendable bone such as the fibula or rib. When the lesion is located in a major bone where resection cannot be carried out without significant functional loss, curettage and bone grafting are used (Figure 20b and c). Radiation is not recommended because of the potential for malignant transformation. The three instances of malignant transformation in our experience occurred after radiation therapy. The overall recurrence rate after treatment of aneurysmal bone cyst in the

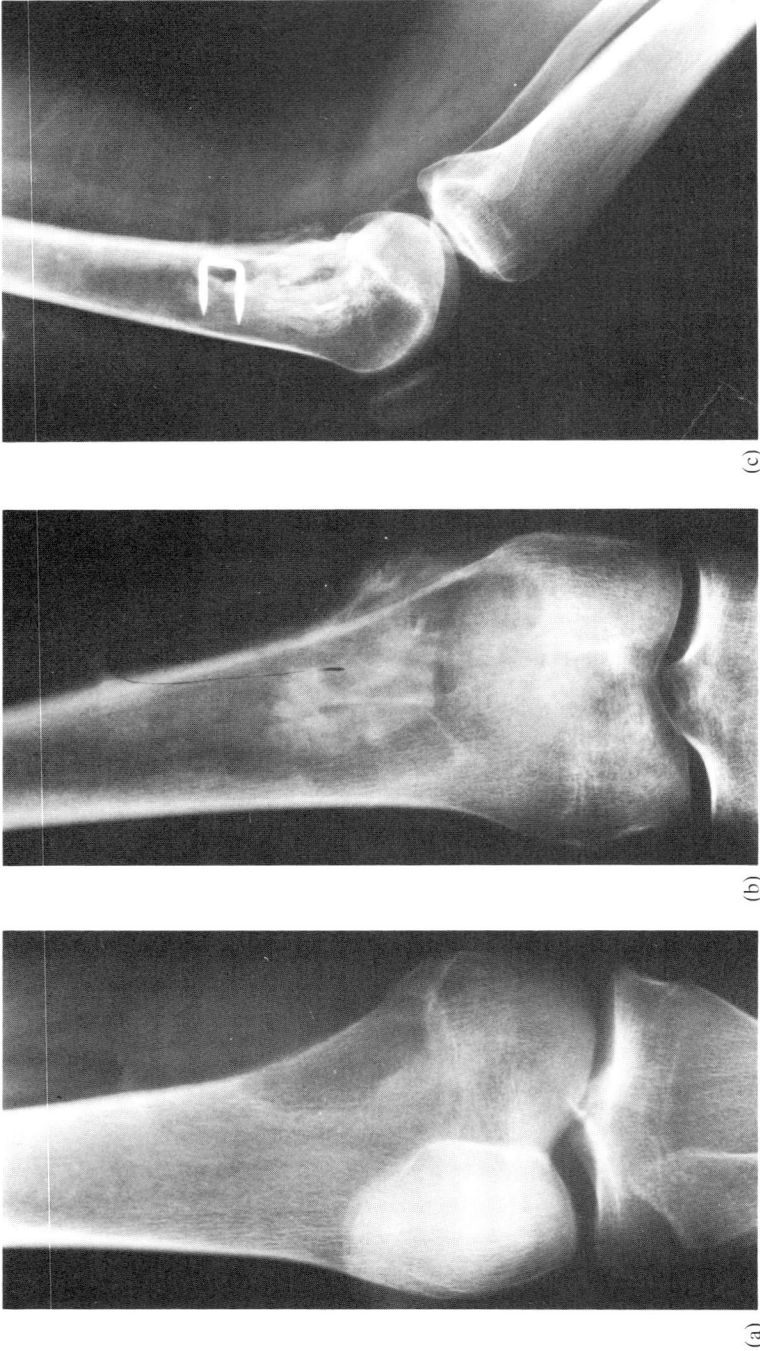

(a)        (b)        (c)

**Figure 20.** Aneurysmal bone cyst. (a) Oblique view of distal femur showing ill-defined lytic lesion, which is poorly marginated. (b) Anteroposterior view of distal femur showing recurrence 3 months after curettage and grafting. (c) Lateral view of distal femur 29 months after recurettage and grafting. From Sim (1984), with permission.

Mayo Clinic series was 21% (Tillman et al, 1968). Twenty-nine per cent of the lesions treated by curettage and grafting developed local recurrence, usually within 2 years. Treatment for the local recurrence is generally the same as that for the primary lesion, but it may involve a more radical procedure such as wide resection and reconstruction. Persistence of a cyst in a portion of a grafted lesion which has not been expanding on serial X-rays and in a patient who is asymptomatic does not demand further treatment. Close observation may be all that is needed.

### Unicameral bone cysts

Unicameral bone cysts are one of the most common tumour-like afflictions of bone manifested in childhood and adolescence. The majority are asymptomatic and the patient presents with a pathological fracture sustained by minor trauma. These fluid-filled cysts represent approximately 3% of all bone lesions and have a definite male predominance (Dahlin and Unni, 1986). They usually arise in the shaft of a long bone; more than one-half of the lesions are located in the proximal shaft of the humerus or femur (Figure 21a; see also Chapter 3, Figure 1).

Because these are frequently multicameral (multiple chambered), the term 'simple bone cyst' is preferred to 'unicameral bone cyst'. Although the lesion is referred to as active if it abuts on the epiphyseal plate and latent if it has migrated away from the epiphysis with growth (Jaffe and Lichtenstein, 1942), the aggressiveness of the lesion does not seem related to the proximity of the growth plate.

The aetiology of simple bone cysts remains unclear. The most plausible theory is that it is due to an aberration of bone growth at the epiphyseal plate resulting from trauma or haemorrhage (Morton, 1964b). Other theories include intramedullary haemorrhage secondary to trauma, inflammatory lesions, osteoblastic proliferation and osseous dystrophy (Morton, 1964b). Others have suggested intraosseous synovial cyst and venous obstruction (Cohen, 1960, 1970, 1977; Mirra et al, 1978).

The radiographic findings are characteristic. The cyst appears as an elongated lucency centred within the medullary cavity. These are wider at the epiphyseal end, but are not wider than the epiphyseal plate itself. Residual ridges of cortex produce a trabeculated appearance. Periosteal new bone formation is not present unless a pathological fracture has occurred.

Pathologically, the cyst contains clear or yellow-green fluid. Histologically, the cyst is lined by a very thin layer of fibrous tissue. The connective tissue contains numerous benign, multinucleated giant cells. Haemosiderin-laden macrophages may be seen in addition to lipid-laden histiocytes and cholesterol clefts.

Until recently, treatment of simple bone cysts has been controversial. Therapeutic intervention, as opposed to watchful waiting, is usually indicated for all but small resolving cysts. Surgical curettage with bone grafting has long been the standard of care for these patients, with approximately 70% cure with the first surgical intervention (Figure 21) (Neer et al, 1966; Boseker et al, 1968). Several factors have been associated with a high

(a)

(b)

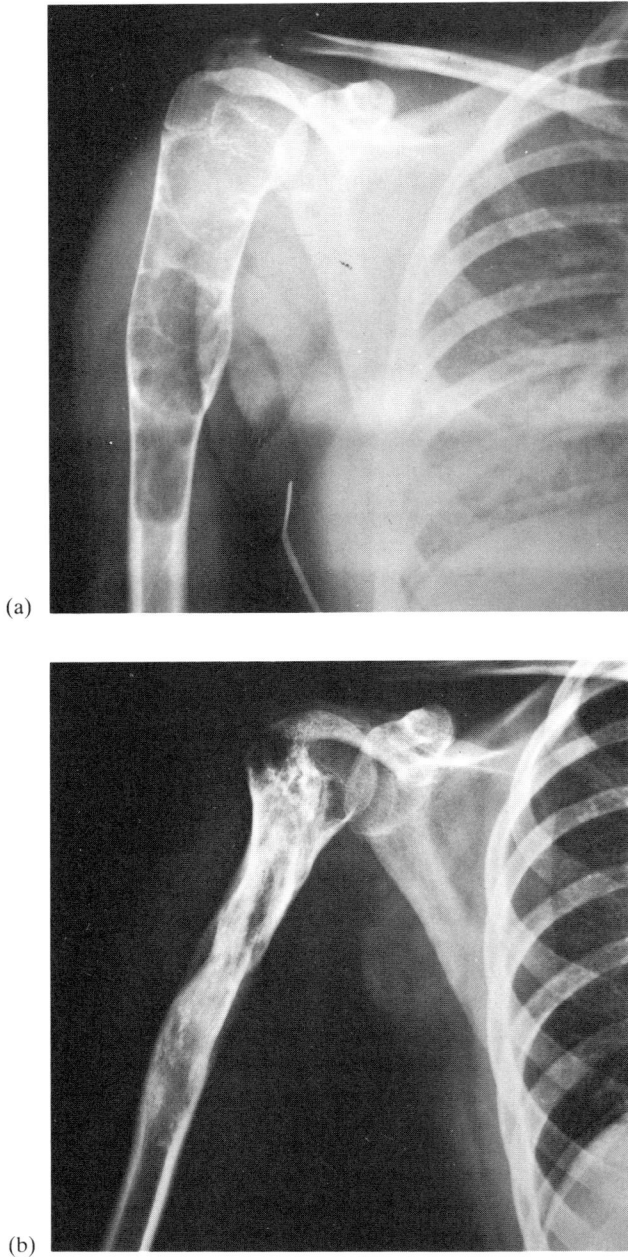

**Figure 21.** (a) Anteroposterior X-ray showing extensive unicameral bone cyst in a 15-year-old girl. (b) Anteroposterior X-ray 4 years after excision and autogenous bone grafting. (Both iliac and tibial bone struts were used.) From Sim et al (1979), with permission.

incidence of recurrence or persistence of the cyst: age less than 10 years, larger lesions, male sex, multilocular lesions and active lesions (Garceau and Gregory, 1954; Spence et al, 1969; Neer et al, 1973; Spence et al, 1976; Campanacci et al, 1986). Since Scaglietti and associates' reports on the effectiveness of steroid injection without significant side-effects (Scaglietti et al, 1979, 1982), this technique has been preferred. In Campanacci and associates' review of 416 cases of simple bone cysts (Campanacci et al, 1986), 78 had been treated with curettage and bone grafting, and 141 were treated by steroid injection. In their series the end results were comparable, but the low risk of complication associated with steroid injections favoured this procedure. Oppenheim and Galleno (1984) reported similar findings. All authors indicate that multiple steroid injections may be necessary. On the other hand, in patients with loss of structural integrity in a weight-bearing bone associated with a large cyst, curettage and grafting are still indicated.

## Benign fibrous lesions of bone

There is a wide spectrum of fibrous lesions in bone. They constitute approximately 5% of all benign bone tumours (Dahlin and Unni, 1986). Considerable confusion often arises because of the terminology used to describe the lesions during the different stages of their development. Fibroma of bone generally includes non-ossifying or non-osteogenic fibroma, metaphyseal fibrous defect, fibrous cortical defect and xanthogranuloma. The periosteal desmoid is another less cellular variant of these fibrous lesions. This benign fibrous lesion probably represents a defect in ossification rather than a true neoplasm.

Fibroma in its classic form is almost exclusively a disease of childhood and has been noted in 30–40% of children aged more than 2 years (Caffey, 1955). Pathologically, the lesion is sharply demarcated from surrounding bone and usually has several distinct lobules. Microscopically, spindle cells are arranged in a storiform pattern. Foci of lipid-laden histiocytes are often noted, with haemosiderin pigment seen within the stromal cells. Mitotic figures are not unusual. The fibrous cortical defect is a small, usually asymptomatic, intracortical lesion; it is usually located on the posteromedial aspect of the distal femoral metaphysis (Figure 22) (Sontag and Pyle, 1941). This site is at the medial supracondylar ridge, which is the attachment site of the aponeurosis of the extensor portion of the great adductor muscle (Barnes and Gwinn, 1974). It is thought that the mechanical stress produces microavulsions of the cortical bone, eliciting hypervascular and fibroblastic responses, which stimulate added osteoblastic activity and bone resorption (Bufkin, 1971). The radiographic findings are seen best when the knee is externally rotated between 20° and 45°, exposing the adductor tubercle. The area of involvement is typically 1–2 cm long and consists of round or ovoid radiolucent region seen in the cortex of the bone. Perpendicular bone spiculation or a lamellar periosteal reaction with irregular ossification may be present during the early phases and may simulate a sarcoma. X-rays in the lateral projection show an area of cortical thickening. An important feature is the lack of soft-tissue mass and preservation of soft-tissue planes. Once the

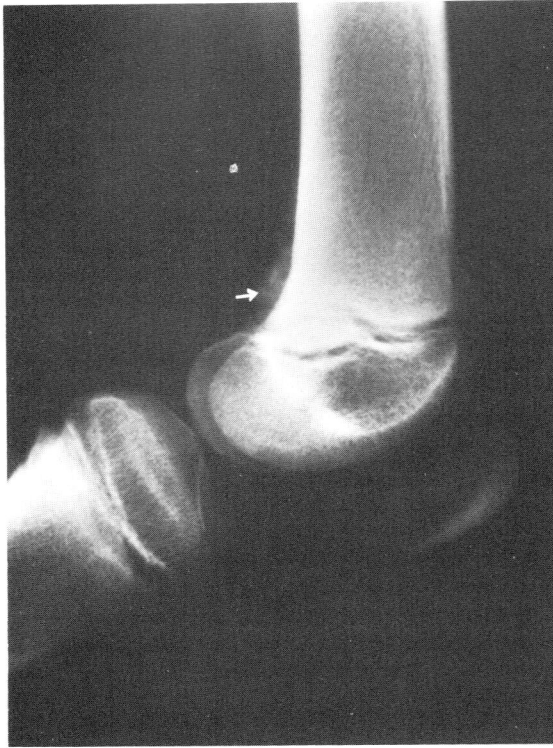

**Figure 22.** Lateral X-ray of left knee showing typical metaphyseal fibrous cortical defect. From Sim et al (1979), with permission.

diagnosis is made, further evaluation is not needed because these lesions regress with skeletal maturity (Greenfield, 1980).

Non-ossifying fibroma is a larger lesion involving the medullary cavity of the bone (Dahlin and Unni, 1986). However, both this lesion and fibrous cortical defects are referred to as metaphyseal fibrous defects. These lesions, which often occur in adolescence and young adulthood, may cause swelling and pain but are usually asymptomatic. They are centrally located in the metaphysis of long bones. They can spontaneously regress, but diaphyseal migration may also occur. The lesion is typically surrounded by a sharp zone of sclerosis, which may be smooth but is usually scalloped. A multiloculated appearance with expansion and cortical thinning of the overlying bone is common (Figure 22). As with fibrous cortical defects, biopsy is usually not necessary for diagnosis. The possibility of pathological fracture occurs in larger lesions, particularly when the transverse plane of the lesion exceeds 50% of the bone in both anteroposterior and lateral X-rays (Figure 23) (Arata et al, 1981).

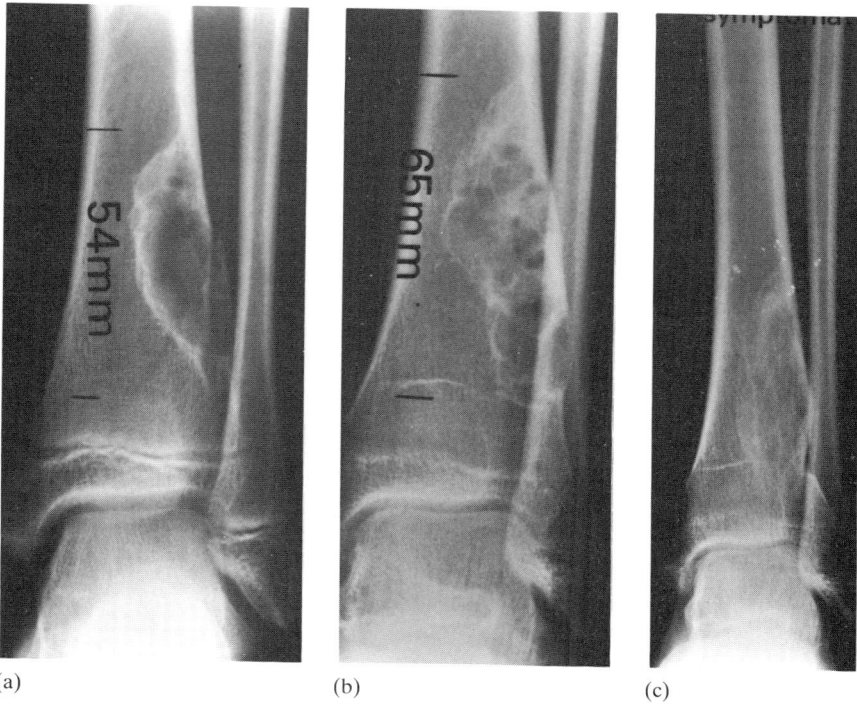

(a)                     (b)                   (c)

**Figure 23.** (a) Pathological fracture through non-ossifying fibroma. Fracture united after cast immobilization. (b) Lesion has persisted and enlarged over a 3½-year period. (c) Patient is asymptomatic 23 months after curettage and bone graft. From Arata et al (1981), with permission.

Treatment of the lesion depends on three factors: (1) the certainty of the diagnosis, (2) the structural integrity of the bone, and (3) the proximity of the lesion to the epiphyseal plate. Usually the diagnosis is certain by X-ray and clinical evidence, and if the lesion does not threaten the strength of the bone, observation alone is indicated. If, however, the lesion is large and occupies more than 50% of the bone diameter, then closer observation or surgical treatment may be indicated (Sim et al, 1984). If surgery is performed, curettage and bone grafting are curative. If fracture occurs through a metaphyseal fibrous defect, conservative treatment of the fracture is usually carried out, but in large defects associated with pathological fractures, curettage and bone grafting may be indicated.

## Desmoplastic fibroma

This is an extremely rare lesion (Dahlin and Unni, 1986). Even though it affects persons of all ages, 60% of the lesions occur in persons aged less than 20 years. It is most commonly found in the metaphyseal region of long bones. The tibia is the most commonly affected, then the femur and humerus. Other rare locations have been the scapula, vertebrae, calcaneus and mandible (Sugiura, 1976).

Radiographically, the rarefying lesion is reasonably well demarcated, but it often has an irregular border producing a trabeculated appearance. The lytic, destructive, indolent nature of the lesion often suggests a low-grade fibrosarcoma.

Pathologically, the lesion can be considered the intraosseous counterpart of the desmoid tumour in the soft tissues. Grossly the tumour is dense, rubbery and grey-white. Histologically, the lesion is hypocellular and composed of slender spindle cells with abundant collagen formation, reminiscent of the soft-tissue desmoid. The fibroblasts with small nuclei without significant pleomorphism and mitotic figures are rare.

Because of the locally aggressive nature of the lesion, curettage or simple excision with a lesional or marginal margin is usually associated with a high incidence of local recurrence. Despite multiple recurrences, the tumour usually retains its benign appearance histologically.

Eradication of the lesion usually requires en bloc resection with a wide margin (Sim et al, 1984). Depending on the location of the lesion, reconstruction after the segmental resection can be carried out by various methods discussed earlier.

## SUMMARY

The management of patients with benign bone tumours remains a challenge. The first hurdle is the recognition of the existence of the lesion. Once the lesion is discovered, a systematic approach to evaluation is important. The problem is magnified by the great diversity of benign bone tumours as well as non-neoplastic lesions that simulate them. After an accurate histological diagnosis based on a carefully planned biopsy, a treatment plan can be formulated and executed. Management of benign bone tumours requires a high degree of teamwork to arrive at a correct diagnosis and effective treatment of the patient.

## REFERENCES

Arata MA, Peterson HA & Dahlin DC (1981) Pathological fractures through non-ossifying fibromas: review of the Mayo Clinic experience. *Journal of Bone and Joint Surgery. American Volume* **63**: 980–988.
Averill RM, Smith RJ & Campbell CJ (1980) Giant-cell tumors of the bones of the hand. *Journal of Hand Surgery* **5**: 39–50.
Baddeley S & Cullen JC (1979) The use of methylmethacrylate in the treatment of giant cell tumours of the proximal tibia. *Australian and New Zealand Journal of Surgery* **49**: 120–122.
Barnes GR Jr & Gwinn JL (1974) Distal irregularities of the femur simulating malignancy. *American Journal of Roentgenology, Radium Therapy and Nuclear Medicine* **122**: 180–185.
Boseker EH, Bickel WH & Dahlin DC (1968) A clinicopathologic study of simple unicameral bone cysts. *Surgery, Gynecology and Obstetrics* **127**: 550–560.
Bufkin WJ (1971) The avulsive cortical irregularity. *American Journal of Roentgenology, Radium Therapy and Nuclear Medicine* **112**: 487–492.

Caffey J (1955) On fibrous defects in cortical walls of growing tubular bones: their radiologic appearance, structure, prevalence, natural course, and diagnostic significance. *Advances in Pediatrics* **7**: 13–51.

Camargo FP & Camargo OP (1985) Surgical treatment of benign cavitary bone lesion employing methylmethacrylate cement and polyethylene prosthesis—an experience with 135 cases. In Enneking WF (Chairman) *Abstracts of the International Symposium on Limb Salvage in Musculoskeletal Oncology*, Orlando, Florida, October 2 to 5, 1985, pp vi–15 (Bristol-Myers/Zimmer Orthopaedic Symposium in cooperation with the Orthopaedic Research and Education Foundation). Published by the American Orthopaedic Association.

Campanacci M, Guinti A & Olmi R (1975) Giant-cell tumours of bone: a study of 209 cases with long-term follow-up in 130. *Italian Journal of Orthopaedics and Traumatology* **1**: 249–277.

Campanacci M, Capanna R & Picci P (1986) Unicameral and aneurysmal bone cysts. *Clinical Orthopaedics and Related Research* **204**: 25–36.

Cohen J (1960) Simple bone cysts: studies of cyst fluid in six cases with a theory of pathogenesis. *Journal of Bone and Joint Surgery. American Volume* **42**: 609–616.

Cohen J (1970) Etiology of simple bone cyst. *Journal of Bone and Joint Surgery. American Volume* **52**: 1493–1497.

Cohen J (1977) Unicameral bone cysts: a current synthesis of reported cases. *Orthopedic Clinics of North America* **8(4)**: 715–736.

Conrad EU, Enneking WF & Springfield DS (1985) Giant cell tumor treatment with curettage and cementation. In Enneking WF (Chairman) *Abstracts of the International Symposium on Limb Salvage in Musculoskeletal Oncology*, Orlando, Florida, October 2 to 5, 1985 (Bristol-Myers/Zimmer Orthopaedic Symposium in cooperation with the Orthopaedic Research and Education Foundation). Published by the American Orthopaedic Association.

Czitrom AA, Langer F, McKee N & Gross AE (1986) Bone and cartilage allotransplantation: a review of 14 years of research and clinical studies. *Clinical Orthopaedics and Related Research* **208**: 141–145.

Dahlin DC (1978) *Bone Tumors: General Aspects and Data on 6221 Cases*, 3rd edn. Springfield, Illinois: Charles C. Thomas.

Dahlin DC (1985) Giant cell tumor of bone: highlights of 407 cases. *American Journal of Roentgenology* **144**: 955–960.

Dahlin DC & Ivins JC (1972) Benign chondroblastoma: a study of 125 cases. *Cancer* **30**: 401–413.

Dahlin DC & Unni KK (1986) *Bone Tumors: General Aspects and Data on 8542 Cases*, 4th edn. Springfield, Illinois: Charles C. Thomas.

Dahlin DC, Cupps RE & Johnson EW Jr (1970) Giant-cell tumor: a study of 195 cases. *Cancer* **25**: 1061–1070.

deSantos LA & Spjut HJ (1981) Periosteal chondroma: a radiographic spectrum. *Skeletal Radiology* **6**: 15–20.

Duncan CP, Morton KS & Arthur JF (1983) Giant cell tumour of bone: its aggressiveness and potential for malignant change. *Canadian Journal of Surgery* **26**: 475–477.

Enneking WF, Spanier SS & Goodman MA (1980) A system for the surgical staging of musculoskeletal sarcoma. *Clinical Orthopaedics and Related Research* **153**: 106–120.

Ewald FC, Poss R, Pugh J, Schiller AL & Sledge CB (1982) Hip cartilage supported by methacrylate in canine arthroplasty. *Clinical Orthopaedics and Related Research* **171**: 273–279.

Garceau GJ & Gregory CF (1954) Solitary unicameral bone cyst. *Journal of Bone and Joint Surgery. American Volume* **36**: 267–280.

Goldenberg RR, Campbell CJ & Bonfiglio M (1970) Giant-cell tumor of bone: an analysis of two hundred and eighteen cases. *Journal of Bone and Joint Surgery. American Volume* **52**: 619–663.

Greenfield GB (1980) *Radiology of Bone Diseases*, 3rd edn. Philadelphia: JB Lippincott.

Harsha WN (1954) The natural history of osteocartilaginous exostoses (osteochondroma). *American Surgeon* **20**: 65–72.

Hudson TM, Hamlin DJ, Enneking WF & Pettersson H (1985) Magnetic resonance imaging of bone and soft tissue tumors: early experience in 31 patients compared with computed tomography. *Skeletal Radiology* **13**: 134–146.

Huvos AG & Marcove RC (1973) Chondroblastoma of bone: a critical review. *Clinical Orthopaedics and Related Research* **95**: 300–312.

Jacobs PA & Clemency RE Jr (1983) Closed cryosurgical treatment of giant cell tumor, aneurysmal bone cyst and other lesions of bone (abstract). *Orthopaedic Transactions* **7**: 195–196.

Jaffe HL (1943) Hereditary multiple exostosis. *Archives of Pathology* **36**: 335–357.

Jaffe HL & Lichtenstein L (1942) Solitary unicameral bone cyst: with emphasis on the roentgen picture, the pathologic appearance and the pathogenesis. *Archives of Surgery* **44**: 1004–1025.

Jaffe HL, Lichtenstein L & Portis RB (1940) Giant cell tumor of bone: its pathologic appearance, grading, supposed variants and treatment. *Archives of Pathology* **30**: 993–1031.

Johnston J (1985) Treatment of giant cell tumor of bone by aggressive curettement and packing with bone cement. In Enneking WF (Chairman) *Abstracts of the International Symposium on Limb Salvage in Musculoskeletal Oncology*, Orlando, Florida, October 2 to 5, 1985, pp vi–13 (Bristol-Myers/Zimmer Orthopaedic Symposium in cooperation with the Orthopaedic Research and Education Foundation). Published by the American Orthopaedic Association.

Larsson S-E, Lorentzon R & Boquist L (1975) Giant-cell tumor of bone: a demographic, clinical, and histopathological study of all cases recorded in the Swedish Cancer Registry for the years 1958 through 1968. *Journal of Bone and Joint Surgery. American Volume* **57**: 167–173.

Levine E (1981) Computed tomography of musculoskeletal tumors. *CRC Critical Reviews in Diagnostic Imaging* **16**: 279–309.

Lewis RJ & Ketcham AS (1973) Maffuci's syndrome: functional and neoplastic significance: case report and review of the literature. *Journal of Bone and Joint Surgery. American Volume* **55**: 1465–1479.

Lichtenstein L & Hall JE (1952) Periosteal chondroma: a distinctive benign cartilage tumor. *Journal of Bone and Joint Surgery. American Volume* **34**: 691–697.

Lukens JA, McLeod RA & Sim FH (1982) Computed tomographic evaluation of primary osseous malignant neoplasms. *American Journal of Roentgenology* **139**: 45–48.

Malawer MM & Zielinski CJ (1983) Giant cell tumor of bone: cryosurgery and 'en-bloc' resection, current concepts and recommendations for treatment. *Orthopaedic Transactions* **7** (abstract): 492.

Mándi A & Kiss I (1976) Ersatz tumoröser Knochensegmente durch Palacos. *Beitrage zur Orthopadie und Traumatologie* **23**: 213–217.

Mankin HJ, Fogelson FS, Thrasher AZ & Jaffer F (1976) Massive resection and allograft transplantation in the treatment of malignant bone tumors. *New England Journal of Medicine* **294**: 1247–1255.

Mankin HJ, Lange TA & Spanier SS (1982) The hazards of biopsy in patients with malignant primary bone and soft-tissue tumors. *Journal of Bone and Joint Surgery. American Volume* **64**: 1121–1127.

Manley PA, McKeown DB, Schatzker J, Palmer NC & Carman S (1982) Replacement of epiphyseal bone with methylmethacrylate: its effect on articular cartilage. *Archives of Orthopaedic and Traumatic Surgery* **100**: 3–10.

Marcove RE (1980) *En bloc* resections for osteogenic sarcoma. *Cancer* **45**: 3040–3044.

Marcove RC, Weiss LD, Vaghaiwalla MR & Pearson R (1978) Cryosurgery in the treatment of giant cell tumors of bone: a report of 52 consecutive cases. *Clinical Orthopaedics and Related Research* **134**: 275–289.

Marsh BW, Bonfiglio M, Brady LP & Enneking WF (1975) Benign osteoblastoma: range of manifestations. *Journal of Bone and Joint Surgery. American Volume* **57**: 1–9.

McDonald DJ, Sim FH, McLeod RA & Dahlin DC (1986) Giant-cell tumor of bone. *Journal of Bone and Joint Surgery. American Volume* **68**: 235–242.

McGrath PJ (1972) Giant-cell tumour of bone: an analysis of fifty-two cases. *Journal of Bone and Joint Surgery. British Volume* **54**: 216–229.

McLeod RA, Gisvold JJ, Stephens DH, Beabout JW & Sheedy PF II (1978) Computed tomography of soft tissues and breast. *Seminars in Roentgenology* **13**: 267–275.

Mirra JM, Bernard GW, Bullough PG, Johnston W & Mink G (1978) Cementum-like bone production in solitary bone cysts (so-called 'cementoma' of long bones): report of three cases. Electron microscopic observations supporting a synovial origin to the simple bone cyst. *Clinical Orthopaedics and Related Research* **135**: 295–307.

Morton KS (1964a) On the question of recurrence of osteochondroma. *Journal of Bone and Joint Surgery. British Volume* **46**: 723–725.

Morton KS (1964b) The pathogenesis of unicameral bone cyst. *Canadian Journal of Surgery* **7**: 140–150.

Neer CS II, Francis KC, Marcove RC, Terz J & Carbonara PN (1966) Treatment of unicameral bone cyst: a follow-up study of one hundred and seventy-five cases. *Journal of Bone and Joint Surgery. American Volume* **48**: 731–745.

Neer CS II, Francis KC, Johnston AD & Kiernan HA Jr (1973) Current concepts on the treatment of solitary unicameral bone cyst. *Clinical Orthopaedics and Related Research* **97**: 40–51.

Oppenheim WL & Galleno H (1984) Operative treatment versus steroid injection in the management of unicameral bone cysts. *Journal of Pediatric Orthopedics* **4**: 1–7.

Parrish FF (1973) Allograft replacement of all or part of the end of a long bone following excision of a tumor: report of twenty-one cases. *Journal of Bone and Joint Surgery. American Volume* **55**: 1–22.

Peimer CA, Schiller AL, Mankin HJ & Smith RJ (1980) Multicentric giant-cell tumor of bone. *Journal of Bone and Joint Surgery. American Volume* **62**: 652–656.

Persson BM & Wouters HW (1976) Curettage and acrylic cementation in surgery of giant cell tumors of bone. *Clinical Orthopaedics and Related Research* **120**: 125–133.

Persson BM, Ekelund L, Lövdahl R & Gunterberg B (1984) Favourable results of acrylic cementation for giant cell tumors. *Acta Orthopaedica Scandinavica* **55**: 209–214.

Radin EL, Orr RB, Kelman JL, Paul IL & Rose RM (1982) Effect of prolonged walking on concrete on the knees of sheep. *Journal of Biomechanics* **15**: 487–492.

Rock MG, Pritchard DJ & Unni KK (1984) Metastases from histologically benign giant-cell tumor of bone. *Journal of Bone and Joint Surgery. American Volume* **66**: 269–274.

Sanerkin NG (1980) Malignancy, aggressiveness, and recurrence in giant cell tumor of bone. *Cancer* **46**: 1641–1649.

Scaglietti O, Marchetti PG & Bartolozzi P (1979) The effects of methylprednisolone acetate in the treatment of bone cysts: results of three years follow-up. *Journal of Bone and Joint Surgery. British Volume* **61**: 200–204.

Scaglietti O, Marchetti PG & Bartolozzi P (1982) Final results obtained in the treatment of bone cysts with methylprednisolone acetate (Depo-Medrol) and a discussion of results achieved in other bone lesions. *Clinical Orthopaedics and Related Research* **165**: 33–42.

Schajowicz F & Gallardo H (1970) Epiphysial chondroblastoma of bone: a clinico-pathological study of sixty-nine cases. *Journal of Bone and Joint Surgery. British Volume* **52**: 205–226.

Sim FH (ed.) (1983) Principles of surgical treatment. In *Diagnosis and Treatment of Bone Tumors: A Team Approach*, pp 23–35. Thorofare, New Jersey: Slack.

Sim FH (1984) Aneurysmal bone cysts. In Uhthoff HK (ed.) *Current Concepts of Diagnosis and Treatment of Bone and Soft Tissue Tumors*, pp 255–260. New York: Springer-Verlag.

Sim FH, Dahlin DC & Beabout JW (1977a) Multicentric giant-cell tumor of bone. *Journal of Bone and Joint Surgery. American Volume* **59**: 1052–1060.

Sim FH, Dahlin DC, Stauffer RN & Laws ER Jr (1977b) Primary bone tumors simulating lumbar disc syndrome. *Spine* **2**: 65–74.

Sim FH, Irwin RB & Dahlin DC (1979) Management of benign bone tumors in children. *Progress in Pediatric Hematology/Oncology* **2**: 233–256.

Sim FH, Unni KK, Wold LE & McLeod RA (1983) Benign tumors. In Sim (ed.) *Diagnosis and Treatment of Bone Tumors: A Team Approach*, pp 107–151. Thorofare, New Jersey: Slack.

Sim FH, Wold LE & Swee RG (1984) Fibrous tumors of bone. *Instructional Course Lectures* **33**: 40–59.

Sim FH, Beauchamp CP & Chao EYS (1987a) Reconstruction of musculoskeletal defects about the knee for tumor. *Clinical Orthopaedics and Related Research* **221**: 188–201.

Sim FH, Beauchamp CP & Chao EYS (1987b) Joint arthrodesis: with particular reference to knee arthrodesis using a porous-coated intercalary prosthesis. In Coombs R (ed.) *Bone Tumour Management*. Borough Green, Kent: Butterworths.

Sirsat MV & Doctor VM (1970) Benign chondroblastoma of bone: report of a case of malignant transformation. *Journal of Bone and Joint Surgery. British Volume* **52**: 741–745.

Solomon L (1964) Hereditary multiple exostosis. *American Journal of Human Genetics* **16**: 351–363.

Sontag LW & Pyle SI (1941) The appearance and nature of cyst-like areas in the distal femoral metaphyses of children. *American Journal of Roentgenology and Radium Therapy* **46**: 185–188.

Spence KF, Sell KW & Brown RH (1969) Solitary bone cyst: treatment with freeze-dried cancellous bone allograft; a study of one hundred and seventy-seven cases. *Journal of Bone and Joint Surgery. American Volume* **51**: 87–96.

Spence KF Jr, Bright RW, Fitzgerald SP & Sell KW (1976) Solitary unicameral bone cyst: treatment with freeze-dried crushed cortical-bone allograft; a review of one hundred and forty-four cases. *Journal of Bone and Joint Surgery. American Volume* **58**: 636–641.

Sugiura I (1976) Desmoplastic fibroma: case report and review of the literature. *Journal of Bone and Joint Surgery. American Volume* **58**: 126–130.

Sung HW, Kuo DP, Shu WP et al (1982) Giant-cell tumor of bone: analysis of two hundred and eight cases in Chinese patients. *Journal of Bone and Joint Surgery. American Volume* **64**: 755–761.

Takigawa K (1971) Chondroma of the bones of the hand: a review of 110 cases. *Journal of Bone and Joint Surgery. American Volume* **53**: 1591–1600.

Taminiau AHM & Wouters HW (1985) Treatment of giant cell tumors by curettage and acrylic cementation. In Enneking WF (Chairman) *Abstracts of the International Symposium on Limb Salvage in Musculoskeletal Oncology*, Orlando, Florida, October 2 to 5, 1985, pp vi–6 (Bristol-Myers/Zimmer Orthopaedic Symposium in cooperation with the Orthopaedic Research and Education Foundation). Published by the American Orthopaedic Association.

Tillman BP, Dahlin DC, Lipscomb PR & Stewart JR (1968) Aneurysmal bone cyst: an analysis of ninety-five cases. *Mayo Clinic Proceedings* **43**: 478–495.

Vidal J, Mimran R, Allieu Y, Jamme M & Goalard G (1969) Plastie de comblement par métacrylate de méthyle traitement de certaines tumeurs osseuses bénignes. *Montpellier Chirurgical* **15**: 389–396.

Wilkins RM, Okada Y, Gorski JP, Sim FH & Chao EY (1985) Methyl methacrylate replacement of subchondral bone: a biomechanical, biochemical, and morphologic analysis. In Enneking WF (Chairman) *Abstracts of the International Symposium on Limb Salvage in Musculoskeletal Oncology*, Orlando, Florida, October 2 to 5, 1985, pp vi–7–vi–8 (Bristol-Myers/Zimmer Orthopaedic Symposium in cooperation with the Orthopaedic Research and Education Foundation). Published by the American Orthopaedic Association.

Willert HG (1985) Clinical results of the temporary acrylic bone cement plug in the treatment of bone tumors: a multicentric study. In Enneking WF (Chairman) *Abstracts of the International Symposium on Limb Salvage in Musculoskeletal Oncology*, Orlando, Florida, October 2 to 5, 1985 (Bristol-Myers/Zimmer Orthopaedic Symposium in cooperation with the Orthopaedic Research and Education Foundation). Published by the American Orthopaedic Association.

Willert HG & Enderle A (1983) Temporary bone cement plug: an alternative treatment of large cystic tumorous bone lesions near the joint. In Kotz R (ed.) *Proceedings of the 2nd International Workshop on the Design and Application of Tumor Prostheses for Bone and Joint Reconstruction*, pp. 69–72. Wien: Egerman.

Wilson PD (1951) Follow-up study of the use of refrigerated homogenous bone transplants in orthopaedic operations. *Journal of Bone and Joint Surgery. American Volume* **33**: 307–322.

Wouters HW (1974) Tumeur à cellules géantes de l'extrémité distale du fémur avec fracture intra-articulaire de genou: traitée par excochléation et remplissage avec du ciment osseux. *Revue de Chirurgie orthopédique et réparatrice de l'Appareil Moteur* **60** (supplement 2): 316.

Zimmer WD, Berquist TH, Sim FH et al (1984) Magnetic resonance imaging of aneurysmal bone cyst. *Mayo Clinic Proceedings* **59**: 633–636.

# 7

# Chemotherapy of operable osteosarcoma

## VIVIEN H. C. BRAMWELL

Osteosarcomas are rare tumours which occur predominantly in children and young adults, and until recently, their prognosis has been dismal. Five-year survival figures published prior to 1972 were remarkably consistent—a mean of 19.7% (range 16–23%) in 1286 cases collected from the world literature (Friedman and Carter, 1972; Carter, 1980). As more than 80% of patients manifest pulmonary metastases after surgical ablation of the primary tumour, systemic micrometastases are presumed to be present at the time of surgery. Historically, 50% of patients developed metastases within 6 months of diagnosis, and 90% of those relapsing, were dead within 2 years (Jeffree et al, 1975). Despite the limited efficacy of most cytotoxic agents in established metastatic disease, impressive 2-year relapse-free survival (RFS) figures ranging from 60 to 90% have been associated with the use of adjuvant chemotherapy (Eilber et al, 1978; Jaffe et al, 1978b; Ettinger et al, 1979; Rosen et al, 1981; Rosen et al, 1982a). However, it has become evident that chemotherapy can delay the appearance of metastases (Jaffe et al, 1978b), and by 5 years, overall survival in most series using adjuvant chemotherapy has fallen to between 40 and 50% (Cortes et al, 1978; Etcubanas and Wilbur, 1978; Pratt et al, 1978; Sutow et al, 1978; Rosenberg et al, 1979; Herson et al, 1980; Ettinger et al, 1981). Jaffe et al (1978a) compared 15 patients receiving adjuvant chemotherapy with ADR and HDMTX with 33 age- and sex-matched controls. The median time to appearance of metastases was 17 months in the adjuvant group compared with 7 months in the control group, while the median number of metastases were 2 and 12 respectively. Bone metastasis (three cases) was seen only in the adjuvant group. Guiliano and Eilber (1983) also commented on the changing pattern of metastases in patients receiving adjuvant chemotherapy. Eighteen out of nineteen (94.7%) relapsing patients, treated by amputation alone at the University of California (UCLA) between 1971 and 1974, metastasized first to the lungs, whereas only 18 out of 40 patients (45%), treated after 1974 with surgery and adjuvant chemotherapy, developed pulmonary metastases alone as the initial site of recurrence. Conversely, no patient treated by surgery alone developed an extrapulmonary metastasis as the first site of recurrence, whereas 11 out of 40 patients (27.5%) treated with adjuvant chemotherapy relapsed initially in an extrapulmonary site, and a further 11 patients developed simultaneous pulmonary and extrapulmonary metastases.

All the early impressive results of adjuvant chemotherapy were generated in single arm studies, in which outcome was compared with that of historical controls. This had provoked enormous controversy, which has only recently been clarified by the results of two randomized studies (Eckardt et al, 1985; Link et al, 1986) demonstrating a clear benefit for patients receiving adjuvant chemotherapy in comparison with those treated with surgery alone. Before these randomized trials, one area of concern was that the selection criteria for admission to uncontrolled studies of adjuvant chemo-therapy were stricter than those applied to historical controls, and this was certainly true for many studies. Patients in such studies may have had smaller tumours, been diagnosed earlier, had better socioeconomic back-grounds with higher motivation, and had more complete diagnostic evaluation, including pulmonary computerized tomography (CT) scanning. Although comparisons with historical controls were usually made between patients in similar age groups, and were restricted to high-grade extremity tumours, this was not always the case, which further confused the issue. Goorin et al (1985) re-examined the records of 333 patients treated by surgery alone at the Dana Faber Institute in Boston before 1972, and found that only 61 (18%) would meet current eligibility criteria for adjuvant chemotherapy trials. Of these patients, 23% had remained disease-free since diagnosis and treatment. It is clear therefore that selection bias may make comparison with historical controls very unreliable.

The following general criteria are used to define eligibility for trials of adjuvant treatment for osteosarcoma:

1.  Histologically confirmed osteosarcoma, of the 'common' high-grade type. Low-grade tumours (e.g. parosteal, intraosseous, well differ-entiated) are excluded. Other rare varieties with better (periosteal) or worse (Pagetoid, radiation-induced) prognosis are also ineligible.
2.  Non-metastatic osteosarcoma of bones of the extremity only. Tumours of axial skeleton including pelvis, scapula, clavicle, jaw, etc., are usually excluded, as are multifocal tumours.
3.  The age range varies but usually excludes patients above the age of 40 years (sometimes 30 years).
4.  Patients must have normal cardiac, renal, hepatic, haematological and pulmonary function.
5.  The patient's general physical (performance status) and mental con-dition usually must meet certain standards, and patients who have had a previous malignancy are ineligible.
6.  Previous chemotherapy (sometimes previous radiotherapy) is not per-mitted.
7.  Chemotherapy usually must commence within a specified time period after histological confirmation of the diagnosis (or definitive surgery).
8.  For trials of preoperative (neoadjuvant) chemotherapy, any surgery other than biopsy generally will exclude the patient.
9.  Informed consent must be obtained according to institutional or national requirements.

An imbalance of prognostic factors between compared groups could skew results. Although in single-arm studies known prognostic factors can be matched in experimental and control groups, it is clear that some variables may as yet be unknown. Large randomized studies are most likely to produce well-matched groups. Taylor et al (1985), reviewing the Mayo Clinic experience of 336 patients with osteosarcoma treated between 1963 and 1981, identified six unfavourable characteristics: age younger than 10 years, male sex, tumour diameter more than 15 cm, cell type osteoblastic or chondroblastic, duration of symptoms 2 months or less, and involvement of the femur or humerus.

## SINGLE AGENT AND COMBINATION CHEMOTHERAPY

Chemotherapy has always produced rather unimpressive results in metastatic disease. Collected data on the most active single agents are presented in Table 1, and the results of several drug combinations are detailed in Table 2. While not exhaustive, these data give a fair indication of the effects of chemotherapy on established metastatic disease. In contrast with the earlier studies evaluating ADR, HDMTX and IFOS, the majority of patients receiving DDP had already received chemotherapy, which may account for the rather low overall response rate documented in Table 1. Results in previously untreated patients are likely to be considerably better, e.g. two partial responses in six patients in the European Organization for Research on Treatment of Cancer Study (Gasparini et al, 1985). There are no data to document the single agent activity of BLEO. Durations of response have

**Table 1.** Single-agent chemotherapy for metastatic osteosarcoma.

| Drug | No. evaluable | Overall response | | References |
|------|------|------|------|------|
| | | No. | % | |
| CPD | 28 | 4 | 14 ⎫ | |
| DACT | 25 | 2 | 8 | |
| L-PAM | 32 | 5 | 16 ⎪ | |
| MIT-C | 76 | 11 | 14 ⎬ | Pratt, 1979 |
| VCR | 21 | 0 | 0 | Bramwell and Pinedo, 1982 |
| DTIC | 14 | 2 | 14 ⎪ | |
| ADR | 183 | 39 | 21 ⎭ | |
| DDP | 115 | 21 | 18 | Pratt, 1979; Samson et al, 1979; Rosen et al, 1980b; Gasparini et al, 1985; Pratt et al, 1985. |
| IFOS | 78 | 19 | 24 | Brade, 1985; Klegar et al, 1986; EORTC, unpublished. |
| HDMTX* | 102 | 26 | 25 | Isacoff et al, 1978; Ambinder et al, 1979; Pratt et al, 1980; Rosen et al, 1980a; Edmonson et al, 1981; Jaffe et al, 1981; Vaughn et al, 1984; Wagener et al, 1986. |

* Often preceded by VCR.

**Table 2.** Combination chemotherapy for metastatic osteosarcoma.

| Combination | No. evaluable | No. of responses | | Overall responses (%) | Reference |
|---|---|---|---|---|---|
| | | Complete | Partial | | |
| ADIC +/− VCR | 46 | 3 | 13 | 35 ⎫ | Benjamin et al, 1978 |
| CYVADIC | 29 | 1 | 6 | 24 ⎬ | |
| CYVADACT | 20 | 2 | 3 | 25 ⎭ | |
| BCD† | 11 | 0 | 4 | '36' | Mosende et al, 1977 |
| VCR/HDMTX/CPD/ADR | 8 | 2 | 2 | '50' | Pratt et al, 1978 |
| ADR/CPD escalating +/− HDMTX | 11 | 1 | 1 | '9' | Levine et al, 1978 |
| MAV/OMAD/ALOMAD | 40 | — | — | 17.5 | Magill et al, 1977 |
| T7 | 10 | 0 | 8 | '80' | Rosen et al, 1979a |
| 5FU/DDP* | 9 | 0 | 0 | 0 | Land et al, 1981 |
| ADR/DDP/CYCLO +/− BLEO | 13 | 6 | | '46' | Edmonson et al, 1983, 1984a |
| ADR/DDP* | 20 | 4 | 3 | 35 | Rosen et al, 1982b |
| ADR/DDP† | 19 | 2 | 3 | 26 | Pratt et al, 1985 |
| DDP/VP-16-213* | 6 | 1 | 1 | '33' | Gasparini et al, 1982 |
| DDP/VCR/HDMTX* | 29 | 2 | 6 | 28 | Morgan et al, 1984 |
| ADR/DDP/MITC | 11 | 5 | | '45' | Edmonson et al, 1985 |
| DDP/VCR/HDMTX† | 15 | 5 | 5 | '66' | Gasparini et al, 1986 |

* Received previous chemotherapy.

† Some had received previous chemotherapy.

Quotation marks indicate that the response rate is derived from very small numbers.

generally been short, although prolonged remissions and probably cures
have been achieved by chemotherapy combined with surgery (Rosen et al,
1978). However, as resection of pulmonary metastases without the addition
of chemotherapy may also be curative, the exact role of chemotherapy in the
management of metastatic disease (palliative versus curative) remains in
doubt.

More recently, interest has focused on the effects of chemotherapy on
primary tumours. In this situation, assessment of response is much more
complex and is based on a combination of clinical, laboratory, radiological
and pathological features. Clinical features include reduction in pain and
swelling, but the latter may be misleading, particularly around a joint where
effusions may occur after biopsy and muscle atrophy may ensue with disuse.
A fall in alkaline phosphatase (if elevated) has been regarded as evidence of
response (Thorpe et al, 1979; Juergens et al, 1981), and a number of
radiological techniques including radio-isotope scanning (Reiman et al,
1981), plain radiography (Smith et al, 1982), CT (Mail et al, 1985) and
angiography (Chuang et al 1982) may be used to evaluate response.
Magnetic resonance imaging is under active investigation.

A number of groups in the USA and Europe (Rosen et al, 1979b;
Salzer-Kuntschik et al, 1983; Picci et al, 1985; Raymond et al, 1986) have
proposed pathological grading systems for determination of response in
patients treated with preoperative chemotherapy, but the accuracy and
reproducibility of these techniques remains to be verified. Data on primary
tumour response to intravenous single agents are available only for
HDMTX, as most adjuvant regimens with a preoperative component have
used HDMTX alone or combinations of drugs. Rosen et al (1980) reported a
clinical response in 38 out of 44 (86%) primary tumours treated with weekly
HDMTX, although Jaffe et al (1985a) were only able to achieve 4 (27%)
responses in 15 patients treated in a similar way. Rosen's group also
reported that BCD (see Appendix 2) had activity against primary osteosarcoma (Mosende et al, 1977). The effects of other drug combinations in
primary osteosarcoma are dealt with in the sections reviewing trials of
adjuvant chemotherapy in operable disease.

## ADJUVANT CHEMOTHERAPY

### Non-randomized studies

The results of 26 non-randomized studies performed between 1969 and 1985
are summarized in Table 3. Only eight of these studies included more than 50
patients, and with the exception of the studies (Rosen et al, 1983) performed
at Memorial Sloan Kettering (MSK) and Paris (Kalifa et al, 1986), chemotherapy was generally given after ablative surgery. Some patients in more
recent studies underwent limb salvage procedures (Campanacci et al, 1981;
Eilber et al, 1984; Eckardt et al, 1985) and/or preoperative chemotherapy
(Lange et al, 1982). Wherever possible, figures for relapse-free (and overall)
survival have been quoted as 5-year actuarial figures (Table 3) where the

**Table 3.** Adjuvant therapy for operable osteosarcoma—non-randomized studies.

| Group (reference) dates of study | Chemotherapy | Treatment of primary tumour | No. of evaluable patients | Local recurrence | Metastases | Follow-up | 5-year RFS (%) | 5-year OS (%) |
|---|---|---|---|---|---|---|---|---|
| *NCI* (Hoover et al, 1978) 1969–1972 | Warfarin | A | 9 | 0 | 4 | 5–8 yr | 44 | 56 |
| *South West Oncology Group* (Herson et al, 1980) | | | | | | | | |
| 1971–1973 | CONPADRI-I† | A | 47 | | 22 | >6 yr | 49 | } NS |
| 1973–1975 | COMPADRI-II† | A | 55 | | 31 | >3 yr | 35 | |
| 1974–1978 | COMPADRI-III† | A | 98 | | 43 | 1–5 yr | 39 | |
| *CALGB* (Cortes et al, 1978, 1981) 1975–1975 | ADR | A | 88 | 3 | 40 | >6 yr | 48 | NS |
| *Boston* (Goorin et al, 1985) | | | | | | | | |
| 1972–1974 | VCR/HDMTX | A | 12 | 0 | 7 | >10 yr | 42 | 67 |
| 1974–1975 | VCR/HDMTX/ADR | A | 22 | 0 | 9 | 8.5–9.8 yr | 59 | 68 |
| 1976–1981 | Intensive VCR/HDMTX/ADR | A26, L20 | 46 | 1(L) | 18 | 4.7–7.8 yr | 60 | 78 |
| *Seattle* (Bleyer et al, 1982) 1972–1977 | ADR/VCR/HDMTX | A | 18 | 1 | 7 | median 5 yr | 61 | 59 |
| *Bologna* (Campanacci et al, 1981) | All heparin | | | | | | | |
| 1972–1976 | VCR/ADR/LDMTX | A102 | 55 | 8 | 27 | 5 yr | } 45 | NS |
| 1976–1977 | ADR | L15 | 35 | 1 | 16 median | 3 yr | | |
| 1978 | VCR/MDMTX/ADR | | 27 | 1 | 9 | 18 mo | | |
| *Roswell Park* (Ettinger et al, 1986) 1976–1980 | ADR/DDP | A20, L2 | 22 | 2 (L1) | 6 | all 5 yr | 64 | 77 |
| *Philadelphia* (Lange et al, 1982) 1975–1979 | ADR/VCR/HDMTX | A16, L2 | 18* | 2 (L) | 12 | median 4 yr | 33 | 33 |

\* Most received preoperative chemotherapy.
† See Appendix 2.
A = amputation.
L = limb salvage.

mo = months.
NS = not stated.
OS = overall survival.
RFS = relapse-free survival.

median follow-up is at least 5 years. However, for many studies (Table 4, except MSK T4, T5 and T7), follow-up is much shorter and the results must be interpreted with caution.

The first multiagent adjuvant regimen used for osteosarcoma was the CONPADRI-I (see Appendix 2) programme initiated by the South-West Oncology Group. Interestingly enough, despite the addition of HDMTX (COMPADRI-II) and later intensification of the ADR dosage (COMPADRI-III) with the intention of preventing relapse, the results of later protocols were slightly (but not significantly) worse (Herson et al, 1980).

It is evident from the results presented in Tables 3 and 4, and also in Tables 5 and 6, that the relapse-free survivals (RFS) at 5 years for most studies with sufficient follow-up lie between 40 and 60%. The results achieved with VCR/HDMTX/ADR have been quite variable, with RFS ranging from 33 to 61%, and it seems unlikely that minor differences in scheduling could account for this discrepancy. The use of DDP instead of HDMTX, in combination with ADR (Ettinger et al, 1986), was associated with an impressive RFS rate of 65% (all patients were followed for more than 5 years). The major criticism of this study is its small accrual.

In Sweden, the results of adjuvant interferon (Strander et al, 1979) (Table 4) were compared with the outcome for contemporary controls taken from the Swedish National Tumour Registry. Life table analysis predicted that 58% of 33 patients given interferon would be free of metastases at 3 years compared with 37% of the 30 contemporary non-randomized controls. Subsequently, Brostrom et al (1980) published a comparison of two groups of Swedish patients treated surgically for osteosarcoma. The historical group (35 patients) were managed at the Karolinska Institute between 1952 and 1972, and the contemporary group (33 patients) were treated at other centres in Sweden between 1972 and 1974 (and represented some of the controls for Strander's study). Clear differences between the two groups, relating to the period of treatment, were evident, e.g. management after the appearance of metastases, and illustrated the problems associated with the use of historical controls. However, other differences between the groups (size, site, grade of malignancy) were apparent, and clearly demonstrate the fallacy of making comparisons with even contemporary non-randomized control subjects.

The series of protocols from MSK (Table 4) demonstrates several unique features. The first regimen (T4) involved the use of postoperative adjuvant chemotherapy with VCR/HDMTX/ADR (Rosen et al, 1983). Refinements in surgical techniques in the early 1970s opened up the possibilities of limb salvage by 'en bloc' resections of primary tumours and replacement by prostheses or allografts. As such implants needed to be custom-fitted, delays in surgery were inevitable, and the advantages of preoperative or 'neo-adjuvant' chemotherapy were evident. A pilot study—T5—using ADR/ VCR/HDMTX preoperatively and the same drugs with CPD postoperatively, demonstrated a high degree of histological necrosis in resected specimens from approximately half of the 31 patients. In the T7 protocol, all patients received preoperative chemotherapy, children aged less than 12 years

**Table 4.** Adjuvant therapy for operable osteosarcoma—non-randomized studies.

| Group (reference) dates of study | Chemotherapy | Treatment of primary tumour | No. of evaluable patients | Local recurrence | Metastases | Follow-up | RFS (%) | OS (%) |
|---|---|---|---|---|---|---|---|---|
| *Milan* (Fossati-Bellani et al, 1979) 1974–1978 | ADR | A | 17 | 0 | 10 | 1–48 mo | 47 | NS |
| *Stockholm* (Strander et al, 1979) 1972–1975 | IFN* | A18, L15 | 33 | NS | NS | 3 yr | 58 | 68 |
| *UCLA* (Eilber et al, 1984; Eckardt et al, 1985) | | | | | | | | |
| 1972–1974 | BCG + autologous cells | A | 9 | 0 | 9 | 1–32 mo | 0 | 0 |
| 1974–1981 | ADR/VCR/HDMTX (preoperative IA ADR + XRT) | L | 57 | 2 | NS | 32 mo | 62 | NS |
| *St Jude* (Pratt et al, 1984) | | | | | | | | |
| 1973–1977 | HDMTX/ADR/CPD Intensive | A | 26 | 0 | 13 | 4–59 mo | 50 | NS |
| 1977–1981 | HDMTX/ADR/CPD | A | 51 | 1 | 25 | 1–30 mo | 51 | NS |
| *NCI* (Rosenberg et al, 1979) 1975–1977 | HDMTX +/– VCR | A | 39 | 22 | | median 27 mo | 38 | NS |

| | ADR/HDMTX | A | 26 | 0 | 9 | 1–4 yr | 65 | 69 |
|---|---|---|---|---|---|---|---|---|
| *Toronto* (Sonley et al, 1979) 1974–1979 | ADR/HDMTX | A | 26 | 0 | 9 | 1–4 yr | 65 | 69 |
| *Memorial* (Rosen et al, 1983) | | | | | | | | |
| 1973–1976 | T4/T5§ | A23, L29 | 52**† | 5 (L) | NS | 80 mo | 48 | ⎱ approx. |
| 1976–1978 | T7§ | A34, L20 | 54**‡ | 4 (L) | NS median | 54 mo | 80 | the same |
| 1978–1981 | T10§ | A42, L37 | 79**‡ | 2 (L) | NS | 22 mo | 92 | ⎰ as RFS |
| (Rosen, 1985) 1981–1985 | T12 | NS | 51 | 6 | NS | median 2 yr | 75 | 76 |
| *Paris* (Kalifa et al, 1986) 1981–1985 | T10 | A8, L41 | 49 | 9 | 9 | median 2 yr | 75 | NS |

\* Leukocyte interferon.
\*\* Only includes patients aged more than 21 years.
† 29 received preoperative chemotherapy.
‡ Most received preoperative chemotherapy.
§ See Appendix 2.
A = amputation.
IA = intra-arterial.
L = limb salvage.
mo = months.
NS = not stated.
OS = overall survival.
RFS = relapse-free survival.
XRT = radiotherapy.

**Table 5.** Adjuvant therapy for operable osteosarcoma—randomized studies.

| Group (reference) dates of study | Adjuvant treatment | Treatment of primary tumour | No. of evaluable patients | Follow-up | RFS (%) | Difference between arms |
|---|---|---|---|---|---|---|
| *MAYO* (Gilchrist et al, 1981) 1969–1972 | Lung XRT + DACT vs 0 | A | 26 27 | median 18 mo | 42 38 | None |
| *EORTC* (Breur et al, 1979) 1970–1975 | lung XRT vs 0 | A | 44 42 | 26–72 mo | 43 28 | Borderline significance P = 0.06 |
| *MAYO* (Gilchrist et al, 1981) 1974–1975 | Transfer factor vs ADR/VCR/HDMTX | A | 17‡ 18 | median 2 yr | 42 33 | None |
| *NCI* (Rosenberg et al, 1979) 1975–1977 | BCG vs 0 (all VCR/HDMTX) | A | 18 20 | median 27 mo | 38 | None P = 0.2 |
| *COSS-80* (Winkler et al, 1984) 1979–1982 | IFN* vs 0 (all ADR/VCR/HDMTX† BCD or DDP) | A53 L54 | 45 63 | median 20 mo | 77 73 | None |

* Fibroblast interferon.
† Received preoperative chemotherapy.
‡ 4 received ADR/VCR/HDMTX.
A = amputation.
L = limb salvage.
mo = months.
RFS = relapse-free survival.
XRT = radiation.

**Table 6.** Adjuvant therapy for operable osteosarcoma—randomized studies.

| Group (reference) dates of study | Adjuvant treatment | Treatment of primary tumour | No. of evaluable patients | Follow-up | RFS (%) | Difference between arms |
|---|---|---|---|---|---|---|
| CALGB (Cortes and Holland, 1981) 1975–1980 | ADR vs ADR/HDMTX | A | 51 / 38 | median 34 mo | 52 / 40 | Significant difference (P = 0.02) for ADR |
| MRC (UK) (MRC, 1986) 1975–1981 | VCR-MDMTX vs ADR/VCR/MDMTX | A | 99 / 95 | 26–94 mo | 27 | None |
| NCI (C) (Jenkin et al, 1981) 1976–1980 | ADR/HDMTX Concurrent vs ADR/HDMTX sequential | A | 60 / 53 | 5–9 yr | 51 / 41 | None |
| EORTC (Burgers et al, 1985) 1978–1983 | Lung XRT vs ADR/VCR/HDMTX + XRT short vs ADR/VCR/HDMTX/CPD prolonged | A | 73 / 67 / 64 | median 43 mo | 30 | None |
| COSS-80 (Winkler et al, 1984) 1979–1983 | BCD vs DDP (all received ADR/VCR/HDMTX +/− IFN) | A53 / L54 | 59 / 49 | median 20 mo | 77 / 73 | None |
| Bologna (Bacci et al, 1985) 1980–1983 | MDMTX/ADR vs HDMTX | A70 / L22 | 51 / 41 | median 34 mo | 63 / 49 | None |

A = amputation.   RFS = relapse-free survival.
L = limb salvage.   XRT = radiotherapy.
mo = months.

receiving higher doses of MTX, and a further group of drugs—BCD (see Appendix 2)—was added. A second innovative measure was the intro- duction of an ADR/DDP combination postoperatively in those patients whose tumours showed a poor degree of necrosis after preoperative chemo- therapy (T10 regimen). This concept, which is based on the assumption that chemotherapy will have a similar effect on the primary tumour and micro- metastatic disease, has been challenged by Simon et al (1986). They found that, in five patients, there were considerable disparities in the percentages of necrosis seen in simultaneously resected primary and metastatic deposits from the same patient.

The results of the T7 and T10 regimens remain unequalled in the literature. Some other studies using chemotherapy based on the T10 regimen are discussed below, and others are in progress. The relapse-free survival (RFS) figure at 2 years for the T10 regimen reported by Kalifa et al (1986) is inferior to the 92% survival figure published by Rosen et al (1983). The latter results have been updated for 87 patients receiving only preoperative chemotherapy, for whom the RFS figure is 77%, with follow-up ranging from 3 to 6 years (Rosen, 1985). The most recent protocol—T12—shortens chemotherapy for those achieving a complete response of the primary tumour on HDMTX/ BCD, so that they receive a total of only 15 weeks of treatment (Rosen, 1985). After a median follow-up period of 2 years, it is stated that the RFS figure (75%) was not significantly different from the T10 protocol. It is not clear whether this comparison takes into account the different follow-up experience of the 2 groups, as the 2-year RFS figure for the T10 regimen was reported as 92% (Rosen et al, 1983). Approximately 50% of the patients (exact number not stated) were able to terminate chemotherapy at 15 weeks.

### Randomized studies

#### Adjuvant immunotherapy and lung irradiation

The results of three studies evaluating the effectiveness of adjuvant *immunotherapy* are summarized in Table 5. Patients receiving adjuvant chemotherapy did not benefit from the addition of bacillus Calmette-Guérin (BCG)(Rosenberg et al, 1979) or interferon (Winkler et al, 1984) in trials from the National Cancer Institute (NCI) US and a German multicentre group (COSS-80) respectively. In a study from the Mayo Clinic (Gilchrist et al, 1981), the RFS and overall survival figures did not differ significantly between groups receiving adjuvant chemotherapy or transfer factor, neither doing better than historical surgical controls. Table 5 also contains the results of two conflicting studies examining the value of lung irradiation. The study from the Mayo Clinic (Gilchrist et al, 1981) was negative but the European Organization for Research on Treatment of Cancer (EORTC) (Breur et al, 1978), using a slightly higher dose of irradiation (2000 rad versus 1500 rad), found an improvement in a 2-year RFS figure of borderline significance but no significant difference in overall survival. Benefit was only apparent in patients aged less than 17 years and in patients treated in three of the collaborating centres, excluding Paris which entered 43% of the total. The reasons for these discrepancies were not clear.

*Comparisons of adjuvant chemotherapy regimens*

The results of five randomized studies comparing different chemotherapy regimens (also lung irradiation in the EORTC study) are shown in Table 6. The Cancer and Acute Leukaemia Group B (CALGB) study (Cortes and Holland, 1981) demonstrated a significant advantage for the intensive use of Adriamycin (30 mg/m² day × 3 every 4 weeks for six courses) compared with two courses of ADR alternating with two courses of HDMTX for a total of six courses of each drug. It is interesting to note that administering HDMTX concurrently with ADR in each 28-day cycle (Jenkin et al, 1981) was as good as giving six cycles of ADR (as in the CALGB study), although this was followed by 11 cycles of HDMTX. In the Medical Research Council trial (1986) it seems likely that both chemotherapy regimens had a minimal effect in delaying or preventing metastasis. In this large study, the chemotherapy was given at a lower dosage and intensity than that used in other protocols.

It is possible that the adjuvant chemotherapy regimens used in the EORTC trial (Burgers et al, 1985) had some effect in delaying the appearance of metastases, as there were early differences in the RFS figure in favour of chemotherapy (unpublished data) which disappeared with longer follow-up. It seems likely that the eventual outcome for all three treatments will be little better than historical controls. The failure of the German multicentre trial to find any difference between BCD and DDP in the context of multi-drug adjuvant chemotherapy (a regimen based on MSK T10) may be attributable to a lack of dose intensity (each given four times at 8-week intervals) rather than to equivalency of the regimens. In addition, the numbers in the study would preclude the detection of small differences. Bacci et al (1985) were unable to demonstrate that HDMTX (2 g/m²) was any more effective than a medium dose of the drug (200 mg/m²), although again the numbers accrued to this study would not permit the detection of small differences in the RFS figures. The dose of methotrexate in the high-dose arm was considerably lower than that advocated by other workers (Jaffe et al, 1974; Rosen et al, 1981).

*Adjuvant chemotherapy compared with control*

The excellent early results of pilot studies of adjuvant chemotherapy (Jaffe et al, 1974; Rosen et al, 1974; Sutow et al, 1974) compared with the grim fate of historical controls were hailed as a therapeutic triumph and 'a milestone in the treatment of this disease' (Burchenal, 1974). Some clouds appeared on the horizon when late relapses occurred, and it became evident that 5-year RFS figures for most studies were of the order of 40–50%. Nevertheless, these results still compared favourably with the corresponding figures of less than 20% for 5-year RFS figures for historical controls. Results reported by the Mayo Clinic (Taylor et al, 1978) then created major doubts about the efficacy of adjuvant chemotherapy and the validity of historical controls. This retrospective analysis revealed significant improvements in 2-year RFS figures for the periods 1969–1971 and 1972–1974, which were 43% and 30% respectively, compared with 13% between 1963 and 1968. This was independent of adjuvant treatment. Corresponding improvements in overall survival were also evident, but an aggressive policy of resection of pulmonary metastases in later years was certainly contributory.

Based on these findings, investigators at the Mayo Clinic initiated in November 1976 the first study of adjuvant chemotherapy (VCR/HDMTX $3–7.5 \, g/m^2$ every 3 weeks $\times$ 1 year) to include a concurrent randomized control group treated by surgery alone. The results of this study, which accrued patients very slowly, were first reported in 1980 (Edmonson et al, 1980), and a definitive paper on the 5-year results (Edmonson et al, 1984b) appeared in 1984 (Table 7). Actuarial analysis estimated 42% of patients remaining continuously relapse-free with no significant difference in outcome between the two arms.

This series of results provoked a spate of editorials and review articles (Frei et al, 1978; Muggia and Loule, 1978; Carter, 1980; Lange and Levine, 1982; Rosen and Nirenberg, 1982; Jaffe et al, 1983; Link and Vietti, 1983; Carter, 1984; Editorial, 1985; Goorin et al, 1985) questioning or defending the value of adjuvant chemotherapy for extremity osteosarcomas. A central issue was the implication from the Mayo Clinic results that the natural history of the disease was changing and that osteosarcoma had become a less aggressive tumour. Some indirect evidence that this was not so is provided by two trials from Europe (Table 6) performed between 1975 and 1983 (Burgers et al, 1985; Medical Research Council (MRC), 1986) which report 4–5 RFS figures of 30% and 27% respectively for large series of patients. Unless one postulates that the adjuvant regimens were detrimental (there were two toxic deaths in 194 patients in the MRC study, and 1 in 204 patients in the EORTC study), it would seem that there have not been major changes in the natural history of osteosarcoma.

In the early 1980s two groups designed studies to resolve this controversial issue. Both compared groups receiving intensive multiagent chemotherapy, based on the MSK T10 regimen, with concurrently randomized surgical control patients, and the results are summarized in Table 7. In the Multi-Institutional Osteosarcoma Study (MIOS) all chemotherapy was given after definitive surgery (Link et al, 1986), whereas 79% of patients in the UCLA study (Eckardt et al, 1985) were managed by limb salvage procedures after preoperative intra-arterial ADR and irradiation (both arms). In both trials, the 2-year RFS figure was significantly better for the groups receiving adjuvant chemotherapy, and the studies were terminated in 1984. After such short follow-up, figures for overall survival were not significantly different. The numbers randomized in these studies were small, and in the MIOS the accrual was exceeded by patients refusing randomization. The results comparing patients who chose their adjuvant treatment paralleled those of the randomized study (Table 7). The very poor results seen in the control group of each of those trials also refute the theory of a change in the

**Table 7.** Adjuvant therapy for operable osteosarcoma—randomized trials with control arm treated by surgery alone.

| Group (reference) dates of study | Chemotherapy | Treatment of primary tumour | No. of evaluable patients | Relapse | Follow-up | RFS (%) | OS (%) | Difference between arms |
|---|---|---|---|---|---|---|---|---|
| *MAYO* (Edmonson et al, 1984b) 1976–1980 | VCR/HDMTX vs 0 | A37 L1 | 20 / 18 | 12 / 10 | median 5 yr | 5 yr 42 | 5 yr 52 | Not significant |
| *UCLA* (Eckardt et al, 1985) 1981–1984 | T10A vs 0 | A11 L41 | 24 / 28 | 10 / 18 | median 15 mo | 2 yr 49 / 21 | 3 yr 71 / 29 | RFS $P < 0.033$ ; OS $P < 0.025$ |
| *MIOS* (Link et al, 1986) 1982–1984 | *Randomized* T10 modified vs 0 | A14 L4 / A14 L4 | 18 / 18* | 15 / 6 | median 2 yr | 66 / 17 | 2 yr approx. 72 | RFS $P < 0.001$ ; OS not significant |
| | *Non-randomized* T10 modified vs 0 | A44 L15 / A17 L1 | 59 / 18 | 16 / 15 | median 2 yr | 67 / 9 | approx. 85 / approx. 70 | NS |

* 3 received immediate chemotherapy.

mo = months.
NS = not stated.
OS = overall survival.
RFS = relapse-free survival.

natural history of osteosarcoma. In December 1984 a consensus development conference on limb sparing treatment of adult soft tissue sarcomas and osteosarcomas was held at the National Institutes of Health, USA. One of the briefs of the review panel was to answer the question 'Are there types of patients with extremity sarcoma for whom adjuvant chemotherapy is indicated?' The conclusion of the panel (National Institutes of Health, Consensus Development Panel, 1985) was that 'although further follow-up . . . is required, the panel is optimistic that adjuvant systemic chemotherapy will ultimately prove beneficial to the well-being and survival of patients with osteosarcoma'.

## CURRENT QUESTIONS

Although the balance of opinion is currently in favour of adjuvant chemotherapy, many questions remain concerning the exact nature of this treatment. Three broad areas are being explored by current trials: intra-arterial chemotherapy, the composition and duration of chemotherapy, and the modification of current combination chemotherapy by the introduction of new agents.

### Intra-arterial chemotherapy

Clear evidence of clinical and pathological tumour response to preoperative chemotherapy, associated with new surgical techniques and more durable prostheses, had led to a dramatic increase in the numbers of patients considered suitable for limb salvage procedures (Benjamin, 1985). Many investigators believe that more direct delivery of active agents to the tumour by the intra-arterial route will increase local tumour destruction and facilitate limb salvage in a larger number of patients. The results of several studies, using intra-arterial DDP, are presented in Table 8. In the two largest series the results of limb salvage are 76% (Picci et al, 1986) and 66% (Benjamin et al, 1986) with low rates of local recurrence. Eckhardt et al (1985), using intra-arterial ADR and irradiation, were able to carry out limb-sparing procedures in 67% of their patients. Two studies using preoperative intravenous chemotherapy describe lower rates of lower salvage of 47% (Rosen et al, 1983) and 50% (Winkler et al, 1984). It is difficult to make comparisons between these studies as they were not all contemporary, the German trial (Winkler et al, 1984) was multicentre and there will be variations in surgical attitudes and expertise between centres. Not surprisingly, the overall outcome in terms of the RFS figures is not dissimilar between studies using intra-arterial and intravenous chemotherapy. A randomized study is needed to determine whether the advantages of intra-arterial chemotherapy outweighs its hazards, expense and inconvenience.

### The composition and duration of chemotherapy

The current German multicentre study, COSS-82 (Winkler et al, 1986),

**Table 8.** Adjuvant therapy for operable osteosarcoma—intra-arterial cisplatin.

| Author (reference) | Chemotherapy | Treatment of primary tumour | No. of evaluable patients | Response (pathological) | Metastases | Follow-up | RFS (%) | OS (%) |
|---|---|---|---|---|---|---|---|---|
| Jaffe et al (1985) | DDP 150 mg/m² every 14–21 d × 2–4 | A6 L7 None 2 | 15 | 7 complete 2 partial | 7 | NS | 53 | 73 |
| Picci et al (1986) | DDP 120–150 mg/m² 72 hr infusion every 5w × 2 + HDMTX i.v. or MDMTX i.v. | A22 L71 | 93 54 39 | 50 good 32 fair 11 poor | 25 (1LR) | 5–29 mo | NS | NS |
| Petrilli et al (1986) | DDP 100 mg/m² every 2w × 2–5 + i.v. ADR/DDP | A39 L19 | 58 | NS | 10 (1LR) | median 20 mo | 59 | 90 |
| Benjamin et al (1984, 1986) | DDP 120–200 mg/m² + i.v. ADR DTIC or BCD | A22 L43 | 65 | approx 55% (>90% necrosis) | NS | 3 yr | 65 | NS |

A = amputation.
d = days.
L = limb salvage.
LR = local recurrence.
mo = months.
NS = not stated.
OS = overall survival.
RFS = relapse-free survival.
w = weeks.

suggests that reserving potent drugs such as ADR and DDP for postoperative treatment in patients showing a poor response to preoperative chemotherapy with HDMTX and BCD is detrimental. The current Children's
Cancer Study Group trial is a single-arm study re-evaluating the MSK T10
regimen in a multicentre setting, and to date has not been reported. Dis-
satisfied with the results of their most recent studies, the British MRC and
the EORTC/International Society for Paediatric Oncology (SIOP) have
joined forces—the European Osteosarcoma Intergroup (EOI)—and have
just completed a pilot study evaluating two short (15 week), intensive
adjuvant regimens—ADR/DDP vs HDMTX/ADR/DDP. Preliminary data
(Bramwell, 1987) suggest an advantage for the two-drug regimen, with
results very similar to the multi-institutional studies using the T10 type of
protocols. A new study (opened September, 1986) therefore seeks to
determine whether such a short intensive treatment is as effective as the
longer, complex, more expensive and toxic T10 regimen pioneered by MSK
(Rosen et al, 1983).

### Modification of current combination chemotherapy by the introduction of new agents

Ifosfamide has shown significant activity in metastatic osteosarcoma (Table
1) and merits evaluation in combination chemotherapy. A pilot study
recently initiated by the EOI introduces ifosfamide into the ADR/DDP
regimen, and will assess the incidence of regression in primary and metastatic disease as well as the adjuvant effect of this new combination. The
Paediatric Oncology Group and their collaborators are also preparing a
study along these lines.

## MANAGEMENT OF PATHOLOGICAL VARIANTS OF OSTEOSARCOMA

### Parosteal osteosarcoma

Parosteal osteosarcoma is generally a well-differentiated tumour which
presents as a dense, lobulated mass arising superficially from the metaphyseal
region of a long bone, and involving the medullary cavity. Occasional foci of
high-grade sarcoma may be found in some tumours (Unni et al, 1976a). These
tumours have a propensity for local recurrence unless radically removed, but
metastasize infrequently, e.g., 4 of 27 cases treated by amputation in the
series reported by Unni et al (1976a). The optimum treatment is radical
resection, and systemic adjuvant chemotherapy would seem to be super-
fluous. However, the importance of adequate margins is emphasized by the
high rate of local recurrence after simple resection and, with increasing
interest in limb-salvage procedures, preoperative chemotherapy—either
intra-arterial or intravenous—may be beneficial for bulky tumours. As these
tumours are rare (< 1% of all osteosarcomas) there have been no series
evaluating the effects of chemotherapy locally or systemically.

## Periosteal osteosarcoma

In contrast with parosteal tumours, periosteal osteogenic sarcomas, which present as small radiolucent lesions at the bone surface, are characteristically high-grade lesions with chondroblastic differentiation. Nevertheless, in the series of 23 cases described by Unni et al (1976b), they seemed to do well when treated by surgery alone. Local recurrences appeared in five out of nine patients treated by excision or resection, but only one patient developed metastases after further resection or amputation. Three of the 13 patients treated by amputation eventually developed metastases. Hall et al (1985) reviewed 61 patients collected from the literature, of whom 10 had died of metastatic disease during a mean follow-up period of 6½ years. Systemic adjuvant chemotherapy does not seem appropriate, particularly in a tumour that frequently shows chondroblastic differentiation.

## Intraosseous, well-differentiated osteosarcoma

These tumours, also very rare, may be confused with benign lesions. They tend to recur after local excision but rarely metastasize [in 3 out of 27 cases described by Unni et al (1977)]. In contrast with periosteal osteosarcomas, they are intramedullary lesions. Management should follow the lines suggested for parosteal and periosteal tumours, radical resection being the definitive treatment.

## Telangiectatic osteosarcoma

These tumours are very different from the preceding three variants. They typically present as large lytic destructive tumours, located in the central metaphysis, often leading to fracture of the bone. Histologically, cystic spaces containing blood are lined by anaplastic spindle cells. Matsuno et al (1976) placed 25 out of 1000 osteosarcomas presenting to the Mayo Clinic in this category, of whom 23 (92%) had died of metastatic disease. In contrast, Huvos et al (1982) at MSK described 124 (11%) cases identified from 1129 cases on file from 1921 to 1979. Compared with 'classical' osteosarcoma, they were unable to demonstrate an adverse prognosis for the telangiectatic variant. A small subgroup of patients received adjuvant chemotherapy between 1975 and 1982 and 12 out of 16 were continuously disease-free. Tumours from 9 out of 11 patients receiving preoperative chemotherapy demonstrated more than 90% histological necrosis, and all of these patients were free of recurrence. In reviewing the cases from the MD Anderson Hospital, Chawla et al (1985) found that 9 out of 10 patients treated by amputation followed by CONPADRI-I (see Appendix 2) had relapsed and died with a median RFS figure of 10 months, whereas 8 patients treated with intra-arterial DDP together with intravenous ADR and DTIC (Table 8—Benjamin et al, 1984, 1986) had not relapsed after a median follow-up period of 19+ months. Histological necrosis of more than 95% was observed in five cases, with pathology pending in two. These tumours are clearly responsive to chemotherapy and should be included in current trials of adjuvant therapy.

## Osteosarcoma arising in Paget's disease (see Chapter 1, p 15)

In keeping with the age incidence of the primary disease, osteosarcomas arising in Paget's disease occur at a median age of 63 years (McKenna et al, 1964; Huvos et al, 1983; Smith et al, 1984), unlike 'classical' osteosarcoma which is commonest in the teenage years. Two large series (McKenna et al, 1964; Huvos et al, 1983) suggest an incidence of approximately 5% of all osteosarcomas. The outlook is appalling with 5-year survivals, in all series, of less than 5%. More than 50% of these tumours occur in the axial skeleton and are often very advanced at presentation precluding radical surgery. These factors, and the poor tolerance of intensive multiagent chemotherapy by an elderly group of patients, may account for the negligible impact of chemotherapy on this disease. The use of intensive adjuvant regimens would certainly be justified in the occasional younger, fitter patient, particularly if the primary tumour was potentially resectable.

## Post-irradiation osteosarcoma (see Chapter 1, p 12)

These tumours have an incidence and age distribution similar to that of Pagetoid osteosarcoma (Huvos et al, 1985). In the series from MSK described by Huvos et al (1985), the 5-year survival was 17%, suggesting that these tumours are not quite as aggressive as osteosarcomas occurring secondary to Paget's disease. Nevertheless, the prognosis is poor and again relates to the difficulty of achieving local eradication of axial primaries. There is insufficient information to judge the effects of chemotherapy, but previous exposure to certain drugs for the primary malignancy may limit the choice, and sclerosis of blood vessels as a late effect of radiation may limit drug access.

### Osteosarcoma of the jaws

Maxillary and mandibular osteosarcomas are locally aggressive tumours which typically occur in patients in their early 30s. Local control is a significant problem, particularly for maxillary tumours where radical resection may not be possible, but metastasis is uncommon (Garrington et al, 1967; Clark et al, 1983). Little information is available on the use of adjuvant chemotherapy, but the use of intra-arterial chemotherapy for bulky tumours may be worth exploring.

### Childhood multifocal osteosarcoma

The simultaneous appearance of two or more tumours at any site in the skeleton may be taken as evidence for this condition, although a single tumour with osseous metastases cannot be excluded. The absence of pulmonary metastases has been cited as evidence for a multicentric origin (Price, 1957). Nine paediatric cases (mean age 11 years) were described by Parham et al (1985), all of whom had multiple, densely sclerotic lesions, usually in metaphysical locations. The serum alkaline phosphatase was raised in all cases—mean 2.4 × normal—and appeared to reflect growth or regression of the tumours. Intensive combination chemotherapy based on HDMTX or ADR/DDP only produced four instances of temporary disease stabilization, and all patients died 6–37 months from diagnosis.

## FUTURE DIRECTIONS

There are many areas in which the management of osteosarcoma needs to be refined. There has always been concern about the durability of prostheses in young, physically active individuals, but considerable progress has already been made in improving the composition of metal alloys and the structural design of prostheses (see Chapter 5).

Despite the exceptional results reported from MSK (Rosen et al, 1983), it is likely that the present generation of large-scale chemotherapy trials will yield 5-year RFS rates of the order of 50–65%, with the possibility of a few late relapses. With an aggressive policy towards resection of pulmonary metastases, a further 10–20% of relapsing patients may be salvaged. There is still considerable room for improvement in current chemotherapy regimens, and the paucity of active drugs remains a problem. Current information suggests that only HDMTX, ADR and DDP have significant efficacy in osteosarcoma, although early data on ifosfamide are promising. A continued search for active new agents should have high priority, examining both analogues of present agents and novel structures.

Current chemotherapy regimens are very intensive and have many toxicities. Without exception they cause nausea, vomiting, alopecia and myelosuppression. Infection and bleeding due to the latter effect are occasionally responsible for chemotherapy-related deaths. Longer term side-effects are equally threatening, with the risks of cardiotoxicity, renal impairment, sterility and second malignancies being particularly important. Some studies are already in progress evaluating brief, intense treatments, and considerable progress has been made in many aspects of supportive care such as anti-emetic regimens, antibiotics and blood components. Intensive research in the field of analogue development has yielded some interesting new compounds such as Epiadriamycin, Carboplatin and Iproplatin. In such rare tumours as osteosarcomas, the adequate evaluation of analogues, particularly those which have been developed for their reduced toxicity rather than for their lack of cross-resistance, is a significant problem. In patients presenting with metastases synchronous with the primary tumour, consideration should be given to using these drugs as initial chemotherapy for one to two courses, with careful monitoring for evidence of progression. Iproplatin is an analogue of cisplatin, which, compared with the parent compound, has reduced renal, oto- and neurotoxicity (Bramwell et al, 1985) although the incidence of thrombocytopenia is significantly increased. This agent is currently being evaluated in a phase II study conducted by the Soft Tissue and Bone Sarcoma Group of the EORTC.

The concept of using monoclonal antibodies directed against antigens on the surface of the cancer cell, for diagnosis or therapy, has universal appeal. Pimm et al (1982) have developed such an antibody which reacts preferentially with human tumour xenografts of osteosarcoma. They have subsequently identified this human osteogenic sarcoma antigen as an integral membrane protein with an apparent molecular weight of 72 000 (Price et al, 1983). A radiolabelled antibody has been used for isotopic imaging of primary osteosarcoma in humans (Armitage et al, 1986). The therapeutic use of monoclonal antibodies may be limited by heterogeneity of antigen expression by the tumour and metastases. A group from the National Institutes of Health (NIH) (Roth et al, 1984), using a panel of four monoclonal antibodies, examined antigen expression by paired primary and autologous metastases from surgically excised osteogenic and soft-tissue sarcomas from 15 patients. They observed marked heterogeneity of binding intensity between primary and metastatic tumours, and of cells expressing antigen within tumours. This occurred even though primary and metastatic tumours demonstrated homogeneous histology and cellular morphology. Differences were noted between patients as well as among metastases taken from an individual. Clearly, more work is needed in this fascinating field before the technology can be applied therapeutically.

The observations of Rosenberg et al (1985), at the National Cancer Institute, of clear regressions of established metastases from generally resistant solid tumours following treatment with interleukin-2 and lymphokine-activated killer cells may offer therapeutic possibilities in the future. Although responses were only noted in melanoma, colon and renal cancer, with no effects on one osteosarcoma and three soft-tissue sarcomas, with further investigation and refinements this technique may have broad applications.

## CONCLUSIONS

There are many lessons to be learnt from a historical perspective of the use of adjuvant chemotherapy in osteosarcoma. The main issue, as to whether metastases could be prevented by intensive chemotherapy, has been clouded by a plethora of small, uncontrolled studies, each using slightly different regimens and reporting results in diverse ways and at different points in time. Comparison with historical controls was invalidated by concomitant advances in diagnostic and surgical techniques and supportive care. Evaluation of chemotherapy proceeded in an uncoordinated fashion and the necessary randomized studies were considered unethical in the early 1970s (Burchenal, 1974) but were eventually performed 10 years later. Research effort can now be directed towards improving results and reducing toxicity. It is generally considered axiomatic that chemotherapy regimens are only suitable as adjuvant treatments if they produce remissions (preferably complete) in more than 50% of patients with evaluable metastatic disease. Although this is not the case for osteosarcoma, there is no doubt that this level of response may be achieved in primary tumours, and possibly future studies in other tumour types should take into consideration activity of the drug regimen on the primary disease. For rare tumours such as osteosarcoma it is imperative that the majority of patients are entered into clinical trials attempting to answer the important remaining questions (which drugs in what sequence, the optimal route and duration of treatment, etc.) and the complexity of the options for limb salvage and adjuvant treatment make referral to specialist centres mandatory. Collaboration between centres (and even between nations as in Europe) is essential to achieve the large numbers of patients necessary for randomized trials. These numbers are essential if survival differences of the order of 5–10% are to be detected with confidence. Differences larger than this are unlikely to be achieved by modification of existing programmes. A steady, small improvement of the results of treatment is likely and each step must be properly validated to avoid the controversies of the past.

## APPENDIX 1: ABBREVIATIONS FOR DRUGS

| | |
|---|---|
| ADR | Adriamycin (doxorubicin hydrochloride) |
| BCG | Bacillus Calmette-Guerin |
| BLEO | Bleomycin |
| CLB | Chlorambucil |
| CPD | Cyclophosphamide |
| DACT | Actinomycin D |
| DDP | Cisplatin |
| DTIC | 5-(3,3 dimethyl-1-triazeno)imidazole carboxamide |
| 5FU | 5-Fluorouracil |
| HDMTX | High dose Methotrexate (M = medium dose, L = low dose) |
| IFN | Interferon |
| IFOS | Ifosfamide |
| L-PAM | Melphalan |
| MeCCNU | 1-(2,chloroethyl)-3-3(4 methyl-cyclohexyl)-1-nitrosourea |
| MITC | Mitomycin C |
| VCR | Vincristine |
| VP-16-213 | 4'dimethylepipodophyllotoxin-9-(4,6,0-ethylidine-B-D-glucopyranoside) |

## APPENDIX 2: ABBREVIATIONS FOR CHEMOTHERAPY REGIMENS

| | |
|---|---|
| ADIC | ADR/DTIC |
| ALOMAD | VCR/MDMTX/ADR/DACT/CLB/DTIC |
| BCD | BLEO/CPD/DACT |
| COMPADRI-II | HDMTX/CPD/VCR/L-PAM/ADR |
| COMPADRI-III | HDMTX/CPD/VCR/L-PAM/ADR (more intensive) |
| CONPADRI-I | CPD/VCR/L-PAM/ADR |
| CYVADACT | CPD/VCR/ADR/DACT |
| CYVADIC | CPD/VCR/ADR/DTIC |
| MAV | MeCCNU/ADR/VCR |
| OMAD | VDR/MDMTX/ADR/DACT |
| T4/5 | VCR/HDMTX/ADR/CPD (postoperatively only, T4; pre- and postoperatively, T5) |
| T7 | BCD/VCR/HDMTX/ADR/CPD (pre- and postoperative chemotherapy) |
| T10 | HDMTX/BCD/ADR +/− VCR (preoperative chemotherapy) **A** If poor (grade I, II) histological necrosis, ADR/DDP postoperatively **B** If good (grade III, IV) histological necrosis, continue HDMTX/BCD/ADR +/− VCR postoperatively |
| T12 | HDMTX/BCD +/− VCR (preoperative chemotherapy) **A** If poor (grade I, II) histological necrosis, ADR/DDP postoperatively × 6 (27 weeks total) **B** If good (grade III, IV) histological necrosis, continue HDMTX/BCD postoperatively (15 weeks total) |

# REFERENCES

Ambinder EP, Perloff M, Ohnuma T et al (1979) High dose Methotrexate followed by Citrovorum factor reversed in patients with advanced cancer. *Cancer* **43**: 1177–1182.

Armitage NC, Perkins AC, Pimm MV et al (1986) Imaging of bone tumors using a monoclonal antibody raised against human osteosarcoma. *Cancer* **58**: 37–42.

Bacci G, Campanacci M, Picci P et al (1985) Adjuvant chemotherapy (AC) with Adriamycin (ADR) with high and moderate dose of Methotrexate (MTX) for osteosarcoma of the extremities (OSE): an evaluation of results and comparison with a concurrent group treated with surgery alone. *Proceedings of the American Society of Clinical Oncology* **4**: 127.

Benjamin RS (Editorial) (1985) Limb salvage surgery for sarcomas: a good idea receives formal blessing. *Journal of the American Medical Association* **254**: 1795–1796.

Benjamin RS, Baker LH, O'Bryan RM et al (1978) Chemotherapy of metastatic osteosarcoma—studies by M.D. Anderson Hospital and the South West Oncology Group. *Cancer Treatment Reports* **62**: 237–238.

Benjamin RS, Murray JA, Wallace S et al (1984) Intra-arterial preoperative chemotherapy for osteosarcoma—a judicious approach to limb salvage. *Cancer Bulletin* **36**: 32–36.

Benjamin RS, Chawla SP, Carrasco CH et al (1986) Primary chemotherapy of patients with osteosarcoma of an extremity. *Proceedings of the American Society of Clinical Oncology* **5**: 139.

Bleyer WA, Haas JE, Feigl P et al (1982) Improved three year disease-free survival in osteogenic sarcoma. *Journal of Bone and Joint Surgery* **64B**: 233–238.

Brade WP, Herdrich K & Varini M (1985) Ifosfamide—pharmacology, safety and therapeutic potential. *Cancer Treatment Reviews* **12**: 1–47.

Bramwell V (1987) *Preliminary report of the first European Osteosarcoma Intergroup Study.* p 232. Abstract 884. Proceedings of the 4th European Conference on Clinical Oncology and Cancer Nursing.

Bramwell VHC & Pinedo HM (1982) Treatment of metastatic bone and soft tissue sarcomas. In Carter et al (eds) *Principles of Cancer Treatment*, pp 718–733. London: McGraw-Hill.

Bramwell VHC, Crowther D, O'Malley S et al (1985) Activity of JM9 in advanced ovarian cancer: a phase I-II trial. *Cancer Treatment Report* **69**: 409–416.

Breur K, Cohen P, Schweisguth O et al (1978) Irradiation of the lungs as an adjuvant therapy in the treatment of osteosarcoma of the limbs: an EORTC randomized study. *European Journal of Cancer* **14**: 461–471.

Brostrom L-A, Aparisi T, Ingimarsson S et al (1980) Can historical controls be used in current clinical trials in osteosarcoma? Analysis of prognostic factors. *International Journal of Radiation Oncology, Biology and Physics* **6**: 1711–1715.

Burchenal JH (1974) A giant step forward—if . . . *New England Journal of Medicine* **291**: 1029–1031.

Burgers JMV, Voute PA & Van Glabbeke M (1985) *Adjuvant Treatment for Osteosarcoma of the Limbs, Trial 20781 of the SIOP and the EORTC Radiotherapy/Chemotherapy Group*, p 65. Proceedings of the 3rd European Conference on Clinical Oncology and Cancer Nursing, Stockholm.

Campanacci M, Bacci G, Bertoni F et al (1981) The treatment of osteosarcoma of the extremities: twenty years experience at the Instituto Ortopedico Rizzoli. *Cancer* **48**: 1569–1581.

Carter SK (1980) The dilemma of adjuvant chemotherapy for osteogenic sarcoma. *Cancer Clinical Trials* **3**: 29–36.

Carter SK (Editorial) (1984) Adjuvant chemotherapy in osteogenic sarcoma: the triumph that isn't. *Journal of Clinical Oncology* **2**: 147–148.

Chawla SP, Raymond AK, Carrasco CH et al (1985) High rates of complete remission, limb salvage, and prolonged survival in telangiectatic osteosarcoma after preoperative chemotherapy with intra-arterial Cisplatinum and systemic Adriamycin. *Proceedings of the American Society of Clinical Oncology* **4**: 152.

Chuang VP, Benjamin R, Jaffe N et al (1982) Radiographic and angiographic changes in osteosarcoma after intra-arterial chemotherapy. *American Journal of Roentgenology* **139**: 1065–1069.

Clark JL, Unni KK, Dahlin DC et al (1983) Osteosarcoma of the jaw. *Cancer* **51:** 2311–2316.
Cortes EP & Holland JF (1981) Adjuvant chemotherapy for primary osteogenic sarcoma. *Surgical Clinics of North America* **61:** 1391–1404.
Cortes EP, Holland TD & Glidewell O (1978) Amputation and Adriamycin in primary osteosarcoma: a 5 year report. *Cancer Treatment Reports* **62:** 271–278.
Eckardt JJ, Eilber FR, Grant TT et al (1985) Management of stage IIB osteogenic sarcoma: experience at the University of California, Los Angeles. *Cancer Treatment Symposia* **3:** 117–130.
Editorial (1985) Osteosarcoma. *Lancet* **ii:** 131–133.
Edmonson JH, Green SJ, Ivins JC et al (1980) Methotrexate as adjuvant treatment for primary osteosarcoma. *New England Journal of Medicine* **303:** 642–643.
Edmonson JH, Creagan ET & Gilchrist GS (1981) Phase II study of high-dose Methotrexate in patients with unresectable metastatic osteosarcoma. *Cancer Treatment Reports* **65:** 538–539.
Edmonson JH, Hahn RG, Schutt AJ et al (1983) Cyclophosphamide, Doxorubicin and Cisplatin combined in the treatment of advanced sarcomas. *Medical and Paediatric Oncology* **11:** 319–321.
Edmonson JH, Creagan ET, Kvols LK et al (1984a) Failure of Bleomycin to improve the therapeutic effects of a combination of Cyclophosphamide, Doxorubicin and Cisplatin (CAP) in advanced sarcomas. *Medical and Paediatric Oncology* **12:** 264–266.
Edmonson JH, Green SJ, Ivins JC et al (1984b) A controlled pilot study of high-dose Methotrexate as post-surgical adjuvant treatment for primary osteosarcoma. *Journal of Clinical Oncology* **2:** 152–156.
Edmonson JH, Long HJ, Richardson RL et al (1985) Phase II study of a combination of Mitomycin, Doxorubicin and Cisplatin in advanced sarcomas. *Cancer Chemotherapy and Pharmacology* **15:** 181–182.
Eilber FR, Grant T & Morton DL (1978) Adjuvant therapy for osteosarcoma: preoperative and postoperative treatment. *Cancer Treatment Reports* **62:** 213–216.
Eilber FR, Eckhardt J & Morton DL (1984) Advances in the treatment of sarcomas of the extremity. Current status of limb salvage. *Cancer* **54:** 2695–2701.
Etcubanas E & Wilbur JR (1978) Adjuvant chemotherapy for osteogenic sarcoma. *Cancer Chemotherapy Reports* **62:** 283–288.
Ettinger LJ, Douglass HO, Higby DJ et al (1979) Adriamycin (ADR) and cis-Diamminedichloroplatinum (DDP) as adjuvant therapy in primary osteosarcoma (OS). *Proceedings of the American Society of Clinical Oncology* **20:** 438.
Ettinger LJ, Douglass HO, Higby DJ et al (1981) Adjuvant Adriamycin and cis-diamminedichloroplatinum (Cisplatinum) in primary osteosarcoma. *Cancer* **47:** 248–254.
Ettinger LJ, Douglass HO, Mindell ER et al (1986) Adjuvant Adriamycin and Cisplatin in newly diagnosed, non-metastatic osteosarcoma of the extremity. *Journal of Clinical Oncology* **4:** 353–362.
Fossati-Bellani F, Gasparini M & Bonadonna G (1979) Adriamycin in the adjuvant treatment of operable osteosarcoma. *Recent Results in Cancer Research* **68:** 25–27.
Frei E, Jaffe N, Gero M et al (1978) Adjuvant chemotherapy of osteogenic sarcoma: progress and perspectives. *Journal of the National Cancer Institute* **60:** 3–10.
Friedman MA & Carter SK (1972) The therapy of osteogenic sarcoma: current status and thoughts for the future. *Journal of Surgical Oncology* **4:** 482–510.
Garrington GE, Scofield HH, Cornyn J et al (1967) Osteosarcoma of the jaws: analysis of 56 cases. *Cancer* **20:** 377–391.
Gasparini M, Santoro A, Fossati-Bellani F et al (1982) Platinum plus Etoposide in the treatment of refractory solid tumors of children and adolescents. *Proceedings of the American Society of Clinical Oncology* **1:** 175.
Gasparini M, Rouesse J, Van Oosterom A et al (1985) Phase II study of Cisplatin in advanced osteogenic sarcoma. *Cancer Treatment Reports* **69:** 211–213.
Gasparini M, Tondini C, Rottoli L et al (1986) CDDP continuous infusion plus HDMTX and VCR in advanced osteosarcoma. *Proceedings of the American Society of Clinical Oncology* **5:** 147.
Gilchrist GS, Pritchard DJ, Dahlin DC et al (1981) Management of osteogenic sarcoma: a perspective based on the Mayo Clinic experience. *National Cancer Institute Monograph* **56:** 193–199.

Goorin AM, Abelson HT & Frei E (1985) Osteosarcoma: fifteen years later. *New England Journal of Medicine* **313**: 1637–1643.

Guiliano AE & Eilber FR (1983) Changing patterns of metastasis of osteosarcoma. *Proceedings of the American Society of Clinical Oncology* **2**: 229.

Hall RB, Robinson LH, Malawar MM et al (1985) Periosteal osteosarcoma. *Cancer* **55**: 165–171.

Herson J, Sutow WW, Elder K et al (1980) Adjuvant chemotherapy in non-metastatic osteosarcoma: a South West Oncology Group study. *Medical and Paediatric Oncology* **8**: 343–352.

Hoover HC, Ketcham AS, Millar RC et al (1978) Osteosarcoma: improved survival with anticoagulation and amputation. *Cancer* **41**: 2475–2480.

Huvos AG, Rosen G, Bretsky SS et al (1982) Telangiectatic osteogenic sarcoma: a clinicopathologic study of 124 cases. *Cancer* **49**: 1679–1689.

Huvos AG, Butler A & Bretsky SS (1983) Osteogenic sarcoma associated with Paget's disease of bone. A clinicopathologic study of 65 patients. *Cancer* **52**: 1489–1495.

Huvos AG, Woodard HQ, Cahan WG et al (1985) Post-radiation osteogenic sarcoma of bone and soft tissues. A clinicopathologic study of 66 patients. *Cancer* **55**: 1244–1255.

Isacoff WH, Eilber F, Tabbarah H et al (1978) Phase II clinical trial with high-dose Methotrexate therapy and citrovorum factor rescue. *Cancer Treatment Reports* **62**: 1295–1304.

Jaffe N, Frei E, Traggis D & Bishop Y (1974) Adjuvant Methotrexate and citrovorum factor treatment of osteogenic sarcoma. *New England Journal of Medicine* **291**: 994–997.

Jaffe N, Frei E, Smith E et al (1978a) A hypothesis for the pattern of pulmonary metastases in osteogenic sarcoma: impact of adjuvant therapy. *Proceedings of the American Society of Clinical Oncology* **19**: 400.

Jaffe N, Frei S, Watts H et al (1978b) High-dose Methotrexate in osteogenic sarcoma: a 5 year experience. *Cancer Treatment Reports* **62**: 259–264.

Jaffe N, Link MP, Cohen D et al (1981) High-dose Methotrexate in osteogenic sarcoma. *National Cancer Institute Monograph* **56**: 201–206.

Jaffe N, Van Eys J & Gehan E (1983) Response to: 'Is it ethical not to conduct a prospectively controlled trial of adjuvant chemotherapy in osteosarcoma?' *Cancer Treatment Reports* **67**: 743–744.

Jaffe N, Robertson R, Ayala A et al (1985) Comparison of intra-arterial cis-diamminedichloroplatinum II with high-dose Methotrexate and Citrovorum factor rescue in the treatment of primary osteosarcoma. *Journal of Clinical Oncology* **3**: 1101–1104.

Jeffree GM, Price CHG & Sissons HA (1975) The metastatic patterns of osteosarcoma. *British Journal of Cancer* **32**: 87–107.

Jenkin R, Bishop A, Bouchard H, Chevalier L & Cruikshank B (1981) Osteosarcoma. A preliminary report of a trial of adjuvant chemotherapy. *Proceedings of the American Society of Clinical Oncology* **22**: 525.

Juergens H, Kosloff C, Nirenberg A et al (1981) Prognostic factors in the response of primary osteogenic sarcoma to preoperative chemotherapy (high-dose Methotrexate with citrovorum factor). *National Cancer Institute Monograph* **56**: 221–226.

Kalifa C, Du Bousset J, Contesso G et al (1986) Experience of the T10 protocol for the treatment of osteosarcomas (OS). SIOP XVIII Annual Meeting, Beograd, 15–20 September.

Klegar K, Ryan L, Elias AD et al (1986) Ifosfamide (IFF) for advanced previously treated sarcomas: phase II. *Proceedings of the American Society of Clinical Oncology* **5**: 132.

Land VJ, Dyment PG, Starling K et al (1981) 5-Fluorouracil and Cisplatinum in the treatment of refractory solid tumours: a Paediatric Oncology Group phase I–II study. *Medical and Paediatric Oncology* **9**: 289–291.

Lange B & Levine AS (1982) Is it ethical not to conduct a prospectively controlled trial of adjuvant chemotherapy in osteosarcoma? *Cancer Treatment Reports* **66**: 1699–1704.

Lange B, Kramer S, Gregg JR et al (1982) High-dose Methotrexate and Adriamycin in osteogenic sarcoma. *American Journal of Clinical Oncology* **5**: 3–8.

Levine AS, Appelbaum FR, Graw RG et al (1978) Sequential combination chemotherapy (containing high-dose Cyclophosphamide) for metastatic osteogenic sarcoma. *Cancer Treatment Reports* **62**: 247–250.

Link MP & Vietti TT (1983) Response to: 'Is it ethical not to conduct a prospectively controlled trial of adjuvant chemotherapy in osteosarcoma?' *Cancer Treatment Reports* **67**: 743–745.

Link MP, Goorin AM, Miser AW et al (1986) The effect of adjuvant chemotherapy on relapse-free survival in patients with osteosarcoma of the extremity. *New England Journal of Medicine* **134**: 1600–1606.

Magill GB, Goldbey RB & Krakoff IH (1977) Chemotherapy combinations in adult sarcomas. *Proceedings of the American Society of Clinical Oncology* **18**: 332.

Mail JT, Cohen MD, Mirkin LD & Provisor AJ (1985) Response of osteosarcoma to pre-operative intravenous high dose methotrexate chemotherapy: CT evaluation. *American Journal of Radiology* **144**: 89–94.

Marcove RC (1978) En bloc resection of osteogenic sarcomas. *Cancer Treatment Reports* **62**: 225.

Matsuno T, Unni KK, McLeod RA et al (1976) Telangiectatic osteogenic sarcoma. *Cancer* **38**: 2538–2547.

McKenna RJ, Schwinn CP, Soong KY et al (1964) Osteogenic sarcoma arising in Paget's disease. *Cancer* **17**: 42–65.

Medical Research Council (MRC) (1986) A trial of chemotherapy in patients with osteo-sarcoma (a report to the Medical Research Council by their working party on bone sarcoma). *British Journal of Cancer* **53**: 513–518.

Morgan E, Baum E, Bleyer WA et al (1984) Treatment of patients with metastatic osteogenic sarcomas: a report from the Children's Cancer Study Group. *Cancer Treatment Reports* **68**: 661–664.

Mosende C, Gutierrez M, Caparros B et al (1977) Combination chemotherapy with Bleomycin, Cyclophosphamide and Dactinomycin for the treatment of osteogenic sarcoma. *Cancer* **40**: 2779–2786.

Muggia FM & Loule AC (1978) Five years of adjuvant treatment of osteosarcoma: more questions than answers. *Cancer Treatment Reports* **62**: 301–305.

National Institutes of Health Consensus Development Panel on Limb Sparing Treatment of Adult Soft Tissue Sarcomas and Osteosarcomas (1985) Introduction and Conclusions. *Cancer Treatment Symposia* **3**: 1–5.

Parham DM, Pratt CB, Parvey LS et al (1985) Childhood multifocal osteosarcoma. Clinico-pathologic and radiologic correlates. *Cancer* **55**: 2653–2658.

Petrilli S, Gentil F, Quadros J et al (1986) Preoperative treatment with intra-arterial (I/A) cis-diamminedichloroplatinum II (CDP) and postoperative adjuvant treatment with CDP and Adriamycin (ADR) for osteosarcoma of the extremities. *Proceedings of the American Society of Clinical Oncology* **5**: 202.

Picci P, Bacci G, Campanacci M et al (1985) Histologic evaluation of necrosis in osteosarcoma induced by chemotherapy. Regional mapping of viable and non-viable tumors. *Cancer* **56**: 1515–1521.

Picci P, Bacci G, Guerra A et al (1986) Neoadjuvant chemotherapy for osteosarcoma (OS). A study on 93 cases. *Proceedings of the American Society of Clinical Oncology* **5**: 127.

Pimm MV, Embleton MJ, Perkins AC et al (1982) In vivo localization of anti-osteogenic sarcoma 791T monoclonal antibody in osteogenic sarcoma xenografts. *International Journal of Cancer* **30**: 75–85.

Pratt DB (1979) Chemotherapy of osteosarcoma—an overview. In Van Oosterom AT et al (eds) *Therapeutic Progress in Ovarian Cancer, Testicular Cancer and the Sarcomas*, pp 329–347. The Hague: Martinus Nijhoff.

Pratt CB, Rivera G, Shanks E et al (1978) Combination chemotherapy for osteosarcoma. *Cancer Treatment Reports* **62**: 251–257.

Pratt CB, Howarth C, Ransom JL et al (1980) High-dose Methotrexate used alone and in combination for measurable primary or metastatic osteosarcoma. *Cancer Treatment Reports* **64**: 11–19.

Pratt CB, Green AA, Fleming ID et al (1984) Results of adjuvant chemotherapy for 77 patients with osteosarcoma of an extremity 1973–1981. *Proceedings of the American Society of Clinical Oncology* **3**: 257.

Pratt CB, Champion JE, Senzer N et al (1985) Treatment of unresectable or metastatic osteosarcoma with Cisplatin or Cisplatin-Doxorubicin. *Cancer* **56**: 1930–1933.

Price CHG (1957) Multifocal osteogenic sarcoma: report of a case. *Journal of Bone and Joint Surgery* **39B**: 524–533.

Price MR, Campbell DG, Robins RA et al (1983) Characteristics of a cell surface antigen defined by an anti-human osteogenic sarcoma monoclonal antibody. *European Journal of Cancer and Clinical Oncology* 19: 81–90.

Raymond AK, Benjamin RS, Carrasco CH et al (1986) Osteosarcoma, preoperative chemotherapy: histological evaluation. *Proceedings of the American Society of Clinical Oncology* 5: 138.

Reiman RE, Huvos AG, Benua RS et al (1981) Quotient imaging with N-13 L-glutamate in osteogenic sarcoma: correlation with tumor viability. *Cancer* 48: 1976–1981.

Rosen G (1985) Preoperative (neoadjuvant) chemotherapy for osteogenic sarcoma: a ten year experience. *Orthopaedics* 8: 659–664.

Rosen G & Nirenberg A (1982) Chemotherapy for osteogenic sarcoma: an investigative method, not a recipe. *Cancer Treatment Reports* 66: 1687–1697.

Rosen G, Suwansirikul S, Kwon C et al (1974) High-dose Methotrexate with citrovorum factor rescue and Adriamycin in childhood osteogenic sarcoma. *Cancer* 33: 1151–1163.

Rosen G, Huvos AG, Mosende C et al (1978) Chemotherapy and thoracotomy for metastatic osteogenic sarcoma: a model for adjuvant chemotherapy and the rationale for the timing of thoracic surgery. *Cancer* 41: 841–849.

Rosen G, Caparros B, Nirenberg A et al (1979a) The successful management of metastatic osteogenic sarcoma: a model for the treatment of primary osteogenic sarcoma. In Van Oosterom AT et al (eds) *Therapeutic Progress in Ovarian Cancer, Testicular Cancer and the Sarcomas*, pp 349–365. The Hague: Martinus Nijhoff.

Rosen G, Marcove RC, Caparros B et al (1979b) Primary osteogenic sarcoma. The rationale for preoperative chemotherapy and delayed surgery. *Cancer* 43: 2163–2177.

Rosen G, Nirenberg A & Caparros B (1980a) Evaluation of high-dose Methotrexate (HDMTX) with citrovorum factor rescue (CFR) single agent chemotherapy. *Proceedings of the American Association for Cancer Research* 21: 177.

Rosen G, Nirenberg A & Caparros B (1980b) Cisplatinum in metastatic osteogenic sarcoma. In Prestayko AW et al (eds) *Cisplatinum: Current Status and New Developments*, pp 465–475. New York: Academic Press.

Rosen G, Nirenberg A, Caparros B et al (1981) Osteogenic sarcoma: eighty-percent, three year, disease free survival with combination chemotherapy (T7). *National Cancer Institute Monographs* 56: 213–220.

Rosen G, Caparros B, Huvos AG et al (1982a) Preoperative chemotherapy for osteogenic sarcoma: selection of postoperative adjuvant chemotherapy based on the response of the primary tumor to preoperative chemotherapy. *Cancer* 49: 1221–1230.

Rosen G, Caparros B, Nirenberg A et al (1982b) Cisplatinum (DDP)—Adriamycin (ADR) combination chemotherapy (CT) in evaluable osteogenic sarcoma. *Proceedings of the American Society of Clinical Oncology* 1: 173.

Rosen G, Marcove RC, Huvos AG et al (1983) Primary osteogenic sarcoma: eight year experience with adjuvant chemotherapy. *Journal of Cancer Research and Clinical Oncology* 106(supplement): 55–67.

Rosenberg SA, Chabner BA, Young RC et al (1979) Treatment of osteogenic sarcoma. I. Effect of adjuvant high-dose Methotrexate after amputation. *Cancer Treatment Reports* 63: 739–751.

Rosenberg SA, Lotze MT, Muul LM et al (1985) Observations on the systemic administration of autologous lymphokine-activated killer cells and recombinant Interleukin-2 to patients with metastatic cancer. *New England Journal of Medicine* 313: 1485–1492.

Roth JA, Restrepo C, Scuderi P et al (1984) Analysis of antigenic expression by primary and autologous metastatic human sarcomas using murine monoclonal antibodies. *Cancer Research* 44: 5320–5325.

Salzer-Kuntschik M, Delling G, Beron G et al (1983) Morphological grades of regression in osteosarcoma after polychemotherapy—study COSS 80. *Journal of Cancer Research and Clinical Oncology* 106(supplement): 21–24.

Samson MK, Baker LH, Benjamin RS et al (1979) cis-Dichlorodiammine platinum (II) in advanced soft tissue and bone sarcomas: a South West Oncology Group study. *Cancer Treatment Reports* 63: 2027–2029.

Simon M, Dean L, Dawson P et al (1986) Diverse response of primary and metastatic osteosarcoma (OS) simultaneously resected following preoperative intravenous chemotherapy (PIC). *Proceedings of the American Society of Clinical Oncology* 5: 203.

Smith J, Heelan RT, Huvos AG et al (1982) Radiographic changes in primary osteogenic sarcoma following intensive chemotherapy: radiological-pathological correlation in 63 patients. *Radiology* **143:** 355–360.

Smith J, Botet JF & Yeh SDJ (1984) Bone sarcomas in Paget's disease: a study of 85 patients. *Radiology* **152:** 583–590.

Sonley MJ, Bobechko WP & Simpson JS (1979) Adjuvant therapy with Adriamycin and Methotrexate in osteogenic sarcoma. *Annual Review of the College of Physicians and Surgeons of Canada* **12**(161): 60–61.

Strander H, Adamson U, Aparisi T et al (1979) Adjuvant Interferon treatment of osteosarcoma. *Recent Results in Cancer Research* **68:** 40–44.

Sutow WW, Sullivan MP & Fernbach DJ (1974) Adjuvant chemotherapy in primary treatment of osteogenic sarcoma. *Proceedings of the American Society of Cancer Research* **15:** 20.

Sutow WW, Gehan EA, Dyment PG et al (1978) Multidrug adjuvant chemotherapy for osteosarcomas: interim report of the South West Oncology Group studies. *Cancer Treatment Reports* **62:** 265–270.

Taylor WF, Ivins JC & Dahlin DC (1978) Trends and variability in survival from osteosarcoma. *Mayo Clinic Proceedings* **53:** 695–700.

Taylor WF, Ivins JC, Pritchard DJ et al (1985) Trends and variability in survival among patients with osteosarcoma: a 7 year update. *Mayo Clinic Proceedings* **60:** 91–104.

Thorpe WP, Reilly JJ & Rosenberg SA (1979) Prognostic significance of alkaline phosphatase measurements in patients with osteogenic sarcoma receiving chemotherapy. *Cancer* **43:** 2178–2181.

Unni KK, Dahlin DC, Beabout JW et al (1976a) Parosteal osteogenic sarcoma. *Cancer* **37:** 2466–2475.

Unni KK, Dahlin DC & Beabout JW (1976b) Periosteal osteogenic sarcoma. *Cancer* **37:** 2476–2485.

Unni KK, Dahlin DC, McLeod RA et al (1977) Intraosseous well-differentiated osteosarcoma. *Cancer* **40:** 1337–1347.

Vaughn CB, McKelvey E, Balcerzak SP et al (1984) High-dose Methotrexate with leucovorin rescue plus Vincristine in advanced sarcoma. A South West Oncology Group study. *Cancer Treatment Reports* **68:** 409–412.

Wagener DJT, Van Oosterom AT, Mulder JH et al (1986) Phase II study of low-dose Methotrexate in advanced osteosarcoma followed by escalation after disease progression: a study of the Soft Tissue and Bone Sarcoma Group of European Organization for Research on Treatment of Cancer. *Cancer Treatment Reports* **70:** 615–618.

Winkler K, Beron G, Kotz R et al (1984) Neoadjuvant chemotherapy for osteogenic sarcoma: results of a cooperative German/Austrian study. *Journal of Clinical Oncology* **2:** 617–624.

Winkler K, Beron G, Delling A et al (1986) Selective postoperative (POP) adjuvant chemotherapy (CT) after aggressive vs mild preoperative (PROP) CT in osteosarcoma (OS). *Proceedings of the American Society of Clinical Oncology* **5:** 128.

# 8

# Chemotherapy of Ewing's sarcoma

ALAN W. CRAFT

Ewing's sarcoma of bone is a rare disease with an annual incidence estimated at 0.6 per million population (Price and Jeffree, 1977). It occurs throughout the world but is extremely uncommon in negro races (Glass and Fraumeni, 1970). Although reports of a similar tumour appeared in the German literature in the nineteenth century (Lucke, 1866; Hildebrand, 1890, it was the description by James Ewing which established the disease as a separate entity. He originally reported a diffuse endothelioma of bone (Ewing, 1924) but controversy continued for many years as to whether this was separate from lymphoma and neuroblastoma. However, it is now generally agreed to be a separate disease and is seen in both children and young adults, with 70% of cases occurring under the age of 20 years and a further 20% before the thirtieth birthday. Any bone can be affected, but the commonest sites are the diaphyseal region of long bones and the pelvic bones. The aetiology is unknown but there is increasing evidence of chromosomal rearrangements which may be specific for this type of tumour. A reciprocal translocation (11–22) (q24–q12) has been demonstrated in both primary tumours, metastases and extraskeletal tumours (Bechet et al, 1984; Becroft et al, 1984; Navas-Palacios et al, 1984).

The management of Ewing's sarcoma depended for many years on either surgical amputation, if this was possible, or radiotherapy. Long-term survival using this approach was poor, with 15% or less patients being cured of their disease. Significant improvements in survival did not occur until the advent of chemotherapy. Figure 1 shows the 5-year survival figures for children with Ewing's sarcoma treated in England and Wales, and demonstrates an improvement since chemotherapy has been used. However, the proportion of survivors is still only 40% when looked at on a national basis. Most of these children will not have been entered into organized clinical studies and will therefore have had a variety of treatments. Rosen (1982) claims that over 75% of patients can be cured when treated with aggressive chemotherapy in a single institution. However, the figures for multi-institutional studies are not so encouraging, with Gasparini et al (1981) reporting from Milan a relapse-free survival of 53% at 4 years and the American Intergroup Ewing's Sarcoma Study (IESS) reporting an overall survival of 56% at 3 years (Nesbit et al, 1981).

The disparity between these figures may not only reflect the difference between single and multi-institutional studies, or indeed whether the patient

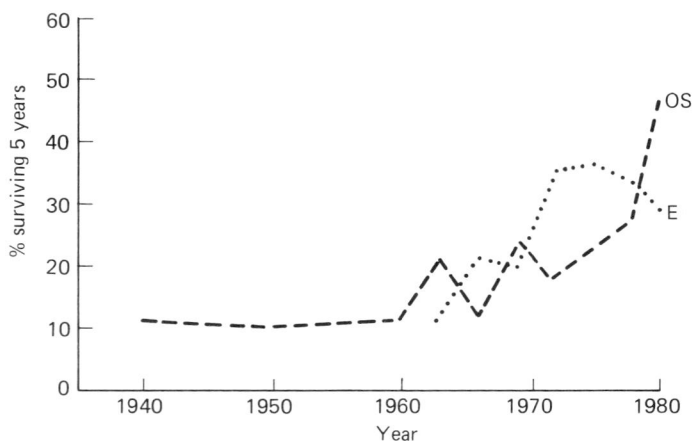

**Figure 1.** Five-year survival figures for children with Ewing's sarcoma and osteosarcoma treated in England and Wales. E = Ewing's sarcoma, O = osteosarcoma.

is in a study at all, but also the fact that there are several important prognostic factors which have to be taken into account when interpreting studies. Bradford Hill (1960) stressed the importance of equal distribution of features which are known to influence outcome, when comparing reports. The concept of prognostic factors is now well established in childhood leukaemia, and indeed treatment regimens are often tailored to the prognostic group. In recent years both the IESS and the German Ewing's Sarcoma Study (CESS) have had different treatment regimens for certain groups of patients. Before considering the chemotherapy of Ewing's sarcoma it is therefore important to consider prognostic factors. These were reviewed by Glaubiger et al (1980) using their experience at the National Cancer Institute (NCI).

## PROGNOSTIC FACTORS

### Metastases at diagnosis

The presence of metastases reduces the chances of long-term survival but death is not inevitable. Pilepich et al (1981) showed that long-term survival could be achieved in such patients in the IESS, and Craft (1985) reported similar findings in the United Kingdom Children's Cancer Study Group (UKCCSG) protocol. Pulmonary irradiation was used in the IESS study but chemotherapy alone achieved the same result in the UKCCSG study. However, Glaubiger reported metastasis to be the most important prognostic determinant, and none of the NCI patients with lung metastases at diagnosis survived.

### Site and size of tumour

Tumours of the axial skeleton, especially those affecting the pelvic bones, are generally accepted to have the worst prognosis (Gehan et al, 1981; Rosen, 1982). However, there is less agreement about the difference in results between distal and proximal long bone tumours, although the balance seems to be in favour of distal long bone primaries having a better outlook than proximal long bone primaries. Axial primaries usually include all bones of the axial skeleton, but it is perhaps important to recognize that primary tumours arising in the vertebrae, especially those of the lumbar spine, have a better prognosis (Pilepich et al, 1981). These differences may simply reflect the different sizes of tumour at different locations, since the sites lose their prognostic significance when tumour volume is taken into account (Gobel et al, 1986a). Tumours arising in the pelvis tend to have larger volumes and present later than those arising in the long bones, and those in the vertebral bodies usually present at a very early stage as soon as neurological function is compromised. Gobel et al (1986a), reporting the results of the CESS 81 study, calculated tumour volume from both plain X-rays and CT scans. The 3-year survival for patients with a tumour volume of greater than $100 \text{ cm}^3$ was only 17% compared with 78% for those with a volume of less than this. Larger tumours tended to be in axial and proximal long bone sites, but the size of tumour was a prognostic factor that was independent of the site.

### Age and sex

The UKCCSG study suggested that older patients had a worse prognosis than those aged 15 years or less (Craft, 1985). This was not seen in the IESS, but only 4% of patients in that study were over the age of 20 years compared to 10% in the UKCCSG study.

### Pathology

The pathological diagnosis of Ewing's sarcoma has always been difficult and it is often a diagnosis of exclusion. Various attempts have been made to define subtypes which could influence outcome. Strattan et al (1982) reported decreased survival in a small number of patients who were found to have intramyofibre skeletal muscle invasion by 'Ewing's cells', and Kissane et al (1983) suggested that a filigree pattern could be associated with a worse prognosis. These findings await substantiation by others. De Stefani et al (1984) report that extensive tumour necrosis is a poor prognostic factor.

### Response to chemotherapy

Any prognostic factor is only valid for a particular protocol of treatment.

However, within any regimen the response of the tumour to that treatment can be a prognostic factor in itself. Oberlin et al (1985) reported on 95 children with Ewing's sarcoma treated on a standard protocol. Response was assessed by clinical measurement of soft-tissue extension and the presence of 'functional' symptoms. Sixty seven could be evaluated and of these 41 (61%) were good responders, with either complete disappearance of soft-tissue mass or only a small residual tumour. Twenty six (31%) were bad responders, with some of the tumours growing during treatment. At 4 years from diagnosis only 9% of the bad responders were disease-free compared with 57% of the good responders. A significant difference in survival according to tumour site was also seen with limb bones having a better outlook than axial primaries, but the response to chemotherapy was independent of this fact.

### Serum lactic dehydrogenase (LDH)

An elevated serum LDH at diagnosis has been reported as a poor prognostic factor (Glaubiger et al, 1980) but this finding has not so far been sub-stantiated by others.

### TREATMENT

Evaluation of the contribution of different modalities of treatment has become very much more complicated in recent years. Surgery, radiotherapy and chemotherapy all have a significant role to play in the management of this disease, but the interrelationships of these factors are complex. There are two major factors to be considered, i.e. control of disease locally and prevention (or treatment) of metastatic spread. Ewing's original patient had local radiotherapy only and relapsed in the primary site 1 year later, followed soon after by metastatic spread. Sixty years later these are still the same problems which confront us. The radiotherapy and surgery of bone tumours has been dealt with in other chapters, so only those aspects which are relevant to the evaluation of multimodality treatment regimens will be discussed here.

### Single agent chemotherapy

Several early studies showed the responsiveness of Ewing's tumour to cyto-toxic drugs, and these were then incorporated into the multi-agent protocols which have been the mainstay of treatment over the past 10 years. The alkylating agents nitrogen mustard (mustine hydrochloride), chlorambucil and cyclophosphamide were all shown to have activity, but the latter seemed to be most effective and was incorporated into future studies (Sutow and Sullivan, 1962; Samuels and Howe, 1967). Selawry et al (1968) reported on the effectiveness of vincristine. Actinomycin D was evaluated by Senyszyn et al (1970) in patients with metastatic Ewing's sarcoma and was shown to be a useful drug.

Adriamycin (doxorubicin hydrochloride) was also shown to be very effective by Wang et al (1971), Oldham and Pomeroy (1972) and Tan et al (1973). These four agents have therefore been combined in therapeutic protocols. However, other agents have been evaluated both several years ago and more recently, as follows:

## BCNU (carmustine)

De Vita et al (1965) and Palma et al (1972) both showed this drug to be effective.

## 5-fluorouracil

Krivit and Bentley (1960) investigated this agent in a variety of advanced malignancies of childhood. In Ewing's sarcoma they found three significant responses out of four treated patients.

## Ifosfamide

This drug, which is an analogue of cyclophosphamide, has become more widely available for study in recent years. Its principal side-effect is that of haemorrhagic cystitis, but this can now be circumvented by the use of mesna (sodium 2-mercaptoethanesulfonate) which protects the bladder epithelium from damage by acrolein formed during the metabolism of ifosfamide. This has enabled much larger doses of this alkylating agent to be given. The response data from some of the studies so far published are shown in Table 1. All of these ifosfamide treatments were given to heavily pre-treated patients with recurrent or metastatic disease.

## Dacarbazine

Gottlieb et al (1976) reported no responses in three treated patients. When combined with rubidazone (zorubicin), one partial response was seen in a patient with previously untreated metastatic Ewing's tumour (Zidar et al, 1983).

Table 1. Ifosfamide in Ewing's sarcoma.

| Author | No. of patients treated | CR | PR | CR and PR | Significant responses (%) |
|---|---|---|---|---|---|
| Magrath et al, 1986 | 20 | | 9 | 9 | 45 |
| Scheulen et al, 1983 | 6 | 1 | 1 | 2 | 33 |
| de Kraker and Voute, 1983 | 4 | | 1 | 1 | 25 |
| Gobel et al, 1986b | 8 | 2 | 3 | 5 | 67 |
| Pinkerton et al, 1985 | 4 | 1 | 1 | 2 | 50 |
| Total | 42 | 4 | 15 | 19 | 45 |

CR = complete remission, PR = partial remission.

*Cisplatin*

Baum et al (1981) reported only two very short-lived responses out of 13 patients given this drug, and Vietti et al (1979) had previously reported no responders out of eight patients given the drug.

*Epipodophyllotoxins*

Bleyer et al (1978), in a preliminary study, reported both VM-26 (teniposide) and VP-16 (etoposide) to be effective agents against recurrent Ewing's tumour. Chard et al (1979) documented one response out of three patients and Hayes et al (1983a) demonstrated complete or partial response in two out of seven patients using VP-16.

In a randomized study, using in addition Adriamycin and DTIC (dacarbazine), etoposide was shown to be as effective as vincristine (Campbell et al, 1983).

*High-dose melphalan*

Floersheim and Torhorst in 1981 reported the ability to eradicate Ewing's tumours in mice by a single supralethal dose of melphalan followed by marrow rescue. Human studies followed and showed initial promise. Two out of three patients with disseminated disease showed a complete remission (Cornbleet et al, 1981) and one out of two patients showed a similar complete remission (Lazarus et al, 1983). Late follow-up of the London patients is disappointing (JS Malpas, TJ McElwain, 1987, personal communication). Jacobsen et al (1984) treated four patients, two in almost complete remission at the time of the procedure. One of these patients remained in complete remission at 44 months from diagnosis (Jacobsen, 1987, personal communication). Graham-Pole et al (1982) reported five partial responses out of seven patients treated in this way and felt that soft tissue responded better to treatment than osseous lesions. Two laboratory studies have recently shown conflicting results with regard to melphalan. An in vitro clonogenic assay of Ewing's sarcoma cells incubated with melphalan showed marked resistance of the cells to the drug, even at a 100-fold higher concentration than that which inhibited neuroblastoma and osteosarcoma cells (Worthington-White et al, 1986). On the other hand, Floersheim et al (1986), using a human tumour xenograft model in immunosuppressed mice, showed very marked activity of Ewing's tumour cells to both melphalan, cyclophosphamide and irradiation.

*Total body irradiation (TBI)*

The use of TBI as an agent to control systemic disease was initially reported in 1982 from Milan by Lombardi et al. Sequential half-body irradiation was used in those with progressive disease. The objective response rate was 50%, and 33% remained alive 4–27 months later. In vitro studies were carried out at the NCI to determine the optimum dose and rate for incorporation into clinical protocols. These studies suggest two 4.0 Gy fractions of 2 cGy per minute separated by 24 hours with autologous marrow rescue (Kinsella et al, 1984). This work has been challenged by Wheldon et al (1985) quoting the linear quadratic model of Alper (1975) on the grounds of optimizing tumour cell kill and normal tissue tolerance. Kinsella et al (1985) agreed that more data on human tissue tolerance to TBI were needed, but in the meantime they felt that their suggested schedule was the best that was currently available. A similar pilot study of this approach was reported from Toronto by Berry et al (1986) and from the Mayo Clinic by Evans et al (1984). Both centres reported the TBI to be tolerable but felt that its place in management needed further evaluation.

## Combination drug studies

There is great difficulty in determining the contribution of an individual drug in a non-randomized study of combination chemotherapy. Most studies have been carried out with large numbers of drugs, but there are some where two drugs have been tried in combination in a phase 2 setting, as follows:

### Cisplatin–ifosfamide

Jurgens et al (1983) studied 14 patients who had relapsed on the CESS 81 protocol. They had all been pretreated with vincristine, actinomycin D, Adriamycin and cyclophosphamide. There were two patients with complete remission and four with partial remission, i.e. 43%, and toxicity was tolerable. This combined complete and partial remission rate is very similar to the overall rate shown in Table 1 for ifosfamide alone, and in view of the poor response to cisplatin, when used as a single agent it seems unlikely that this combination of the two drugs has anything to offer over the use of the clearly active agent ifosfamide. Nierderle et al (1983), using the same combination, reported two partial and one marginal response out of six treated patients.

### Ifosfamide–vincristine

In Amsterdam, de Kraker and Voute (1984) have used this combination to treat 25 children with various relapsed solid tumours. Four of these children had Ewing's tumour and one showed a temporary partial response.

### Ifosfamide–etoposide (VP-16)

Miser et al (1986), in studies carried out at the National Cancer Institute, utilized these two drugs in 19 patients with recurrent childhood tumours. Eight of these patients were Ewing's sarcoma patients. All 19 patients had an objective response. A more recent follow-up (Magrath, 1987, personal communication) indicates a 90% response rate in Ewing's sarcoma, with some complete responses. They are sufficiently impressed with these results that this combination of drugs is now being used as first-line chemotherapy in previously untreated patients.

*Adriamycin–cyclophosphamide*

In an attempt to evaluate which elements of a multidrug regimen are beneficial, Hayes et al (1983), working at St Jude Hospital in Memphis, assessed the response of newly diagnosed patients with Ewing's sarcoma to sequential cyclophosphamide and Adriamycin induction therapy. Twenty-four children were entered into the protocol, and at the completion of five courses of this combination they were fully restaged. Patients achieving a complete or partial remission were then referred for surgery for either biopsy or resection, and a pathological response to the induction chemotherapy could therefore be made. Of 14 patients without metastases at diagnosis, 10 achieved a clinical complete remission and three a partial remission, and one was not evaluable. In 12 patients it was possible to determine the response pathologically, and in six there was no tumour present. In the remainder there was only microscopic residual tumour. A further 10 patients had metastases at diagnosis. Of these, seven achieved a complete remission in the primary tumour, two a partial remission and only one had no response. In addition, eight of these patients had a complete remission and one a partial remission of the metastatic disease. Five had no tumour present pathologically. Nineteen out of 23 evaluable patients therefore achieved a complete remission with a two-drug induction chemotherapy alone.

## Multidrug regimens

Several groups have used multidrug regimens over the past 15 years, many of them utilizing identical agents but often being administered in a different schedule. These different groups will be considered separately.

*Memorial Sloan-Kettering Cancer Center (MSKCC)*

In 1981, Rosen et al reported 10 years of experience of chemotherapy containing protocols for patients with Ewing's sarcoma treated in one medical centre in New York. A total of 67 patients without metastases at diagnosis had been treated with regimens which also included radiotherapy and, where feasible, surgery to the primary tumour. The first 19 patients were treated with the T2 protocol (Rosen et al, 1974) which employed vincristine, Adriamycin, actinomycin D and cyclophosphamide for a total period of 18–24 months. The next protocol, T6, was used for 30 patients and was similar to T2 but included three additional drugs during the induction phase, i.e. bleomycin, BCNU and low-dose oral methotrexate ($18\,mg/m^2$). The final 18 patients were managed on the T9 protocol, which included the same drugs as in the induction phase of T6, apart from BCNU, but these were continued for 9 months rather than just a short induction phase. There was then no maintenance therapy. Seventy per cent of the patients had axial or proximal long bone primaries, so they were not a selected group of good prognosis patients. At the time of the report in 1981, 79% were surviving free of disease from 12 to 118 months, with a median follow-up of 41 months from the start of treatment. The disease-free survival figures for the different sites were: axial—65%, proximal—79%, and distal—95%. They conclude that aggressive preoperative (or preradiotherapy) chemotherapy dramatically reduces the bulk of the tumour and allows the bone to heal before institution of the definitive treatment for the primary lesion. A later publication by Rosen (1982) gives disease-free survival rates of 65%, 76% and 90% for axial, proximal and distal lesions respectively. These single-institution survival figures have never been matched by a multicentre study.

*Intergroup Ewing's Sarcoma Study (IESS)*

In 1973 the Children's Cancer Study Group, the South West Oncology Group and the Cancer and Leukaemia Group B combined together, and up to 1978, 264 children with Ewing's sarcoma, from 83 separate institutions, were entered into a randomized three-arm study designed to determine the efficacy of the addition of Adriamycin or pulmonary irradiation to the three-drug combination of vincristine, actinomycin and cyclophosphamide (VAC) and irradiation of the primary tumour. The overall survival rate at 3 years was 56%. The regimen with Adriamycin was the most effective, with 74% of the patients being disease-free at 2 years. Adriamycin was not significantly more effective than pulmonary irradiation in prolonging survival, but both were more effective than VAC on its own. Pulmonary irradiation and Adriamycin were equally effective in preventing pulmonary metastases (Nesbit et al, 1981). A concurrent study of patients who had metastatic disease at diagnosis was also carried out. VAC and Adriamycin was given to all patients with irradiation both to the primary tumour and metastases. Thirty-one out of 44 treated patients showed a complete response to this treatment. Eighteen remained free of disease at a median follow-up time of 34 months, but four patients died of therapy-related complications (Pilepich et al, 1981). The addition of Adriamycin to VAC improves local tumour control, i.e. 96% vs 86% (Perez et al, 1977; Razek et al, 1980).

*National Cancer Institute (NCI)*

In 1975 Pomeroy and Johnson reported on 66 consecutive patients who had been treated with increasingly intensive chemotherapeutic regimens. Forty-three patients who had no metastases at diagnosis had 2- and 4-year survival rates of 64% and 52% respectively. The regimens included vincristine, Adriamycin and cyclophosphamide. A more recent report (Tepper et al, 1980) indicated that 19%, 33% and 57% of patients with central, proximal and distal lesions respectively were alive and well. They reported a local control rate of 93% but they stressed the importance of biopsy of the primary lesions in those who develop metastases. Some of these patients have evidence of occult local recurrence. More recent studies at the NCI have concentrated on therapy with vincristine, Adriamycin and cyclo-phosphamide with TBI and autologous bone marrow rescue (Kinsella et al, 1983; Miser, 1986).

## St Jude Hospital, Memphis

An early study from St Jude reported on 70 patients with localized Ewing's sarcoma, and all but four received combination chemotherapy with vincristine, Adriamycin, actinomycin and cyclophosphamide. The disease-free survival figures at 1, 2 and 3 years were 79%, 44% and 40% respectively (Hayes, 1986, personal communication). Hayes et al (1983b) reported the initial results of sequential cyclophosphamide and Adriamycin induction therapy, and 19 out of 23 patients had no evidence of residual disease after this therapy. Definitive treatment was then given to the primary tumour. This approach to treatment has now been adopted by the Paediatric Oncology Group, who are studying the effect of standard or 'tailored' radiotherapy to the primary tumour after cyclophosphamide/Adriamycin induction and following it with the addition of vincristine and actinomycin D (Hayes, 1986, personal communication).

## European studies

The United Kingdom Children's Cancer Study Group (UKCCSG), using the four commonly used drugs, vincristine, Adriamycin, actinomycin and cyclophosphamide, has shown an overall survival of only 39% at 4 years, but the poor result may be due to an excess of poor prognosis patients or indeed the reporting at a later stage than many of the previous studies (Craft, 1985). The current UKCCSG Ewing's tumour protocol consists of preoperative chemotherapy with ifosfamide, vincristine and Adriamycin (IVAD) with the substitution of actinomycin for Adriamycin (IVA) after definitive treatment of the primary tumour with surgery and or radiotherapy.

The French Paediatric Oncology Society reported on a very similar regimen. The 4-year survival was 56.2% and disease-free survival was 52.1% (Oberlin et al, 1985). More recently they have also been exploring the use of ifosfamide in place of the cyclophosphamide used in the previous study (Demeocq et al, 1984).

A separate French group, le Groupe d'Étude des Tumeurs Osseuses (GETO), reported on 24 patients with Ewing's sarcoma treated on two different protocols containing the four commonly used drugs alone or with the addition of low-dose oral methotrexate ($18 \, mg/m^2$) and/or procarbazine. Disease-free survival was 50% for the early protocol and over 80% at 2 years for the more recent regimen. However, there were very small numbers of patients and follow-up was very short for the more recent study (Le Mevel et al, 1980).

In Italy, results have been reported from two groups. Bacci et al (1985), reporting from Bologna, described the use of 2 years of chemotherapy with vincristine, Adriamycin and cyclophosphamide in 37 patients with Ewing's sarcoma. Follow-up ranged from 12 to 62 months. Only nine of these had developed either metastases or local recurrence at the time of follow-up compared with 38 out of 40 patients in a historical control series from the same centre. From the chemotherapy series they later concluded that the number of patients remaining disease-free was greater when local treatment of the primary was performed with surgery alone, or surgery plus radio-therapy, rather than radiotherapy alone, i.e. 63% vs 32%. Their present study therefore utilizes the same drugs with surgery to the primary lesion whenever possible (Bacci et al, 1986).

Gasparini and his group from Milan reported on 34 patients with localized disease treated with Adriamycin, vincristine and cyclophosphamide. Actuarial relapse-free survival at 4 years was 53%. Local recurrence was responsible for treatment failure in two patients and distant metastases in 12 patients. They suggested that incomplete eradication of the primary tumour might be responsible for metastatic seeding before, or even without, clinical evidence of local reactivation (Gasparini et al, 1981). This group have also studied the use of sequential half-body irradiation in relapsing patients, with an objective response rate of 50% and 6 out of 18 patients being alive from 4–27 months (Lombardi et al, 1982).

In 1981, a German cooperative group, Cooperative Ewing-Sarkome Studie (CESS), was established under the auspices of the German Society of Paediatric Oncology. The CESS 81 study again used the same four active agents as most other protocols of the period, i.e. vincristine, Adriamycin, actinomycin D and cyclophosphamide. Eighteen weeks of 'induction' therapy was given before surgery and/or radiotherapy and this was followed by a further 18 weeks of similar treatment. With this protocol there was a low systemic failure rate, i.e. 11 out of 68 patients (16%), but an apparently increased rate of local recurrence, i.e. 18 out of 68 patients (26%). However, of these local failures, 17 had incomplete surgery with radio-therapy being relied upon as the main modality of definitive treatment (Jurgens et al, 1985). As already stated, the survival was closely related to tumour volume, and Jurgens suggested that the CESS 81 data support the Goldie-Coldman hypothesis that if a tumour has grown to a large volume then resistant cell lines are likely to have developed (Goldie and Coldman, 1979; de Vita, 1983). However, it is difficult to disentangle the effects of surgery and tumour volume as smaller tumours are likely to occur in surgically accessible sites. A 5-year follow up was reported by Jurgens et al (1986) and a Kaplan-Meier disease-free survival figure was 51%. Based on the findings of their first study CESS 86 has now been designed. This divides patients into good and bad prognosis groups depending on the tumour volume at diagnosis. The good risk patients with tumours of less than $100 \, cm^3$ received conventional four-drug chemotherapy, but in the high risk group, ifosfamide is substituted for cyclophosphamide (Jurgens, 1986, personal communication).

**Supralethal chemo/radiotherapy with autologous bone marrow transplant (ABMT)**

As discussed earlier, both melphalan and TBI have been shown to be very effective agents for the management of disease refractory to conventional treatment. Initially these agents were used in relapsed patients, but recently attempts have been made to utilize this approach earlier in the course of the disease. Baumgartner et al (1984) treated three patients with TBI and

ABMT after preconditioning them with vincristine, Adriamycin and cyclo-phosphamide. The treatment was tolerated but response was not reported. Graham-Pole et al (1984) used high-dose melphalan and ABMT in eight relapsed patients. A partial remission was seen in six patients but the median survival after the procedure was only 3 months. Two patients had fatal complications of the procedure. Ninane et al (1985) achieved two complete remissions out of two patients with relapsed Ewing's sarcoma using high-dose melphalan and TBI. Kinsella et al (1983) at the NCI gave ABMT after a treatment consisting of chemotherapy alone or one including TBI. Twenty-four patients, who were in complete remission following induction chemo-therapy, were treated with vincristine, cyclophosphamide, DTIC and Adriamycin as high-dose therapy, and nine of these patients were alive with no evidence of disease from 22 to 72 months later. A subsequent regimen added TBI to Adriamycin and cyclophosphamide in 10 patients. The combined results of the NCI's massive therapy and ABMT regimens in this disease were reported by Miser (1986). Out of a group of 57 selected very bad risk patients, 26 were alive 2 years following the therapy. In Europe, Philip (1984) reviewed the experience in 35 patients for the European Bone Marrow Transplant (EBMT) group. A response rate of 66% was seen in evaluable patients. However, the results depend on the stage of the disease at which the procedure was carried out. Figure 2 shows that those patients receiving ABMT whilst in complete remission have a survival figure of 80% at 1 year, whereas those treated at a stage of progressive disease were all dead by 7 months (Pinkerton et al, 1986).

From the previous studies it can be seen that up to 50% long-term survival can probably be achieved using a combination of the four active drugs—vincristine, Adriamycin, actinomycin and cyclophosphamide—with either

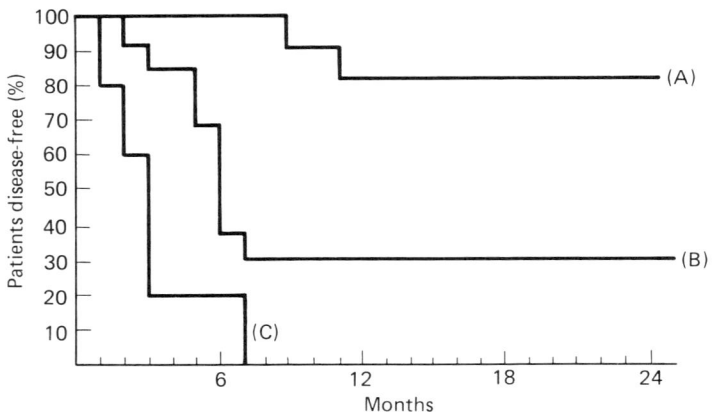

**Figure 2.** Thirty four cases of Ewing's sarcoma receiving ABMT in Europe (EBMT review, 1984, unpublished data). (A) bad-risk patients. ABMT in CR (n = 11); (B) non-resistant PR or relapses (n = 13); (C) resistant relapses (n = 10).

surgery and/or radiotherapy to the primary tumour. Long-term survival is also occasionally seen in those who have metastases at diagnosis. The survival rate is even higher in selected groups of patients, and the tumour volume and site of tumour seem to be significantly associated with prognosis. It is unlikely that any further improvement in survival will be seen with these four drugs and, of the newer agents, ifosfamide and etoposide appear to be those which have shown most promise. It is too early to know whether the novel approach of very high dose therapy with ABMT will improve survival, and, in view of its high rate of toxicity, it should probably be reserved for those patients who have responding tumours but who can be predicted to have a poor prognosis, and in those centres able to provide the high level of supportive care.

## SUMMARY

Long-term survival rates for patients with Ewing's sarcoma treated with surgery and/or radiotherapy alone are 10% or less. The addition of adjuvant chemotherapy has led to a significant improvement, and up to 50% of such patients may now be cured. The four most active agents used in most studies over the past decade are vincristine, Adriamycin, actinomycin D and cyclophosphamide, and these are combined with surgery and/or radiotherapy to the primary tumour. Long-term survival may also be seen in patients who present with advanced and metastatic disease. Even higher survival rates can be seen in selected groups of patients. Tumour volume and the site of the tumour seem to be significantly associated with outcome. Smaller tumours fare better than those larger than 100 cubic centimetres, and axial bone primaries have the worst prognosis followed by proximal and then distal long bone tumours. Of the newer agents, ifosfamide and etoposide show most promise. Novel approaches of supralethal chemo/radiotherapy regimens with autologous marrow rescue are being used, but it is too soon to evaluate them.

## REFERENCES

Alper T (1975) Cell survival after low doses of radiation. London: Institute of Physics and John Wiley.

Bacci G, Picci P, Gherlinzoni F et al (1985) Localized Ewing's sarcoma of bone: ten years' experience at the Instituto Orthopedico Rizzoli in 124 cases treated with multimodal therapy. *European Journal of Cancer and Clinical Oncology* **21**(2): 163–173.

Bacci G, Picci P, Frezza G et al (1986) *Neoadjuvant Chemotherapy for Ewing's Sarcoma (ES) of the Extremities: Preliminary Results of a New Protocol which Largely Uses Surgery for Local Control.* Abstracts of the American Society of Clinical Oncology, C792.

Baum ES, Gaynon P, Greenberg L, Krivit W & Hammond D (1981) Phase II trial of cisplatin in refractory childhood cancer: Children's Cancer Study Group report. *Cancer Treatment Reports* **65**: 815–822.

Baumgartner C, Bleher EA, del Re GB et al (1984) Autologous bone marrow transplantation in the treatment of children and adolescents with advanced malignant tumors. *Medical and Pediatric Oncology* **12**: 104.

Bechet JM, Bornkamm G, Freese UK & Lenoir G (1984) The c-cis oncogene is not activated in Ewing's sarcoma. *New England Journal of Medicine* **310**(6): 393.

Becroft DMO, Pearson A, Shaw RL & Zwi LJ (1984) Chromosome translocation in extra-skeletal Ewing's tumour. *Lancet* **ii**: 400.

Berry MP, Jenkin RDT, Harwood AR et al (1986) Ewing's sarcoma: a trial of adjuvant chemotherapy and sequential half-body irradiation. *International Journal of Radiation Oncology, Biology, Physics* **12**: 19–24.

Bleyer WA, Chard RL, Krivit W & Hammond D (1978) Epipodophyllotoxin therapy of childhood neoplasia: a comparative phase II analysis of VM26 and VP 16-213. *Proceedings of the American Society of Clinical Oncology* **19**: 373.

Campbell AM, Ekert H & Waters KD (1983) VM-26 and dimethyl triazenoimidazole carboxamide in Ewing's sarcoma. *Australian Paediatric Journal* **19**: 30–33.

Chard RL, Krivit W, Bleyer WA & Hammond D (1979) Phase II study of VP-16-213 in childhood malignant disease: a Children's Cancer Study Group Report. *Cancer Treatment Reports* **63**: 1755–1759.

Cornbleet MA, Corringham RET, Prentice HG, Boesen EM & McElwain TJ (1981) Treatment of Ewing's sarcoma with high dose melphalan and autologous bone marrow transplantation. *Cancer Treatment Reports* **65**: 241–244.

Craft AW (1985) Controversies in the management of bone tumours. *Cancer Surveys* **3**: 733–750.

de Kraker J & Voute PA (1983) Ifosfamide, mesna and vincristine in paediatric oncology. *Cancer Treatment Reviews* **10** (supplement A): 165–166.

de Kraker J & Voute PA (1984) Ifosfamide and vincristine in paediatric tumours. A phase II study. *European Paediatric Haematology and Oncology* **1**: 47–50.

Demeocq F, Carton P, Pattie C et al (1984) Traitement du sarcome d'Ewing par chimiothérapie initiale intensive. *Presse Medicale* **13**: 717–721.

de Stefani E, Carzoglio J, Deneo-Pellegrini H et al (1984) Ewing's sarcoma: value of tumor necrosis as a predictive factor. *Bulletin du Cancer* **71**: 16.

de Vita VT (1983) The relationship between tumor mass and resistance to chemotherapy. *Cancer* **51**: 1209–1220.

de Vita VT, Carbone PP, Owens AH et al (1965) Clinical trials with 1, 3-Bis (2-chlorethyl)-1-nitrosourea, NSC-409962. *Cancer Research* **25**: 1876–1881.

Evans RG, Burgert EO, Gilchrist GS et al (1984) Sequential half-body irradiation (SHBI) and combination chemotherapy as salvage treatment for failed Ewing's sarcoma—a pilot study. *International Journal of Radiation Oncology, Biology, Physics* **10**: 2363–2368.

Ewing J (1924) Further report of endothelial myeloma of bone. *Proceedings of the New York Pathological Society* **24**: 93–100.

Floersheim GL & Torhorst J (1981) Control of a human tumour (Ewing's sarcoma) in mice by a single lethal dose of dimethyl-myleran and bone marrow. *International Journal of Cancer* **27**: 743–748.

Floersheim GL, Bieri A & Chiodetti N (1986) Xenografts in pharmacologically immuno-suppressed mice as a model to test the chemotherapeutic sensitivity of human tumors. *International Journal of Cancer* **37**: 109–114.

Gasparini M, Lombardi F, Gianni C & Fossati-Bellani F (1981) Localised Ewing's sarcoma: results of integrated therapy and analysis of failures. *European Journal of Cancer and Clinical Oncology* **17**: 1205–1209.

Gehan EA, Nesbit ME, Burgert OE et al (1981) Prognostic factors in children with Ewing's sarcoma. *National Cancer Institute Monographs* **56**: 273–278.

Glass AG & Fraumeni JF Jr (1970) Epidemiology of bone cancer in children. *Journal of the National Cancer Institute* **44**: 187–199.

Glaubiger DL, Makuch R, Schwarz J, Levine AS & Johnson RE (1980) Determination of prognostic factors and their influence on therapeutic results in patients with Ewing's sarcoma. *Cancer* **45**: 2213–2219.

Gobel V, Jurgens H, Etspuler G et al (1986a) Prognostic significance of tumor volume in localized Ewing's sarcoma of bone in children and adolescents. *Cancer Research and Clinical Oncology* (in press).

Gobel V, Jurgens H, Etspuler G et al (1986b) Effectiveness of ifosfamide (IFO) alone and in combination with cisplatinum (DDP) in patients with recurrent Ewing's sarcoma. *Cancer Research and Clinical Oncology* **111** (supplement) S: 30.

Goldie JH & Coldman AJ (1979) A mathematical model for relating the drug sensitivity of tumors to their spontaneous mutation rate. *Cancer Treatment Reports* **63:** 1727–1733.

Gottlieb JA, Benjamin RS, Baker LH et al (1976) Role of DTIC (NSC-45388) in the chemotherapy of sarcomas. *Cancer Treatment Reports* **60:** 199–203.

Graham-Pole J, Gross S, Herzig R et al (1982) High dose melphalan (L-Pam) and bone marrow autografting for refractory neuroblastoma and Ewing's sarcoma. *Clinical Research* **30**(5): 900A (abstract).

Graham-Pole J, Lazarus HM, Herzig RH et al (1984) High dose melphalan therapy for the treatment of children with refractory neuroblastoma and Ewing's sarcoma. *American Journal of Pediatric Hematology and Oncology* **6:** 17–26.

Hayes FA, Green A & Thompson E (1983a) Phase II trial of VP 16-213 in pediatric solid tumors. *Proceedings of the American Society of Clinical Oncology:* c-256.

Hayes FA, Thompson EI, Hustu HO et al (1983b) The response of Ewing's sarcoma to sequential cyclophosphamide and adriamycin induction therapy. *Journal of Clinical Oncology* **1:** 45–51.

Hildebrand (1890) Über das tubulare Angiosarkom oder Endotheliom des Knochens. *Deutsche Zeitschrift für Chirurgie* **31:** 262–281.

Hill AB (1960) *Controlled Clinical Trials.* Oxford: Blackwell Scientific Publications.

Jacobsen A-B, Wist EA & Solheim OP (1984) Treatment of Ewing's sarcoma with high-dose melphalan and autologous bone marrow rescue. In McVie JG et al (eds) *Autologous Bone Marrow Transplantation and Solid Tumours*, pp 157–160. New York: Raven Press.

Jurgens H, Etspuler G, Beck J et al (1983) Prognostic value of local therapy in patients with primary Ewing's sarcoma: results of a cooperative study. In *Second European Conference on Clinical Oncology*, Amsterdam, Abstract 11–31.

Jurgens H, Gobel V, Michaelis J et al (1985) Die co-operative Ewing-Sarkom Studie CESS 81 der GPO—analyse nach 4 jahren. *Klinische Padiatrie* **197:** 225–232.

Jurgens H, Exner U, Ramach W et al (1986) Co-operative Ewing's sarcoma study (CESS 81) of the German Society of Pediatric Oncology (GPO): report after five years. *Abstract of the American Society of Pediatric Oncology* 811.

Kinsella TJ, Glaubiger D, Diesseroth A et al (1983) Intensive combined modality therapy including low dose TBI in high-risk Ewing's sarcoma patients. *International Journal of Radiation Oncology, Biology, Physics* **9:** 1955.

Kinsella TJ, Mitchell JB, McPherson S et al (1984) In vitro radiation studies on Ewing's sarcoma cell lines and human bone marrow: application to the clinical use of total body irradiation. *International Journal of Radiation Oncology, Biology, Physics* **10:** 1005–1011.

Kinsella TJ, Mitchell JB & Glatstein E (1985) Rebuttal. *International Journal of Radiation Oncology, Biology, Physics* **11**(8): 1570.

Kissane JM, Askin FB, Foulkes M, Strattan LB & Shirley SF (1983) Ewing's sarcoma of bone: clinico pathological aspects of 303 cases from the Intergroup Ewing's Sarcoma Study. *Human Pathology* **14:** 773–779.

Krivit W & Bentley HP (1960) Use of 5-fluorouracil in the management of advanced malignancies of childhood. *American Journal of Disease in Children* **100:** 217–227.

Lazarus HM, Herzig RH, Graham-Pole J et al (1983) Intensive melphalan chemotherapy and cryopreserved autologous bone marrow transplantation for the treatment of refractory cancer. *Journal of Clinical Oncology* **1:** 359–367.

Le Mevel B, Mathe G, Jasmin C et al (1980) Traitement du sarcome d'Ewing par radiothérapie et chimiothérapie adjuvante: résultats à 3 et 5 ans. *La Nouvelle Presse Médicale* **9:** 359–362.

Lombardi L, Lattuada A, Gasparini M, Gianni C & Marchesini R (1982) Sequential half body irradiation as systemic treatment of progressive Ewing's sarcoma. *International Journal of Radiation Oncology, Biology, Physics* **8:** 1679–1682.

Lucke A (1866) Beiträge zur geschwulstlehre: III lympho-sarcom der achseldrusen: embolische geschwulste der lungen; allgemeine Leukämie. *Virchows Archiv. Pathologischen Anat* **35:** 524–539.

Magrath I, Sandlund J, Raynor A et al (1986) A phase II study of ifosfamide in the treatment of recurrent sarcomas in young people. *Cancer Chemotherapy and Pharmacology* (in press).

Miser J (1986) High-dose therapy and ABMT in pediatric solid tumour. In de Bernardi B (ed.) *Novel Therapeutic Approaches in Pediatric Oncology* (in press). Boston: Martinus Nijhoff.

Miser J, Kinsella R, Tsokos M et al (1986) High response rate of recurrent childhood tumors to etoposide (VP16), ifosfamide (IFOS) and mesna (MES) uroprotection. *Proceedings of the American Society of Clinical Oncology* **5**: 820.

Navas-Palacios YY, Aparicio-Duque R & Valdes MD (1984) On the histogenesis of Ewing's sarcoma: an ultrastructural, immunohistochemical and cytochemical study. *Cancer* **53**: 1882.

Nesbit ME, Perez CA, Tefft M et al (1981) Multimodal therapy for the management of primary non metastatic Ewing's sarcoma of bone: an Intergroup Study. *National Cancer Institute Monographs* **56**: 255–262.

Niederle N, Scheulen ME, Cremer M et al (1983) Ifosfamide in combination chemotherapy for sarcomas and testicular carcinomas. *Cancer Treatment Reviews* **10**(supplement A): 129–135.

Ninane J, Baurain R, de Selys A, Trouet A & Cornu G (1985) High dose melphalan in children with advanced malignant disease. *Cancer Chemotherapy and Pharmacology* **15**: 263–267.

Oberlin I, Patte C, Demeocq F et al (1985) The response to initial chemotherapy as a prognostic factor in localized Ewing's sarcoma. *European Journal of Cancer and Clinical Oncology* **21**: 463–467.

Oldham RK & Pomeroy RC (1972) Treatment of Ewing's sarcoma with adriamycin (NSC-123127). *Cancer Chemotherapy Reports* **56**(5): 635–639.

Palma J, Gailani S, Freeman A, Sinks L & Holland J (1972) Treatment of metastatic Ewing's sarcoma with BCNU. *Cancer* **30**: 909–913.

Perez CA, Razek A, Tefft M et al (1977) Analysis of local tumor control in Ewing's sarcoma. Preliminary results of a cooperative intergroup study. *Cancer* **40**: 2864–2873.

Philip T (1984) *Status of the Role of ABMT in Solid Tumours in Europe*. Proceedings of the European Bone Marrow Transplant Group, Granada.

Pilepich VM, Vietti TJ, Nesbit ME et al (1981) Radiotherapy and combination chemotherapy in advanced Ewing's sarcoma: intergroup study. *Cancer* **47**: 1930–1936.

Pinkerton CR, Rogers H, James C et al (1985) A phase II study of ifosfamide in children with recurrent solid tumours. *Cancer Chemotherapy and Pharmacology* **15**: 258–262.

Pinkerton R, Philip T, Bouffet E, Lashford L & Kemshead J (1986) Autologous bone marrow transplantation in paediatric solid tumours. *Clinics in Haematology* **15**: 187–203.

Pomeroy TC & Johnson RE (1975) Prognostic factors for survival in Ewing's sarcoma. *American Journal of Roentgenology, Radium Therapy and Nuclear Medicine* **123**: 598–606.

Price CHG & Jeffree GM (1977) Incidence of bone sarcoma in SW England, 1946–74, in relation to age, sex, tumour site and histology. *British Journal of Cancer* **36**: 511–522.

Razek A, Perez CA, Tefft M et al (1980) Intergroup Ewing's sarcoma study. Local control related to radiation dose, volume and site of primary lesion in Ewing's sarcoma. *Cancer* **46**: 516–521.

Rosen G (1982) Current management of Ewing's sarcoma. *Progress in Clinical Cancer* **8**: 267–282.

Rosen G, Wollner N, Tan C et al (1974) Disease-free survival in children with Ewing's sarcoma treated with radiation therapy and adjuvant four-drug sequential chemotherapy. *Cancer* **33**: 384–393.

Rosen G, Caparros B, Nirenberg A et al (1981) Ewing's sarcoma: ten-year experience with adjuvant chemotherapy. *Cancer* **47**: 2204–2213.

Samuels ML & Howe CD (1967) Cyclophosphamide in the management of Ewing's sarcoma. *Cancer* **20**: 961–966.

Scheulen ME, Niederle N & Bremer K (1983) Efficacy of ifosfamide in refractory malignant diseases and uroprotection by mesna: results of a clinical phase II-study with 151 patients. *Cancer Treatment Reviews* **10**(A): 93–101.

Selawry OS, Holland JF & Wolman IJ (1968) Effect of vincristine on malignant solid tumors in children. *Cancer Chemotherapy Reports* **53**: 497–500.

Senyszyn JJ, Johnson RE & Curran RE (1970) Treatment of metastatic Ewing's sarcoma with Actinomycin DD (NSC-3053). *Cancer Chemotherapy Reports* **54**: 103–107.

Strattan B, Askin FB & Kissane JM (1982) Intramyofiber skeletal muscle invasion in Ewing's sarcoma of bone: clinicopathological observations from the intergroup Ewing's sarcoma study. *American Journal of Pediatric Hematology and Oncology* **4**: 231–235.

Sutow WW & Sullivan MP (1962) Cyclophosphamide therapy in children with Ewing's sarcoma. *Cancer Chemotherapy Reports* **23**: 55–60.

Tan C, Etcubanas E, Wollner N et al (1973) Adriamycin—an antitumor antibiotic in the treatment of neoplastic disease. *Cancer* **32:** 9–17.

Tepper J, Glaubiger D, Lichter A, Wackenhut J & Glatstein E (1980) Local control of Ewing's sarcoma of bone with radiotherapy and combination chemotherapy. *Cancer* **46:** 1969–1973.

Vietti TJ, Nitschke R, Starling KA & van Eys J (1979) Evaluation of cis Dichlorodiammine-platinum (11) in children with advanced malignant diseases: South West Oncology Group Studies. *Cancer Treatment Reports* **63:** 1611–1614.

Wang JJ, Cortes E, Sinks L & Holland JF (1971) Therapeutic effect and toxicity of adriamycin in patients with neoplastic disease. *Cancer* **28:** 837–843.

Wheldon TE, O'Donoghue J & Gregor A (1985) Optimal scheduling of total body irradiation in the treatment of Ewing's sarcoma. *International Journal of Radiation Oncology, Biology, Physics* **11:** 1569–1570.

Worthington-White DA, Graham-Pole JR, Stout SA & Riley CM (1986) In vitro studies with melphalan and pediatric neoplastic and normal bone marrow cells. *International Journal of Cancer* **37:** 819–823.

Zidar BL, Benjamin RS, Frank J, Lane M & Baker LH (1983) Combination chemotherapy for advanced sarcomas of bone and mesothelioma utilizing rubidazone and DTIC: A South West Oncology Group Study. *American Journal of Clinical Oncology* **6:** 71–74.

# 9

# Chemotherapy of rare malignant bone tumours

## HELENA M. EARL

The use of chemotherapy in osteosarcomas and Ewing's sarcomas is now clearly defined, but its role in other, rare, malignant bone tumours, apart from primary non-Hodgkin's lymphoma of bone, is more difficult to define. In this chapter I review the available information on the use of chemo-therapy in other malignant bone tumours, in an attempt to provide some guidelines for the use of cytotoxic drugs in patients with these tumours.

## CHONDROSARCOMA

Chondrosarcomas are malignant cartilage tumours containing fully developed cartilage without tumour osteoid being formed by the sarcomatous stroma. The frequency of chondrosarcomas is second only to osteogenic sarcomas, and accounts for approximately 20% of all primary bone tumours. Chondrosarcoma can occur as a primary malignant tumour of bone, or as chondrosarcomatous change in benign lesions such as enchondromas. Patients with Ollier's disease (multiple enchondromatosis) are more at risk of developing chondrosarcomas than are the general population. Chondro-sarcoma is rare under the age of 30 years, and most cases are in the 40–60 year age group. The affected sites are as follows: pelvis—31%, femur—21%, ribs—9%, craniofacial bones—9%, proximal humerus and shoulder girdle—13%. Radiographic appearances are of central, lucent, destructive lesions with blotchy calcification present throughout the lesion, both within the central area of the bone and in the surrounding soft tissue.

### Treatment

Prognosis for patients with chondrosarcoma depends on the histological grade of the tumour. Dahlin and Henderson (1956) graded a series of chondrosarcomas as grade 1–3, the most undifferentiated being grade 3. Marcove and Huvos (1971) developed a similar grading system, and in 1972 they analysed factors which influenced survival in patients with chondro-sarcoma of the pelvis and proximal femur. Cure rate and length of survival were directly related to histopathological grading, with a significant difference between grade 3 and the lower two grades. Evans et al (1977) reported on 71 cases of chondrosarcoma from the M. D. Anderson

Hospital, and also found histopathological grade related directly to prognosis. Grade 1, 2 and 3 chondrosarcomas had 5-year survival rates of 90%, 81% and 43% and 10-year survival rates of 83%, 64% and 29% respectively.

The treatment of chondrosarcomas is principally surgical, and it is an essential part of clinical management to gain control of the primary tumour. The role of chemotherapy in the treatment of chondrosarcoma is not well defined, although chemotherapy has been used in high-grade tumours in an adjuvant setting and in patients with metastatic disease. In some centres, patients with chondrosarcomas have been treated with adjuvant chemotherapy similar to that used for osteosarcomas.

There are few reports of the use of chemotherapy in chondrosarcomas. In 1979, Ryall et al reported on the use of a combination of radiotherapy and razoxane (ICRF 159) in eight patients with 12 chondrosarcomas. The dose of radiotherapy was between 20 and 60 Gy, and razoxane was given usually at 125 mg twice a day on the days of radiotherapy. The authors report that tumours in five patients had complete or partial regressions, three tumours showed no change, and two tumours in one patient progressed. This method of treatment certainly afforded local control in patients with inoperable tumours.

A report from the Children's Hospital in Boston (Aprin et al, 1982) of 12 childhood chondrosarcomas described the use of chemotherapy, mostly in the adjuvant situation. This included actinomycin D alone (three patients), actinomycin D with vincristine (one patient), high-dose methotrexate and Adriamycin (doxorubicin hydrochloride) with or without vincristine (two patients). It is not possible to obtain any information on chemotherapy response from this report except that one patient who received high-dose methotrexate, Adriamycin and vincristine after the resection of a pulmonary metastasis is alive and disease-free 65 months later.

In a report from the M. D. Anderson Hospital (McNaney et al, 1982), describing radiotherapy experience with inoperable chondrosarcomas of bone, five of the 20 cases also had chemotherapy, although it is not clear why these particular cases were selected for chemotherapy. Two cases were treated with Adriamycin and DTIC (dacarbazine), one with six courses prior to irradiation and one with 10 courses after irradiation, and these patients are alive at 77 months and 29 months respectively. One patient received intra-arterial cisplatin before irradiation for a sacral lesion, and is alive, and one patient received intra-arterial actinomycin D and melphalan at the same time as irradiation, for a distal lesion. This patient had residual primary tumour, developed metastasis at 25 months and died of disease 27 months after diagnosis. The fifth patient received chemotherapy and immunotherapy (cyclophosphamide, vincristine, Adriamycin, DTIC, with chondrosarcoma lysates and BCG scarifications) after radiotherapy to a grade III chondrosarcoma of a vertebra, and is alive at 52 months, free of disease. Again, it is not possible to draw firm conclusions from this report about the chemosensitivity of chondrosarcomas.

Krochak et al (1983) report seven cases of well- and moderately differentiated inoperable chondrosarcomas treated with a combination of radiotherapy and chemotherapy [cyclophosphamide $500 \, mg/m^2$, vincristine

1.4 mg/m$^2$ (maximum 2 mg) and Adriamycin 50 mg/m$^2$ on day 1, with DTIC 250 mg/m$^2$ daily on days 1 to 5]. Chemotherapy was given either concomitantly with split-course irradiation, or at the start of irradiation, with subsequent courses after completion of irradiation. Only one of these seven patients has died, but follow-up is short (8–83 months). These results of combined radiotherapy and chemotherapy in inoperable chondrosarcoma, either well or moderately differentiated, are very encouraging.

In conclusion, the role of chemotherapy in the treatment of chondrosarcomas remains ill-defined, although some recent results are encouraging. There is a need for well-designed studies in inoperable and metastatic cases, particularly of a higher grade.

**Mesenchymal chondrosarcoma**

Mesenchymal chondrosarcoma was first described by Lichtenstein and Bernstein (1959) and is a rare type of chondrosarcoma characterized histopathologically by a bimorphic pattern of islands of chondroid tissue in various stages of differentiation mixed with areas of small, anaplastic, frequently spindle-shaped cells, often in a perivascular arrangement. These tumours may arise in bone or, less commonly, in soft tissue.

Mesenchymal chondrosarcomas occur as commonly in males as in females, in the age range of 5–74 years, with 58% of tumours occurring in the second and third decades of life. The usual sites of origin of this rare tumour are as follows: leg—26%, craniofacial bones—23%, vertebral bodies or sacrum—16%, ribs or clavicle—14%, pelvis—13%, arm—8%. The clinical presentation is with pain, swelling, neurological involvement or instability of the affected bone. Radiographs typically show a lytic and destructive lesion, with mottled calcification similar to conventional chondrosarcomas.

The prognosis for mesenchymal chondrosarcoma is poor. Some groups have defined two histological subgroups: the first is a small cell undifferentiated variety, and the second consists of tumours with a predominant haemangiopericytomatoid pattern of growth (Huvos et al, 1983). These histopathological subgroups were primarily defined to establish whether the two different groups have a different prognosis and whether different chemotherapeutic approaches would be applicable.

The cornerstone of treatment for mesenchymal chondrosarcomas is surgical excision. Intralesional excision (i.e. curettage for bone lesions) was followed by a 44% incidence of local recurrence (Nakashima et al, 1986) and an 88% incidence of distant metastases. Wide local excision or amputation both achieved the low local recurrence rate of approximately 10%. In the large series reported from the Mayo Clinic (Nakashima et al, 1986) of 111 patients, 60% went on to develop metastatic disease, with pulmonary metastases being the commonest site, followed by regional and distant lymph node metastases and occasional bone metastases. Survival rates for 23 patients at the Mayo Clinic were a 57% 5-year survival rate and a 26% 10-year survival rate, whilst Huvos et al (1983) report a 43% 5-year survival rate and a 28% 10-year survival rate.

In the Mayo Clinic report, chemotherapy was used as an adjuvant to surgery in 19 patients, 17 (89.5%) of whom eventually died of disease. More details on the cases are not available, so it is not possible to judge whether chemotherapy was used because of the presence of other poor prognostic factors (e.g. incomplete local excision). Irradiation with or without chemotherapy was the initial treatment in seven patients with inoperable disease, six of whom died of their disease.

A clinicopathological analysis of 35 patients with mesenchymal chondrosarcoma from Huvos et al (1983) includes a detailed description of 13 patients diagnosed after 1976 whose treatment included chemotherapy. This report separated the patients into those with predominantly small undifferentiated cell tumours (five patients) and those with a predominant haemangiopericytomatoid growth (eight patients). Two patients with localized disease of the small cell, undifferentiated variant were treated with high-dose methotrexate (HDMTX), but operative specimens showed no evidence of response. These patients went on to receive chemotherapy on the T10 protocol (Rosen et al, 1982); one patient is alive, disease-free, at 27 months and the other is alive with bone metastases. One patient with the small cell, undifferentiated variant with multiple bone metastases was treated with HDMTX with no response, and then with Rosen's T10 protocol, and gained a complete response which lasted for 1 year, terminated by relapse at one of the original bone sites. A further patient in this group who had metastatic pulmonary disease showed no response to the T10 protocol. Therefore, in these patients with the small cell, undifferentiated variant there were *no* responses to HDMTX, whilst three out of four patients responded to T10 chemotherapy [HDMTX with Adriamycin, and the combination of bleomycin, cyclophosphamide and actinomycin D (BCD)].

Eight patients with mesenchymal chondrosarcoma of the haemangiopericytomatoid variant were reported. Two patients had femoral lesions, with chest wall and breast metastases. They received T11 chemotherapy preoperatively and then had the primary and metastases resected. Both had partial responses and postoperatively received T10 chemotherapy (cisplatin and Adriamycin, with BCD). Both are alive without evidence of disease at 8 and 15 months. Two patients with skull lesions were treated with T11 chemotherapy and radiotherapy; one patient had a complete response, and the other a partial response followed by surgical removal of the residual primary tumour. Both patients are alive and disease-free at 27 and 23 months respectively. One patient with inoperable pelvic disease was treated by radiotherapy and had a complete response for 4 years, and on relapse had a partial response to T11 chemotherapy. Another patient with an inoperable pelvic lesion had a complete response to T10 chemotherapy, although she developed local recurrence and metastatic disease 6 months after treatment. One patient with multiple bone involvement at presentation had no response to HDMTX, but a further patient with a tibial lesion treated only by T9 chemotherapy (Rosen et al, 1981) is alive and disease-free 49 months after presentation.

In summary, chemotherapy for mesenchymal chondrosarcoma shows *no* response to HDMTX (five patients), but 9 out of 11 patients responded to multi-agent chemotherapy as described above. Mesenchymal chondrosarcoma is a chemosensitive tumour, and efforts to improve the survival rates in this disease should include adjuvant chemotherapy.

## MALIGNANT FIBROUS HISTIOCYTOMA OF BONE

Malignant fibrous histiocytoma of bone (MFHB) is a distinct clinicopathological entity first described by Feldman and Norman in 1972 which accounts for at least 5% of all primary malignant bone tumours. MFHB is thought to arise from a primitive fixed mesenchymal cell (Roholl et al, 1985) and exhibits both histiocytic and fibrous properties. The criteria for the histopathological diagnosis of MFHB are now well established (Kempson and Kyriakos, 1972; Soule and Enriquez, 1972; Dahlin et al, 1977 and Capanna et al, 1984).

It is more common in men than in women (M:F ratio = 1.5:1) and may arise at any age, although the peak incidence is in middle age. It is interesting that the peak incidence in women is the second decade, whilst in men the peak incidence of tumours is in the 40–60 year age group (Capanna et al, 1984). In up to 20% of patients MFHB arises in an area of abnormal bone, in particular in areas of previous bone infarction (Dahlin et al, 1977; McCarthy et al, 1979), Paget's disease, fibrous dysplasia and as a complication of radiation therapy (Capanna et al, 1984). The main sites of tumour at presentation are as follows: femur—47%, tibia—22%, humerus—9.5%, pelvis—9% (Capanna et al, 1984). This analysis excludes 15 cases reported in the world literature in the craniofacial bones and nine cases arising in the ribs. The majority of tumours arise around the knee (47%), either in the lower metaphysis of the femur or in the upper metaphysis of the tibia. The commonest initial metastatic site is pulmonary (85%) followed by bone (12%), lymph node metastases being extremely rare [1 in 52 cases reported from the Rizzoli Institute (Capanna et al, 1984)].

Traditionally, treatment for MFHB has been surgery sometimes combined with radiation therapy. However, local recurrence or distant metastases will occur in approximately 70% of patients within 5 years when treated in this way. Table 1 gives a summary of the survival data in this group of patients. The largest single group are the 48 patients reported from the Rizzoli Institute, who have 2- and 3-year survival rates of 45% and 32% respectively.

More recently, adjuvant chemotherapy has been used in either pre- and post-radical surgery, or post-surgery alone (Table 2). The chemotherapy used has been largely based on that used for the adjuvant chemotherapeutic treatment of osteosarcomas. Most regimens have therefore included high-dose methotrexate, with citrovorum rescue, vincristine and Adriamycin, with the addition of bleomycin, cyclophosphamide and actinomycin D in patients treated more recently (Rosen et al, 1982). Eight reported cases (Urban et al, 1983; Weiner et al, 1983; den Heeten et al, 1985) have received preoperative chemotherapy for several months, and all of these received high-dose methotrexate. Histopathological examination in these eight patients revealed that seven had a complete response, with no viable tumour

**Table 1.** Survival in patients with malignant fibrous histiocytoma of bone treated by surgery and/or radiotherapy.

| Survival of patients (with long follow-up) | Survival | Reference |
|---|---|---|
| 11 | 7 DOD at 8 mo to 8 yr<br>4 AWD | Feldman and Lattes, 1977 |
| 13 | 11 DOD by 4 yr<br>2 A/W at 4 yr | Spanier et al, 1975, 1977 |
| 12 | 7 DOD at 2 mo to 8 yr<br>1 AWD at 5 yr<br>4 A/W at 5 yr+ | Huvos, 1976 |
| 28 | 33% DFS at 5 yr+ | Dahlin et al, 1977 |
| 21 | 10 DOD by 3 yr<br>2 AWD at 3 yr<br>9 A/W at 3 yr+ | McCarthy et al, 1979 |
| 48 | 2-yr survival: 45%<br>3-yr survival: 32%<br>10-yr survival: 25% | Capanna et al, 1984 |
| Total: 133 | Long-term survivors:<br>30% (39 out of 133) | |

DOD = dead of disease.
AWD = alive with disease.
A/W = alive and well, no relapse.
DFS = disease-free survival.
mo = months.

tissue present in the resected specimen. The eighth patient had tumour necrosis of just under 90% of the resected specimen. These response data demonstrate that MFHB is a tumour which is chemosensitive. The 2-year survival rate for the 32 patients included in Table 2 is 71%, which compares favourably with the 2-year survival rate of 45% in the 48 patients treated at the Rizzoli Institute ($P = 0.02$). Long-term follow-up on the majority of patients is not yet available.

There is one report in the literature (Shuman et al, 1982) of intra-arterial chemotherapy in three patients with malignant fibrous histiocytomas of the pelvis. Three young patients, aged 21, 30 and 41 years, presented with osteolytic pelvic lesions, and were treated at first with intra-arterial cisplatin 120–140 mg/m$^2$ over a 2-hour period. In the two patients who did not respond completely, a combination of Adriamycin 60 mg/m$^2$ in 4 days with 5-(dimethyltriazeno)-imidazole-4-carboxomide (dacarbazine) (1000 mg/m$^2$/4 days) was infused intra-arterially, whilst cyclophosphamide 600 mg/m$^2$ was given intravenously on day 1 (CYADIC). Two patients had complete responses, one to cisplatin and the other to CYADIC, and these were both confirmed on histopathology of the resected primary tumour. These patients are alive 9 months and 2 years after diagnosis.

Malignant fibrous histiocytoma of bone has been shown to be chemosensitive to high-dose methotrexate, Adriamycin, vincristine and BCD.

**Table 2.** Chemotherapy for localized MFHB.

| Chemotherapy | No. of patients | Other treatment | Chemotherapy response | Follow-up | Reference |
|---|---|---|---|---|---|
| HDMTX, VINC, ADM—18 month treatment | 1 | Tumour resection post-chemotherapy | Histopath. CR | A/W 48 mo | Weiner et al, 1983 |
| | 1 | Tumour resection pre-chemotherapy | — | A/W 42 mo | |
| | 1 | Radiotherapy 25 Gy, and tumour resection, pre-chemotherapy | — | A/W 42 mo | |
| T5 protocol (Rosen, 1979) HDMTX, ADM, VINC, CTX | 1 | Resection post-chemotherapy | Histopath. CR | A/W 78 mo | Urban et al, 1983 |
| T7 protocol (Rosen, 1979) HDMTX, ADM, VINC, BCD, CTX | 1 | Resection post-chemotherapy | Histopath. CR | A/W 51 mo | |
| T10 protocol (Rosen, 1982) | 2 | 2, Resection post-chemotherapy | 1, histopath. CR; 1, histopath. 90% tumour necrosis | A/W 24 mo; A/W 18 mo | |
| ADM HDMTX, VINC, ADM | 9 / 11 | Resection pre-chemotherapy | — | 2 yr survival 66%; 5- and 10-yr survival: 36% | Capanna et al, 1984 |
| VINC, ADM, CTX, DTIC | 1 | Resection post-chemotherapy | — | A/W 58 mo | |
| HDMTX, VINC, ADM, BCD | 1 | Resection pre-chemotherapy | — | A/W 41 mo | |
| T10 protocol (Rosen, 1982) HDMTX, VINC, ADM, BCD | 1 | Endoprosthesis, post-chemotherapy | Histopath. CR | A/W 56 mo | den Heeten et al, 1985 |
| T10 protocol | 1 | Curettage, post-chemotherapy | Histopath. CR | A/W 46 mo | |
| T10 protocol | 1 | Inoperable | Histopath. CR | A/W 25 mo | |
| TOTAL | 32 | | 7, histopath. CR | 2-yr DFS: 71% | |

HDMTX = high-dose methotrexate, VINC = vincristine, ADM = Adriamycin, CTX = cyclophosphamide, BCD = bleomycin, cyclophosphamide and actinomycin D, histopath. = histopath. CR = no viable tumour tissue in resection specimen, A/W = alive with no disease, DFS = disease-free survival, mo = months.

This fact, together with the poor long-term survival figures after surgery alone, have encouraged the use of adjuvant chemotherapy in this disease. However, the rarity of this tumour will make it difficult to be sure of the degree of benefit conferred by adjuvant chemotherapy unless collaborative trials are undertaken.

## PRIMARY NON-HODGKIN'S LYMPHOMA OF BONE

Primary non-Hodgkin's lymphoma of bone (PNHLB), formerly referred to as 'reticulum cell sarcoma' of bone, accounts for approximately 5% of primary bone tumours. It is an unusual extranodal presentation of diffuse 'histiocytic' non-Hodgkin's lymphoma, and is the primary site in 5% of all extra-nodal lymphomas (Freeman et al, 1972). One of the earliest reports by Parker and Jackson (1939) described 17 patients with primary reticulum cell sarcomas of bone who had slow-growing tumours and good long-term survival after amputation or local radiotherapy alone.

A review of reported cases of PNHLB from 1972 to the present day includes 119 cases with treatment details and 422 patients reported from the Mayo Clinic with predominantly histopathological data only (Ostrowski et al, 1986). Patients with PNHLB have an age range of 9–91 years, with an increasing incidence up to the age of 70 years, and a male predominance (64% male to 36% female). These reported cases of PNHLB date back to 1907 (Dosoretz et al, 1982; Ostrowski et al, 1986), but the majority have been treated in major centres since 1970 (Reimer et al, 1977; Bacci et al, 1982; Parvinen et al, 1983; Bacci et al, 1986; Loeffler et al, 1986). The commonest sites of disease at presentation are as follows: femur—22%, craniofacial bones—18%, spine—15%, pelvis—14%, humerus—8%; tibia—7%, ribs—6%, scapula—5%.

There seems little doubt that the cornerstone of local treatment for PNHLB is radiotherapy. A report from Dosoretz et al (1983), of 30 patients treated with radiation therapy alone showed that there were only three local failures following treatment, and the cumulative incidence of local recurrence was 14% at 5 years. There were no local failures at radiation doses higher than 50 Gy, or a complementary time-dose-fractionation calculation (Orton and Ellis, 1973) of greater than 70. The three local recurrences occurred in five patients with PNHLB of non-cleaved and pleomorphic cell types who received doses of less than 50 Gy. In a complementary paper (Dosoretz et al, 1982) these authors draw attention to the relationship of histopathological morphological diversity and clinical behaviour, associating the non-cleaved cell tumour group and the pleomorphic cell subgroup with a poorer prognosis. Thirty patients with PNHLB were reported from the Rizzoli Institute (Bacci et al, 1986), 26 treated with radiotherapy and chemotherapy, and four with radiotherapy alone. Three patients receiving combined treatment have relapsed, but not within the irradiated areas, whilst one of the four patients treated with radiotherapy alone had relapsed locally and also with disseminated disease. In this report side-effects due to radiation therapy were moderate, including the 26 patients treated concurrently with chemotherapy.

In only two cases were severe, treatment-related, local complications observed. These consisted of delayed pathological fracture in one patient (treated successfully by internal fixation) and leg-shortening in another. These complications occurred with a radiation dose of 45 Gy and 60 Gy respectively. No secondary tumours developed within the irradiated site (median follow-up time = 87 months). The paper on 31 patients from the Memorial Sloan-Kettering (Parvinen et al, 1983) does not report any cases of radiation-induced problems in local lesions. The reported radiation doses vary more widely, with doses of 40–50 Gy in patients with stage I and stage II disease, and doses of 20–30 Gy in those with stage IV disease. Loeffler et al (1986) report the results of combination treatment in childhood PNHLB, combining local radiotherapy with chemotherapy and prophylactic cranial irradiation. The results are excellent, but the occurrence of two second bone tumours (malignant fibrous histiocytomas of bone), both clearly within the primary irradiated site at 5 and 7 years following diagnosis, is a worrying development.

The majority of patients with PNHLB reported in the literature have been staged using detailed staging methods. The report from the National Cancer Institute (Reimer et al, 1977) on 14 patients presenting between 1970 and 1975 showed that although all patients had clinically localized disease at presentation, after staging, 12 out of 14 were found to have stage IV disease. Staging investigations included chest X-ray, bipedal lymphangiograms, intravenous pyelogram, technetium-99 diphosphonate bone scan and gallium scan, with percutaneous bone marrow and liver biopsies. This study points to the importance of staging investigations to define accurately the extent of disease at presentation.

Since the early 1970s, patients with stage III and stage IV PNHLB have been treated with a combination of radiotherapy to the primary site, together with chemotherapy. Eighteen per cent (21 out of 119) of patients reported in the literature had stage III and stage IV disease, but this is probably not a true reflection of the proportion of patients with PNHLB presenting with disseminated disease because those with stage IV disease are often excluded from analysis (see Bacci et al, 1986, Rizzoli Institute Report). In the report from the Mayo Clinic, 25% of patients (106 out of 422) had or developed nodal and/or soft tissue involvement within 6 months of diagnosis. The chemotherapy of 21 patients with stage III and stage IV PNHLB has been detailed in the literature (see Table 3) and has included cyclophosphamide alone, C-MOPP (Schein et al, 1974), BACOP (Schein et al, 1976) and $L_2$ protocol (Koziner et al, 1982), with some intensive non-Hodgkin's lymphoma (NHL) protocols including CNS prophylaxis. At the time of analysis 11 out of 21 (52%) had died of disease at 3–24 months from diagnosis (median = 19 months). The disease-free survival (DFS) rate at 2 years from diagnosis was 38% (7 out of 18), with three patients alive and free of disease from 11 to 19 months after diagnosis. These results compare favourably with the results of chemotherapy for advanced diffuse histiocytic lymphomas presenting with nodal disease, where DFS rates at 2 years are approximately 40% for all stages and median survival is 11 months in stage IV diffuse histiocytic lymphoma (Fisher et al, 1981).

**Table 3.** Primary non-Hodgkin's lymphoma of bone—stages III and IV.

| Chemotherapy | No. of patients | Stage | Other treatment | Follow-up | Reference |
|---|---|---|---|---|---|
| CTX alone | 2 | IV | RT to primary | DOD 11 mo   DOD 19 mo | Reimer et al, 1977 |
| C-MOPP (Schein, 1974) CTX, VINC, PROC, PRED | 4 | IV | 1, RT to primary site | DOD 8 mo / DOD 16 mo   No RT / DOD 20 mo   (RT) / A/W 24 mo | Reimer et al, 1977 |
| CAV CTX, ADM, VINC | 1 | IV | No RT | DOD 3 mo | Reimer et al, 1977 |
| BACOP (Schein, 1976) BLEO, ADM, CTX, VINC, PRED | 4 | IV | 2, RT to primary site | A/W 32 mo / A/W 19 mo   RT / A/W 19 mo   No RT / A/W 11 mo | Reimer et al, 1977 |
| CVP (Schein, 1974) CTX, VINC, PRED | 1 | IV | RT to primary site | DOD 14 mo | Reimer et al, 1977 |
| CTX or CTX, VINC, PRED | 3 | IV | 2, RT to primary site. 1, RT and surgery to primary site | 1 patient A/W at 5 yr / 2 patients DOD by 2 yr | Parvinen et al, 1983 |
| L₂ protocol (Koziner, 1982) CTX, VINC, PRED, DAUNO with IT MTX or ARA-C. Consolidation with maintenance for 3 years. | 3 | IV | 3, RT to primary site | 1 patient A/W at 5 yr / 2 patients DOD by 2 yr | Parvinen et al, 1983 |
| NHL-3 protocol ADM, CTX, VINC, ARA-C, MTX with IT MTX or ARA-C | 1 | IV | RT to primary site | A/W at 5 yr | Parvinen et al, 1983 |
| APO ADM, PRED, VINC for 2 years. CNS-cranial RT, IT MTX | 2 | III | 1, RT to primary site | A/W 26 mo (+RT) / A/W 84 mo | Loeffler et al, 1986 |
| Total | 21 | 2 III / 19 IV | 13 out of 21 RT to primary site | DF at 2 yr = 38% (7 out of 18) / 3 patients A/W, 11–19 mo after diagnosis | |

CTX = cyclophosphamide, VINC = vincristine, PROC = procarbazine, PRED = prednisolone, ADM = Adriamycin, BLEO = bleomycin, DAUNO = daunorubicin, IT = intrathecal, MTX = methotrexate, ARA-C = cytosine arabinoside, RT = radiotherapy. DOD = dead of disease, A/W = alive and free of disease, mo = months, DF = disease free.

Patients with stage I and stage II PNHLB have been treated in major centres either by radiotherapy and adjuvant chemotherapy or by radiotherapy alone. Summaries of the results of treatment are shown in Tables 4 and 5, comparing patients who received radiotherapy alone with those who received both modalities of treatment. Comparing 51 patients who were treated only by radiotherapy with 45 patients who received both radiotherapy and chemotherapy (Table 6), the 2- and 5-year DFS rates are better for those receiving combined treatment [2-year DFS rate: 84% vs 66% (combined vs single treatment), $P < 0.1 > 0.5$; 5-year DFS rate: 82% vs 54% (combined vs single treatment), $P = 0.01$]. However, the largest group of patients receiving radiotherapy alone (33 patients) was reported by Dosoretz et al in 1982 in a group of patients dating back to 1950. Twenty of these patients would by present day standards be considered to have been inadequately staged, and it is possible that this group includes some patients with unrecognized stage III and stage IV disease. If patients with inadequately staged disease are excluded from the analysis, stage I and stage II patients treated by radiotherapy and chemotherapy still have a better 5-year DFS rate than patients treated by radiotherapy alone [82% (33 out of 40 patients—combined treatment) vs 58% (14 out of 24 patients—single treatment; $P = 0.05$) Table 6]. Analysing DFS rates for patients with localized PNHLB, i.e. stage I disease, also shows that 5-year DFS is higher in patients treated with combined radiotherapy and chemotherapy than with radiotherapy alone [78% (29 out of 37 patients—combined treatment) vs 54% (12 out of 22 patients—single treatment), $P = 0.05$].

Comparisons of this nature which analyse groups from many different centres are of course open to criticism. Patients with stage I disease who have been treated more recently with chemotherapy have been accurately staged, and in the patients from the Rizzoli Institute and Loeffler's group, they form a much younger group of patients. However, the 5-year disease-free survival rates of 82% are very impressive for patients receiving both chemotherapy and radiotherapy for stage I and stage II PNHLB. Ideally, a prospectively randomized trial should be conducted to assess the benefits of combined chemotherapy and radiotherapy at presentation in the patients, but the rarity of this condition would make it difficult. However, in patients with localized nodal diffuse histiocytic lymphoma, Bonnadonna et al (1977) has reported a randomized clinical trial comparing cyclophosphamide, vincristine and prednisone (CVP) chemotherapy plus radiotherapy to radiotherapy alone. He reports a highly significant survival advantage for the use of the combined programme in patients with localized diffuse histiocytic lymphomas.

This evidence, together with that from the published data, lead one to conclude that local radiotherapy and intensive combination chemotherapy are the treatments of choice for younger patients presenting with localized primary non-Hodgkin's lymphoma of bone. Loeffler et al (1986), who reported on children with this disease, also included prophylactic cranial irradiation, and no patients suffered CNS metastases. Interestingly, in the other group of patients treated intensively (not including CNS prophylaxis) at the Rizzoli Institute, 2 out of 30 (6%) patients developed meningeal

**Table 4.** PNHLB—stage I and stage II disease treated without chemotherapy.

| No. of patients | Stage | Other treatment | Follow-up | Reference |
|---|---|---|---|---|
| 2 | IE, IIE | 1, surgery; 1, RT to primary site | A/W: 70 mo (surgery)<br>A/W: 62 mo (RT) | Reimer et al, 1977 |
| 16 | 15I, III | 14, RT to primary site; 2 RT and surgery of primary site | 9 out of 16 A/W at 5 yr<br>7 out of 16 DOD at 2 yr | Parvinen et al, 1983 |
| 4 | I(IAS) | Surgery only | A/W: 264 mo. DOD: 28 mo, 9 mo, 38 mo | Dosoretz et al, 1982 |
| 6 | I(AS) | RT alone | DOD: 12 mo, 11 mo, 29 mo<br>A/W: 66 mo, 36 mo<br>AWD: 29 mo | Dosoretz et al, 1982 |
| 19 | I(IAS) | RT alone | DOD: 26 mo, 10 mo, 6 mo, 100 mo, 3 mo, 5 mo, 16 mo, 15 mo, 14 mo<br>DID: 111 mo, 97 mo, 112 mo<br>A/W: 192 mo, 180 mo, 72 mo, 120 mo 252 mo, 159 mo<br>AWD: 96 mo | Dosoretz et al, 1982 |
| 4 | I(AS) | RT alone | A/W: 42 mo, 48 mo, 72 mo<br>DOD: 101 mo | Bacci et al, 1982 |
| Total: 51 | I(49) II(2) | 25 out of 51 dead (50%) 3–111 mo (med. 24 mo)<br>2-yr DFS: 34 out of 51 (66%)<br>5-yr DFS: 26 out of 48 (54%) | | |

AS = adequately staged, IAS = inadequately staged, RT = radiotherapy, DFS = disease-free survival, A/W = alive and well, AWD = alive with disease, DOD = dead of disease, DID = dead of intercurrent disease, AWR = alive with treated relapse, mo = months.

**Table 5.** PNHLB—stage I and stage II disease treated with chemotherapy.

| Chemotherapy | No. of patients | Stage | Other treatment | Follow-up | Reference |
|---|---|---|---|---|---|
| CTX, MTX, ACD; ADM, PRED, VINC; CTX, VINC, PRED; CTX, VINC, PRED, PROC | 4 | I(AS) | RT to primary site | DOD: 88 mo, 6 mo<br>A/W: 51 mo, 90 mo | Dosoretz et al, 1982 |
| CTX, or CTX, VINC, PRED | 5 | I(AS) | RT to primary site | 2 out of 5 A/W at 5 yr<br>3 out of 5 DOD at 2 yr | Parvinen et al, 1983 |
| NHL-3 protocol | 1 | I(AS) | RT to primary site | DOD at 2 yr | Parvinen et al, 1983 |
| ADM, VINC, CTX for 2 years | 26 | I(AS) | RT to primary site | 20 A/W > 5 yr<br>3 A/W > 2 yr < 5 yr<br>DOD: 11 mo, 12 mo<br>AWR: 35 mo | Bacci et al, 1986 |
| ADM, PRED, ONCO and CNS prophylaxis | 9 | I(5), II(4) | RT to primary site | A/W: 135 mo, 129 mo, 107 mo, 109 mo, 114 mo, 94 mo, 95 mo, 87 mo<br>DID*: 96 mo | Loeffler et al, 1986 |
| Total | 45 | I(41), II(4) | | 2-yr DFS: 84% (38 out of 45)<br>5-yr DFS: 82% (33 out of 40)<br>9 out of 45 (20%) dead<br>6 mo–96 mo (median 24 mo) | |

CTX = cyclophosphamide, MTX = methotrexate, ACD = actinomycin D, ADM = Adriamycin, PRED = prednisolone, VINC = vincristine, PROC = procarbazine, ONCO = Oncovin (vincristine sulphate). AS = adequately staged, RT = radiotherapy, IAS = inadequately staged, AWD = alive with disease, DID* dead of intercurrent disease, a malignant fibrous histiocytoma of bone, in original radiation field, AWR = alive with treated relapse, mo = months.

Table 6. Disease-free survival in patients with stage I and stage II PNHLB.

| | DFS at 2 years (%) | DFS at 5 years (%) |
|---|---|---|
| Stage I and II radiotherapy and chemotherapy | 84% (38 out of 45)[NS] | 82% (33 out of 40)[S] |
| Stage I and II radiotherapy alone (all patients) | 66% (34 out of 51)[NS] | 54% (26 out of 48)[S] |
| Stage I and II radiotherapy alone (staging complete) | 70% (19 out of 27)[NS] | 58% (14 out of 24)[S] |
| Stage I radiotherapy and chemotherapy | 83% (34 out of 41)[NS] | 78% (29 out of 37)[S] |
| Stage I radiotherapy alone (all patients) | 66% (31 out of 47)[NS] | 53% (24 out of 45)[S] |
| Stage I radiotherapy alone (staging complete) | 65% (17 out of 26)[NS] | 54% (12 out of 22)[S] |

NS = $P = > 0.05$ = no significant difference.
S = $P = 0.05$ = significant difference.

lymphoma at 10 and 12 months after diagnosis. However, the overall incidence of CNS relapse is probably not high enough to consider CNS prophylaxis routinely at the present time.

## CHEMOTHERAPY OF OTHER BONE SARCOMAS

Other primary malignant sarcomas of bone are rare, and there is little published work on their treatment. Rosen (1982) has therefore suggested that the rare bone sarcomas be classified according to their histopathological appearance, as either what he calls spindle cell sarcomas of low or high grade (e.g. osteosarcomas and chondrosarcomas) or as small cell sarcomas (e.g. Ewing's sarcomas or mesenchymal chondrosarcoma), and treated accordingly. Using this terminology, haemangioendotheliomas, adamantinomas and malignant schwannomas are called spindle cell sarcomas of low-grade histology. Fibrosarcomas and haemangiopericytomas are spindle cell sarcomas of low- and high-grade histology, and angiosarcomas and primitive neuroectodermal tumours are regarded as small cell sarcomas.

### Epithelioid haemangioendothelioma of bone

This tumour is characterized histopathologically by the presence of epithelioid or 'histiocytoid' endothelial cells that are either round or spindle-shaped. The majority are multicentric bone tumours. These patients have a protracted clinical course, and indeed the multicentric tumours appear to follow an even less aggressive course. Treatment is local only with curettage or tumour resection being adequate in the majority, with the occasional patient requiring the addition of radiotherapy (Tsuneyoshi et al, 1986).

## Adamantinoma of the long bone

Adamantinoma is a malignant tumour of long bones that has a prolonged clinical course. It is an extremely rare, low grade, spindle cell sarcoma of bone, of which there are about 100 cases in the world literature. Electron microscopic studies have suggested that the tumour appears to be composed of cells which differentiate along both mesenchymal and epithelial cell lines. In a report from the Rizzoli Institute (Campanacci et al, 1981) on nine cases, it appears that adequate local surgery is the treatment of choice, only one patient requiring radiotherapy in addition. Although several of the patients developed local recurrence after initial surgery, none have to date developed metastatic disease. The development of metastases in other series (Huvos et al, 1975; Spjut et al, 1971; Unni et al, 1974) has ranged from 15 to 40%. Where isolated pulmonary metastasis develops, thoracotomy with metastasectomy is probably indicated because of the slow growth rate of these tumours.

## Haemangioendothelial sarcomas of bone

Haemangioendothelial sarcomas of bone are of endothelial origin and are clinically malignant. Wold et al (1982) report on 112 cases from the Mayo Clinic, and divide them histopathologically into grade 1, 2 or 3 lesions. DFS for these three tumour grades were: grade 1—95%, grade 2—62% and grade 3—20%, and histological grade was the single feature that correlated best with DFS. The treatment was essentially by local surgical control of the tumour, with occasional radiotherapy for inoperable lesions. Adjuvant chemotherapy was given to patients with a grade 2 lesion, and to three patients with grade 3 lesions, but the effectiveness of this additional treatment is difficult to assess in this rare tumour. It would appear that adjuvant chemotherapy should be considered in grade 3 haemangioendo-thelial sarcomas of bone, as the prognosis with local therapy alone is poor.

## Haemangiopericytoma of bone

Haemangiopericytoma of bone is a rare vascular neoplasm believed to arise from cells surrounding capillaries and post-capillary venules. About one-half of the reported cases show malignant histopathological features. Fifteen cases are reported from the Mayo Clinic (Wold et al, 1982) of which nine were of malignant histology. These patients were treated by surgery in seven cases, with or without irradiation. Two patients also received chemotherapy. The prognosis for this condition appears to be very poor: six out of nine of these patients have died from disease, and two patients are alive but with recurrence.

A report from Beadle and Hillcoat (1983) details the use of Adriamycin ($50\,mg/m^2$) and DTIC ($600$–$700\,mg/m^2$) intravenously every 4 weeks in four patients with advanced haemangiopericytomas. Two patients had good responses, a third had less than a partial response, and the fourth had no response.

Haemangiopericytoma of bone of malignant histological type seems to carry a poor prognosis, so that as well as good local control by surgical measures or radiotherapy, these patients should be considered for chemotherapy along the lines of treatment for spindle cell sarcoma of bone (e.g. osteogenic sarcomas).

### Fibrosarcoma of bone

Fibrosarcomas of bone are most common in the third, fourth and fifth decades of life. Most lesions occur in the distal femur, proximal tibia or proximal humerus, with the next commonest site being the pelvis. They may arise in sites of previous radiotherapy.

In a report from Huvos and Higginbotham (1975) of 130 patients, the periosteal variety of fibrosarcoma had a better prognosis than the medullary lesions, with 10-year survival rates of 50% and 25% respectively following surgical treatment alone. The treatment of fibrosarcoma of bone is the same as for other spindle cell sarcomas of bone. Low-grade fibrosarcomas should be treated by local surgical measures. It is probable that high-grade tumours should be treated by adequate local surgery with the addition of systemic chemotherapy along the lines of that used for osteosarcomas (Rosen et al, 1982).

### Angiosarcoma

Angiosarcomas of bone are very rare, accounting for less than 0.5% of primary malignant bone tumours. They are undifferentiated, small cell sarcomas, arising in vascular structures, that tend to metastasize in the majority of patients. The most widely adopted therapeutic approach to these patients is similar to that used in patients with Ewing's sarcoma, using combination chemotherapy (Rosen et al, 1981) with local control by surgical measures or radiotherapy.

## SUMMARY

Worldwide experience of chemotherapy in bone tumours other than osteosarcomas or Ewing's sarcomas is very limited. Chemotherapy has an important role in the treatment of primary non-Hodgkin's lymphoma of bone, and the treatment of stage I and stage II disease with chemotherapy as well as with radiotherapy does appear to improve the prognosis. Malignant fibrous histiocytoma of bone has been shown to be sensitive to high-dose methotrexate, Adriamycin, vincristine and BCD, and trials of the use of adjuvant chemotherapy should be encouraged in this disease to try and improve long-term survival figures. Mesenchymal chondrosarcomas have been demonstrated to be chemosensitive, not to high-dose methotrexate, but to cisplatin, Adriamycin and BCD, and the adjuvant use of such chemotherapy should be more fully assessed in the disease. The role of chemotherapy in the treatment of the more common and more indolent chondrosarcomas, however, remains ill-defined, although some recent results are encouraging. Amongst the very rare bone tumours, epithelioid haemangioendotheliomas, adamantinomas and grade 1 haemangioendothelial sarcomas do not require adjuvant chemotherapy. However, malignant haemangiopericytomas, fibrosarcomas, grade 2 or 3 haemangioendothelial sarcomas and angiosarcomas have a very poor prognosis which may be improved by the use of adjuvant or preoperative chemotherapy.

## REFERENCES

Aprin H, Riseborough EJ & Hall JE (1982) Chondrosarcoma in children and adolescents. *Clinical Orthopaedics and Related Research* **156**: 329–331.

Bacci G, Picci P, Beroni F et al (1982) Primary lymphoma of bone: results in 15 patients treated by radiotherapy combined with systematic chemotherapy. *Cancer Treatment Reports* **66**(10): 1859–1862.

Bacci G, Jaffe N, Emilian E et al (1986) Therapy for primary non-Hodgkin's lymphoma of bone and a comparison of results with Ewing's sarcoma. Ten years experience at the Instituto Orthopedico Rizzoli. *Cancer* **57**(8): 1468–1472.

Beadle GF & Hillcoat BL (1983) Treatment of advanced malignant haemangiopericytoma with combination Adriamycin and DTIC: a report of four cases. *Journal of Surgical Oncology* **22**: 167–170.

Bonnadonna G, Lattnada A, Manfarddine S et al (1977) Combined radiotherapy-chemotherapy in localised non-Hodgkin's lymphomas: 5 year results of a randomised study. In Jones SE & Salman SE (eds) *Adjuvant Therapy of Cancer*, pp 145–153, 2nd edn. New York: Grune and Stratton.

Campanacci M, Lans M, Giunti A et al (1981) Adamantinoma of the long bones. The experience at the Instituto Orthopaedio Rizzoli. *American Journal of Surgical Pathology* **5**: 533–542.

Capanna R, Bertoni F, Bacchini P et al (1984) Malignant fibrous histiocytoma of bone. The experience of the Rizzoli Institute: report of 90 cases. *Cancer* **54**: 177–187.

Dahlin DC & Henderson ED (1956) Chondrosarcoma, a surgical and pathological problem: review of 12 cases. *Bone and Joint Surgery* **38**A: 1025–1038.

Dahlin DC, Unni KK & Matsuno T (1977) Malignant (fibrous) histiocytoma of bone: fact or fancy? *Cancer* **39**: 1508–1516.

den Heeten GJ, Schraffordt-Koops H, Kamps WA et al (1985) Treatment of malignant fibrous histiocytoma of bone. A plea for primary chemotherapy. *Cancer* **56**(1): 37–40.

Dosoretz DE, Raymond AK, Murphy GF et al (1982) Primary lymphoma of bone. The relationship of morphologic diversity to clinical behaviour. *Cancer* **50**: 1009–1014.

Dosoretz DE, Murphy GF, Raymond K et al (1983) Radiation therapy for primary lymphoma of bone. *Cancer* **51**: 44–46.

Evans HL, Ayala AG & Romsdahl MM (1977) Prognostic factors in chondrosarcoma of bone. A clinicopathologic analysis with emphasis on histologic grading. *Cancer* **40**: 818–831.

Feldman F & Lattes R (1977) Primary malignant fibrous histiocytoma (fibrous xanthoma) of bone. *Skeletal Radiology* **1**: 145–160.

Feldman F & Norman D (1972) Intra- and extraosseous malignant histiocytoma (malignant fibrous xanthoma). *Radiology* **104**: 497–508.

Fisher RI, Hubbard S, DeVita VT et al (1981) Factors predicting long term survival in diffuse mixed, histiocytic or undifferentiated lymphoma. *Blood* **58**: 45–51.

Freeman C, Berg JW & Cutler SJ (1972) Occurrence and prognosis of extranodal lymphomas. *Cancer* **29**: 252–260.

Huvos AG (1976) Primary malignant fibrous histiocytoma of bone: clinicopathologic study of 18 patients. *New York State Journal of Medicine* **76**: 552–559.

Huvos AG & Higginbotham NL (1975) Primary fibrosarcoma of bone—a clinical pathologic study of 130 patients. *Cancer* **35**: 837–847.

Huvos AG & Marcove RC (1975) Adamantinoma of long bones: a clinicopathological study of fourteen cases with vascular origin suggested. *Journal of Bone and Joint Surgery* **57**A: 148–154.

Huvos AG, Rosen G, Dabska M et al (1983) Mesenchymal chondrosarcoma. A clinicopathologic analysis of 35 patients with emphasis on treatment. *Cancer* **51**: 1230–1237.

Kempson RL & Kyriakos M (1972) Fibroxanthosarcoma of the soft tissues: a type of malignant fibrous histiocytoma. *Cancer* **29**: 961–976.

Koziner B, Little C, Passe S et al (1982) Treatment of advanced histiocytic lymphoma. An analysis of prognostic variables. *Cancer* **49**: 1571–1579.

Krochak R, Harwood AR, Cummings BJ et al (1983) Results of radical radiation for chondrosarcoma of bone. *Radiotherapy and Oncology* **1**: 109–115.

Lichtenstein L & Bernstein D (1959) Unusual benign and malignant chondroid tumours of bone. Survey of some mesenchymal cartilage tumours and malignant chondroblastic tumours, including a few multicentric ones, as well as many atypical benign chondroblastomas and chondromyxoid fibromas. *Cancer* **12**: 1142–1157.

Loeffler JS, Tarbell NJ, Kozakewich H et al (1986) Primary lymphoma of bone in children: analysis of treatment results with Adriamycin, Oncovin, Prednisone (AOP) and local radiation therapy. *Journal of Clinical Oncology* **4**(4): 496–501.

Marcove RC & Huvos AG (1971) Cartilaginous tumours of the ribs. *Cancer* **27**: 794–801.

McCarthy EF, Matsuno T & Dorfman HD (1979) Malignant fibrous histiocytoma of bone: a study of 35 cases. *Human Pathology* **10**: 57–70.

McNaney D, Lindberg RD, Ayala AG et al (1982) Fifteen year radiotherapy experience with chondrosarcoma of bone. *International Journal of Radiation, Oncology, Biology and Physiology* **8**: 191–196.

Nakashima Y, Unni KK, Shires TC et al (1986) Mesenchymal chondrosarcoma of bone and soft tissue. A review of 11 cases. *Cancer* **57**: 2444–2453.

Orton CG & Ellis F (1973) A simplification in the use of the NSD concept in practical radiotherapy. *British Journal of Radiology* **46**: 529–537.

Ostrowski ML, Unni KK, Banks PM et al (1986) Malignant lymphoma of bone. *Cancer* **58**: 2646–2655.

Parker F Jr & Jackson H Jr (1939) Primary reticulum cell sarcoma of bone. *Surgical Gynaecology and Obstetrics* **68**: 45–53.

Parvinen LM, Jereb B & Nisce L (1983) Primary non-Hodgkin's lymphoma (reticulum cell sarcoma) of bone in adults. *Acta Radiologica* (Oncology) **22**(6): 449–454.

Reimer RR, Chabner BA, Young RC et al (1977) Lymphoma presenting in bone. Results of histopathology, staging and therapy. *Annals of Internal Medicine* **87**: 50–55.

Roholl PJM, Kleijne J, van Basten CDH et al (1985) A study to analyze the origin of tumour cells in malignant fibrous histiocytomas. *Cancer* **56**: 2809–2815.

Rosen G (1982) Sarcomas of the soft tissue and bone. In DeVita VT et al (eds) *Cancer. Principles and Practice of Oncology*, p 1072. Philadelphia and Toronto: Lippincott.

Rosen G, Marcove R, Caparros B et al (1979) Primary osteogenic sarcoma: the rationale for preoperative chemotherapy and delayed surgery. *Cancer* **43**: 2163–2177.

Rosen G, Caparrus B, Nirenberg A et al (1981) Ewing's sarcoma. Ten-year experience with adjuvant chemotherapy. *Cancer* **47**: 2204–2213.

Rosen G, Caparros B, Huvos AG et al (1982) Preoperative chemotherapy for osteogenic sarcoma: selection of postoperative adjuvant chemotherapy based on the response of the primary tumour to preoperative chemotherapy. *Cancer* **49**: 1221–1230.

Ryall KHD, Bates T, Newton RA et al (1979) Combination of radiotherapy and razoxane (ICRF 159) for chondrosarcoma. *Cancer* **14**: 891–895.

Schein PS, Chabner BA, Canellos GP et al (1974) Potential for prolonged disease-free survival following combination chemotherapy of non-Hodgkin's lymphoma. *Blood* **43**: 181–189.

Schein PS, DeVita VT Jr, Hubbard S et al (1976) Bleomycin, adriamycin, cyclophosphamide, vincristine and prednisolone (BACOP) combination chemotherapy in the treatment of advanced diffuse histiocytic lymphoma. *Annals of Internal Medicine* **85**: 417–422.

Shuman LS, Chuang VP, Wallace S et al (1982) Intra-arterial chemotherapy of malignant fibrous histiocytoma of the pelvis. *Radiology* **142**: 343–346.

Soule EH & Enriquez P (1972) Atypical fibrous histiocytoma, malignant fibrous histiocytoma, malignant histiocytoma and epithelioid sarcoma: a comparative study of 65 tumours. *Cancer* **30**: 128–143.

Spanier SS (1977) Malignant fibrous histiocytoma of bone. *Orthopedic Clinic of North America* **8:** 947–961.

Spanier SS, Enneking WF & Enriques P (1975) Primary malignant fibrous histiocytoma of bone. *Cancer* **36:** 2084–2098.

Spjut HJ, Dorfman HD, Fechner RE et al (1971) *Tumors of Bone and Cartilage.* Washington DC: Armed Forces Institute of Pathology.

Tsuneyoshi M, Dorfman HD & Baner TW (1986) Epithelioid haemangioendothelioma of bone. A clinicopathologic, ultrastructural and immunohistochemical study. *American Journal of Surgical Pathology* **10**(11): 754–764.

Unni KK, Dahlin DC, Beabout JW et al (1974) Adamantinoma of long bones. *Cancer* **34:** 1796–1805.

Urban C, Rosen C, Huvos AG et al (1983) Chemotherapy of malignant fibrous histiocytoma of bone. A report of five cases. *Cancer* **51**(5): 795–802.

Weiner M, Sedlis M, Johnston AD et al (1983) Adjuvant chemotherapy of malignant fibrous histiocytoma of bone. *Cancer* **51**(1): 25–29.

Wold LE, Sim FH, Unni KK et al (1982) Haemangiopericytoma of bone. *American Journal of Surgical Pathology* **6:** 53–58.

# 10

The role of radiotherapy in the management of
primary bone tumours

DAVID SPOONER

Since the advent of megavoltage apparatus, there has been an increased role
for radiation therapy in the treatment of both primary and secondary bone
tumours. Localization techniques have become more refined due to
improved imaging facilities and, for metastatic disease, wide field treatment
techniques have been developed using hemi-body irradiation (HBI) and
total body irradiation (TBI). Primary bone tumours are rare in comparison
to secondary osseous lesions, but megavoltage radiation therapy has produced good local control with limb preservation in the malignant round cell
tumours of bone (Ewing's sarcoma and primary non-Hodgkin's lymphoma).
   This chapter will try to define the importance of dose, fractionation and
treatment volume, with respect to tumour control and late complications, in
the management of primary bone tumours.

## EWING'S SARCOMA

This tumour is particularly sensitive to radiation and therefore megavoltage
radiotherapy has become the treatment of choice for producing good primary tumour control with acceptable function. Amputation of limbs can
now be avoided and good function maintained if careful attention is paid to
treatment planning and fractionation (Suit, 1975). Since the widespread
adoption of systemic cytotoxic chemotherapy, which has accounted for the
improved survival in this disease, the importance of sustained local control
and good long-term function following radiation has become more evident
(Rosen et al, 1974).
   In an attempt to prevent or treat local recurrence and metastatic disease,
radiotherapy has been given in the following ways:

1.  to the local regional sites
2.  to sites of metastatic disease at diagnosis
3.  preoperatively—often by a split course technique to allow removal of a
    dispensable bone or the insertion of a prosthesis followed by further
    radiotherapy if histologically indicated
4.  total body radiotherapy

5.  prophylactic CNS radiation
6.  prophylactic pulmonary radiotherapy

*Loco-regional sites*

The standard conventional guidelines widely accepted are as follows (Suit, 1975; Thomas et al, 1984):

*Shrinkage volume technique.* This initially encompasses the whole bone and soft tissue component with at least a 5 cm margin from 'gross disease' to 3500–4000 cGy in daily fractionation doses of less than 200 cGy. Local tumour boosts of 1000–2000 cGy with the same fraction size have been employed.

*Meticulous planning.* This is essential with (i) megavoltage radiotherapy equipment, (ii) immobilization techniques, (iii) shaped fields to conform to the lesion and custom-built compensators for sloping surfaces, (iv) leaving a strip of non-irradiated tissue for lymphatic drainage, (v) avoidance of joints and epiphyses whenever possible, (vi) avoidance during radiotherapy of cytotoxic drugs which have known radiation sensitization effects (Adriamycin, actinomycin D), (vii) physiotherapy during and after radiotherapy, and (viii) avoidance or reduction of weight bearing in affected limbs considered at risk for pathological fracture. Shielding of the contralateral epiphysis in a long bone is not associated with increased local recurrence (Thomas et al, 1984).

   Current prospective randomized trials are exploring the feasibility of limiting treatment portals further following initial cytotoxic reduction of tumour, but it remains to be seen whether chemotherapy alone is sufficient to control gross soft tissue disease.

*Tumour dose.* It is widely agreed there is no clear dose–response benefit in excess of 5000 cGy over 25 fractions over 5 weeks to the primary tumour (Kinsella et al, 1984; Thomas et al, 1984). Higher doses are associated with increased soft-tissue wasting, late fibrosis, pathological fracture and second primaries (Tables 1 and 2). It is possible that lower doses (3000 cGy in 15 fractions over 3 weeks) may control microscopic residual disease following chemotherapy (Jereb et al, 1986), with larger doses employed for residual bulky soft-tissue disease following primary cytotoxic chemotherapy. This is currently being assessed prospectively by the UKCCSG in Great Britain.

*Metastatic disease at diagnosis*

Rapid but temporary palliation can be produced by radiation therapy, probably the most important of which are the prevention of imminent spinal cord compression and the relief of bone pain.

**Table 1.** Ewing's sarcoma: incidence of pathological fracture (after therapy).

| Reference | No. of humerus fractures | No. of femoral fractures | No. of tibial fractures |
|---|---|---|---|
| Springfield and Paglia-rulo (1985) 5000–6000 cGy 6/52 | 3/8 | 5/9 | |
| Rosenstok et al (1978) 4500 cGy 3/52 | 2/6 | 2/3 | 1/4 |
| Jentzche et al (1981) 5000 cGy 5/52 | | 7/13 | 2/11 |
| Bacci et al (1982) 5500 cGy 6/52 | 0/1 | 2/12 | 4/8 |
| | 5/15 (33%) | 16/37 (43%) | 7/21 (33%) |

**Table 2.** Ewing's sarcoma: development of second primary osteosarcoma.

| Reference | No. | Fractionation dose |
|---|---|---|
| Strong et al (1979) | 4/24 | 6000 cGy + |
| Thomas et al (1984) | 3/247 | 5000–5500 cGy |

## Preoperative radiotherapy

Prior to the advent of cytotoxic chemotherapy, tumour bulk could be dramatically reduced by using a split course of radiotherapy (2500 cGy in 3 weeks), and this is still used in some centres to consolidate initial cytotoxic chemotherapy before proceeding to local surgical resection, and followed by the second half of the radical course should there be detectable metastatic residual disease.

## Total body radiotherapy

Initial studies, prior to the advent of effective cytotoxic chemotherapy, suggested that this radiosensitive tumour may permanently respond to low doses of irradiation capable of being administered as TBI (Millburn et al, 1986; Jenkin 1970). Unfortunately the cumulative toxicity of employing this together with systemic chemotherapy is considerable, and small studies show no improvement in the pattern of metastatic relapse or survival advantage despite initial complete response rates of 80% (Kinsella et al, 1983; Berry et al, 1986). However HBI may produce rapid pain relief within 24 hours and this is a useful palliative treatment for widespread metastases (Evans et al, 1984).

## Prophylactic CNS radiotherapy

Reports of late CNS meningeal relapse (Mehta and Hendrickson, 1974) suggested a parallel in the natural history of Ewing's sarcoma after chemotherapy that was similar to that of acute lymphoblastic leukaemia. However, the numbers that might benefit have proved to be too small (less than 2%) to justify the significant toxicity of routine CNS prophylaxis and its late sequelae.

*Prophylactic pulmonary radiotherapy*

Prior to the introduction of effective chemotherapy, prophylactic pulmonary radiation could significantly delay, and possibly control, the appearance of pulmonary metastatic disease. Combination cytotoxic chemotherapy with an Adriamycin-containing four-drug regimen has been shown to be as effective as a three-drug regimen and pulmonary radiotherapy by the cooperative American Intergroup Ewing's Sarcoma Study (IESS) (Nesbit et al, 1981) and therefore the radiation-induced complications of impaired pulmonary function and chest wall development are not considered to be worthwhile.

**Local recurrence**

There are now a number of factors that are known to affect the risk of local recurrence:

*Inadequate radiotherapy volume*

Careful attention to detailed planning (as above) can reduce the rates of local recurrence. In the initial IESS study, inadequate local tumour volume irradiation was associated with local recurrence rates of 23–26% compared with 10% which were thought to be adequate, with little difference between major and minor protocol violations (Thomas et al, 1984).

*Cytotoxic chemotherapy regimen*

Adriamycin-containing combinations of cytotoxic chemotherapy may possibly reduce the increased local recurrence rate seen with minor treatment planning violations as above. In an Italian series the local recurrence rates were 5% and 8% for adequate and inadequate treatment volumes for patients treated with Adriamycin, cyclophosphamide and vincristine, but there appeared to be a significant improvement in survival in favour of the patients receiving adequate volume therapy (Bacci et al, 1982). Similarly, the difference in local recurrence rates in the IESS 1 study above was only seen in the group of patients receiving vincristine, actinomycin D and cyclophosphamide. In the patients receiving Adriamycin in addition to the above drug combination there was no difference in the local relapse rate, irrespective of the adequacy of the protocol treatment volume (Thomas et al, 1984).

These are preliminary observations on small patient numbers, and great care must be taken to ensure accurate localization of the accepted treatment volume as defined earlier.

*Site of primary disease*

Local recurrence rates vary as a function of the primary site. The highest local control rates are observed in patients with distal primaries compared with proximal or central lesions (Perez et al, 1981).

*Bulky tumour site*

Recent analyses emphasize that tumour volume has more influence than site on the local control rate than can be achieved by radiation (Marcus and Milton, 1984; Brown et al, 1987). Initial primary tumour volumes in excess of 100 millilitres locally recurred in 74% of patients compared with 21% in the smaller tumours (Globel et al, 1987). Bulk is probably the more important effect rather than soft-tissue extension by itself (Mendenhall et al, 1983). This could explain the difference in prognosis between sites where the tumours are bulky such as the pelvis (Evans et al, 1984) compared with other sites such as the rib (Thomas et al, 1983; Demeocq et al, 1984) and the foot or hand (Kinsella et al, 1983), where the lesions are usually smaller.

*Total radiotherapy dose*

There are no reliable data for dose–response relationships for Ewing's sarcoma (Kinsella et al, 1984; Thomas et al, 1984) and no benefit for previously recommended doses of 60–65 Gray with the higher morbidity. In the light of the above multiple factors, which probably influence local recurrence rate, the importance of critical doses is unknown. Many retrospective studies alleging inferior results for lower doses of radiation or superior results for complete resection of tumours may reflect the different aggressive biology of large and small lesions, and care must be taken in stratifying for bulk in prospective studies of local therapy. Smaller tumours or tumours debulked by prior chemotherapy may permit a smaller sterilizing dose of radiation with reduced associated toxicity.

## Radiation therapy versus surgery for local control

*Significance of local tumour control* (Table 3)

Local recurrence after radiotherapy and chemotherapy varies between 6 and 30% and is often associated with concurrent distant metastases and is usually fatal. Occasionally, local recurrence occurs alone and there are a few patients who had peripheral lesions treated by local radiation only in the pre-chemotherapy era in which surgical salvage was possible (Lewis et al, 1977; Kliman et al, 1982). Following local radiation and chemotherapy, solitary local recurrence is also uncommon and is unlikely to be salvaged (Bacci et al, 1982).

Any attempt to avoid local radiotherapy to reduce toxicity may well compromise local tumour control which is associated with an extremely poor

**Table 3.** Local salvage of solitary local recurrences in Ewing's sarcoma.

| | No. | Solitary local recurrence | 5-year survival (NED) |
|---|---|---|---|
| After surgery and chemotherapy only (no local radiation) | 11 | 1 | 0/1 Jereb et al (1986) |
| After radiation and chemotherapy (no surgery) | 70 | 2 | 1/2 Bacci et al (1982) |
| After radiation therapy alone | 22 | 2 | 2/2 Kliman et al (1982) |
| After radiation therapy alone | ? | 3 | 2/3 Lewis et al (1977) |

NED = no evidence of disease.

prognosis. Studies are currently being performed treating small primary tumours, which have an inherently better prognosis, with cytotoxic chemotherapy and surgical resection alone. Small, expendable bones (fibula, foot, hand, rib and clavicle), with very little or minimal soft-tissue component, can be excised in toto. There is no evidence that chemotherapy alone can permanently control soft-tissue disease, and this should therefore be removed completely or irradiated.

Preliminary data from the Memorial Hospital suggests a high local recurrence rate for patients who had no local radiotherapy but who received chemotherapy and local bone resection alone (Jereb et al, 1986). Furthermore, this study illustrates the unreliability of basing a decision to omit radiotherapy on the basis of no viable tumour being seen either in the resected bone or its margins, since local recurrence occurred even in this situation (Table 4).

Conservation surgery and the avoidance of radiotherapy in any other than small lesions, with complete excision of the soft-tissue component (Bacci et al, 1982), remains to be cautiously explored. The addition of lower doses of radiation such as 3000 cGy in 15 daily fractions to the above volume may be effective in the absence of residual macroscopic disease after chemotherapy (Jereb et al, 1986).

The following questions therefore need to be asked about the addition of surgery:

1. What is the clinical significance of histological negative margins following resections?
2. To what extent does inadequate surgery, requiring postoperative radiotherapy which delays effective chemotherapy, compromise survival?
3. Is function following surgery/endoprosthetic replacement as good as after radiation therapy and at what cost? The site may be an important factor here, the results of prosthetic replacement in the humerus being less good than in the lower femur.

**Table 4.** Ewing's sarcoma: failure of surgical resection after chemotherapy and before irradiation to produce negative margins histologically.

| Reference | No. of failures |
|---|---|
| Bacci et al (1982) | 18/28 |
| Jereb et al (1986) | 7/58 |

4. Can local control of bulky pelvic masses be improved with combination modality treatment?
5. What is the optimal timing of each modality?
6. What are the criteria for using endoprosthetic replacements for femoral, humeral and tibial lesions in order to reduce functional impairment, second malignancy and pathological fracture?

**Toxicity**

*Limb function.* Limb function is remarkably well preserved, especially in the upper limb after radical radiotherapy and cytotoxic chemotherapy. Late effects include soft-tissue fibrosis, wasting and impaired function of the lower limb, often associated with limb shortening in children of less than 12 years (Figure 1). Thirty per cent of children who were under 12 years developed severe shortening and functional disability after irradiation to the leg, compared with 17% of older children (Lewis et al, 1977). Fourteen out of 29 patients who survived for longer than 2 years after radical radiation to the lower limb had good function, walking unaided and with less than 2.5 centimetres of shortening (Jentzche et al, 1981).

*Pathological fractures.* The intensification of cytotoxic chemotherapy doses given together with modest radiation therapy produce pathological fractures and avascular necrosis of bone (Prurutz et al, 1981). Pathological fractures of the femur, humerus and tibia are now being increasingly reported after combining adriamycin to 5000 cGy to long bones (Table 1).

*Second malignancy* (Table 2). The problem of second malignancy, usually a poorly differentiated osteosarcoma or fibrosarcoma of bone developing within the irradiated bone, has probably been overstated. The formation of second malignancies is related to high total dose and the increased bone absorption of orthovoltage radiation. This problem is likely to fall as doses of less than 6000 cGy are now used and orthovoltage irradiation is now inappropriate for this tumour.

Toxicity should be reduced in the future if current ongoing studies show a reduction in dose to be safe, especially in tumours which have responded well to previous chemotherapy.

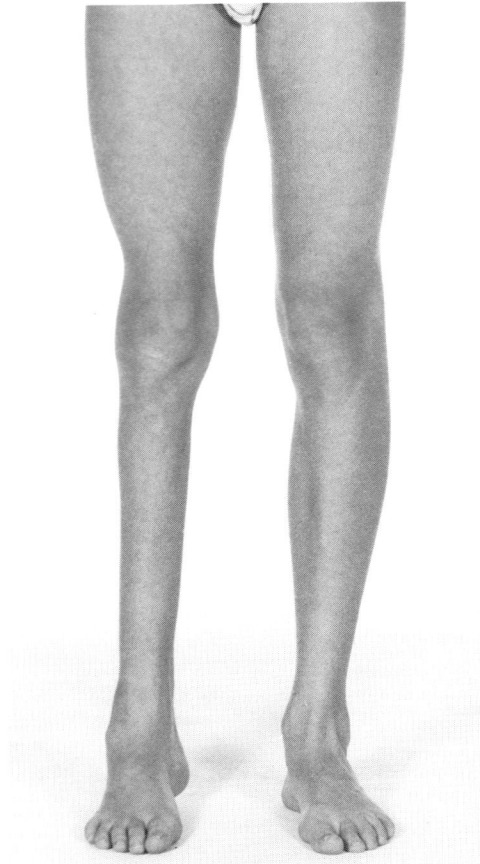

**Figure 1.** Soft tissue atrophy and 5 cm shortening of right lower leg 8 years after radiotherapy (5000 cGy in 25 daily fractions) at the age of 7 years.

*Conclusion*

Radical radiotherapy is the established local treatment for Ewing's sarcoma and its use has dramatically reduced the need for amputation. Any modification of treatment volume or reduction of treatment dose in order to reduce normal soft-tissue toxicity or allow endoprosthetic replacement has to be compared with undoubted achievements of megavoltage radiotherapy.

**MYELOMA**

Palliative radiotherapy rapidly improves bone pain associated with myeloma. Paradoxically, there may be an acute intensification of pain within hours of irradiation, but pain relief is noticed within 24 hours. Great care must be taken of irradiated bones for there is a higher risk of developing a pathological fracture within the following 24-hour period than for other metastatic tumour cell types.

Total body irradiation is well tolerated in patients who have failed first-line cytotoxic chemotherapy. The optimal dose remains to be determined but should be less than 6 Gray to avoid troublesome pneumonitis with heavily pretreated patients. Complete remission has been seen in 40% of patients, with universal improvement in pain and minimal myelo-suppression. Sequential hemi-body irradiation is probably less toxic than total body irradiation (Coleman et al, 1982; Rostom et al, 1984).

### Solitary plasmacytoma

Both medullary and extramedullary plasmacytoma are sensitive to radiation therapy which is the initial treatment of choice. Early administration of cytotoxic chemotherapy has not influenced the natural history, and 2–10% of patients will progress to develop generalized disease.

Doses in excess of 4000 cGy in 20 daily fractions over 4 weeks are recommended. In a retrospective review of 81 patients, lower doses were associated with a local failure rate of 31%, whereas similar or greater doses had a local failure rate of less than 6% (Mendenhall et al, 1982). If a paraprotein is present, the effect of local treatment can be monitored by following serum levels.

## PRIMARY NON-HODGKIN'S LYMPHOMA OF BONE

With the advent of monoclonal antibody stains which recognize leukocyte antigen and accurate, non-invasive, staging techniques, the diagnosis of this rare round malignant cell tumour can be more confidently made than in the past. The chemotherapy of this disease is discussed in Chapter 9.

In the middle and older adult age ranges this tends to be a low-grade malignancy, and disease-free survival rates of 48–62% have been reported (Francis et al, 1954; Wang and Fleischi, 1968; Shoji and Miller, 1971; Bacci et al, 1986).

The treatment volume should include the whole bone and any soft-tissue extension along the guidelines for limb irradiation as outlined above in the Ewing's section. There is no value in exceeding 4500 cGy in 25 daily fractions over 5 weeks on megavoltage equipment. Any subsequent boost will not improve local recurrence but will increase the risk of pathological fracture, especially if chemotherapy is used in addition (Stokes and Waiz, 1983).

Bone lymphomas occurring in the younger age groups have higher grade cell types and should therefore be treated with combination chemotherapy. Meningeal relapse was seen in six out of eight children, and prophylactic CNS therapy should be added to systemic chemotherapy (Wollner et al, 1975).

## OSTEOGENIC SARCOMA

### Primary tumour

Surgical ablation or resection is the local treatment of choice. High doses of radiation of 6000 cGy in 30 fractions over 6 weeks are required to sterilize this radio-resistant tumour with the severe soft-tissue deformity and limb dysfunction that follow (Figure 2). Early work at the Westminster Hospital showed that a high radiation dose could control the tumour for many months, but amputations were performed 6 months following treatment in patients without pulmonary metastases as the primary tumour often recurred later and late radiation damage to the knee produced a painful and fibrosed joint (Cade, 1951).

Preoperative high-dose radiation failed to improve the operability or subsequent survival and therefore has been abandoned (Francis et al, 1954). High total dose and the increased bone absorption of orthovoltage radiation are related to second malignancy formation (Sweetnam et al, 1971), and orthovoltage radiation is now obsolete for this disorder.

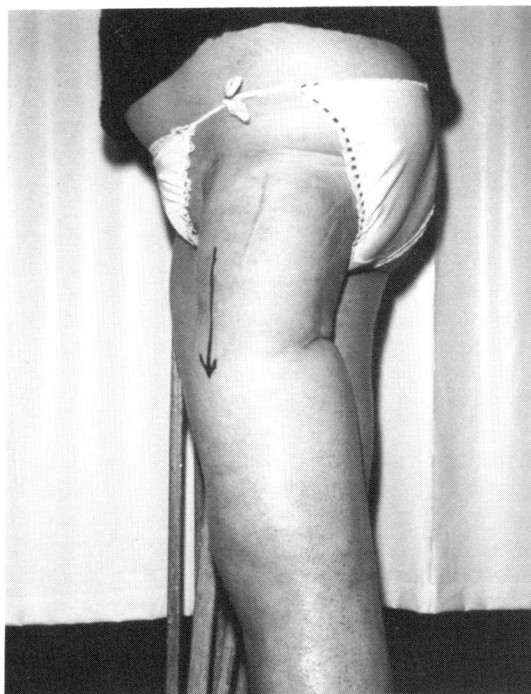

**Figure 2.** Left thigh 18 years after radical radiotherapy for osteogenic sarcoma of the femur.

High-dose radiation is reserved for radical therapy in inoperable sites, e.g. facial skeleton, vertebra and pelvis. Great care must be exercised with the histological differential diagnosis between fibrous dysplasia and low-grade osteogenic sarcoma of the facial skeleton in young people. Good results claimed by high dose preoperative radiation at this site (Chambers and Mahoney, 1970) may be due to the inclusion of patients with fibrous dysplasia which in time will develop a malignant potential if not completely removed after therapy (Tanner et al, 1961). Alteration in radiation frac-tionation by hypofractionation and using the radiosensitizer, Budr, has sterilized local tumours but with severe normal tissue damage producing negligible benefit in the therapeutic ratio (Martinez et al, 1985).

High-dose palliative radiotherapy is still useful for painful bone metastases from osteogenic sarcoma, often with useful reduction in volume. High doses in the region of 4000 cGy in 15 daily fractions over 3 weeks are indicated.

## Pulmonary irradiation

Before the development of adjuvant cytotoxic chemotherapy, prophylactic pulmonary radiation therapy (2000 cGy mpd in 10 daily fractions) was shown to reduce the pulmonary metastatic rate in a number of small series (Rab et al, 1976) with little impairment of pulmonary function (Carcelen et al, 1980). Subsequent phase II (Zaharia et al, 1986) and phase III studies (Breuer et al, 1978) showed that this effect was not superior to the addition of Adriamycin to the cytotoxic regimen, and prophylactic pulmonary irradi-ation is not now usually incorporated into treatment protocols.

## Osteogenic sarcoma arising in Paget's disease

The severe pain associated with this rapidly progressing malignancy can rarely be satisfactorily palliated by radiation therapy. Patients often are too elderly and frail to withstand high dose, local palliative radiotherapy to an inevitably large tumour volume.

## CHONDROSARCOMA

The radical local treatment of choice of chondrosarcoma is surgical resection or ablation. Radical dose radiation therapy has been used for inoperable lesions or for postoperative therapy after incomplete histological removal.

External beam radiotherapy must be considered to be palliative to large inoperable lesions, but it may be associated with significant tumour growth delay locally which has been difficult to monitor satisfactorily before the recent development of sophisticated imaging techniques. The advent of CT scanning of the pelvis will facilitate assessment of tumour response and progression which, until recently, was assessed by the development of pain, and adjacent structures became involved. The failure of significant shrink-age of tumour probably reflects its low cellular content.

High doses have been traditionally given (in excess of 5000 cGy in 25 fractions over 5 weeks) but there is no good evidence of a dose–response relationship, especially for doses greater than this. Dramatic tumour regression has been reported using high radiation doses with the radio-sensitizer, Razoxane, in particular with soft-tissue extension (Ryall et al, 1979).

Careful beam-directed treatment planning should be instituted as often these tumours are adjacent to sensitive bowel or spinal cord. Since they are slow to metastasize, the chronic normal toxicity must be anticipated and minimized as median survival may be 46 months or longer (Harwood et al, 1980; Krochak et al, 1983; McNaney et al, 1982).

Using the physical characteristics of both proton and helium ion beams, high doses of up to an equivalent of 76 cobalt Gray have been delivered to chondrosarcoma without severe acute CNS toxicity. Five patients have been treated by the helium ion beam and 3 chondrosarcomata of the clivus on the proton beam, but it is too early to comment on results (Suit et al, 1982; Sanders et al, 1985). Neutrons have also been employed with no striking benefit over protons. In a report from Houston, one of four patients was controlled locally (Salinas, 1980).

## CHORDOMA

Complete resection of chordomas is unusual except for occasional early lesions in the sacrococcygeal region, and therefore many patients are referred for radiation therapy after biopsy or sub-total resection. These tumours have been termed 'radio-resistant', probably because the rate of response of chordoma masses to irradiation may be slow (Heffelfinger et al, 1973). However, a relatively small decrease in overall tumour volume may be sufficient to relieve pressure on local tissues producing symptomatic pain relief. Radiation therapy alone cannot permanently sterilize macroscopic tumours alone, and the majority of these patients will experience eventual local tumour progression.

The 5-year uncorrected survival rate varies from 40 to 65% in the reported series, with a 10-year uncorrected survival rate of 20% (Cummings et al, 1983; Chetiyawardana, 1984; Amendola et al, 1986; Pearlman and Friedman, 1970).

There is disagreement about the optimal dose. Historically, extremely high doses of 6000–8000 cGy were used, often on orthovoltage machine [for a report of the literature prior to 1970 see Pearlman and Friedman (1970)]. However, a more recent analysis of dose–symptomatic response rate shows no significant dependence on increasing dose within a range of 3500–8500 cGy (Cummings et al, 1983). Using the lower dose, repeated courses of treatment can be given.

Preoperative radiation is unlikely to improve resectability but radiotherapy may be a useful postoperative adjuvant, even after total macroscopic removal. In a small series, 4 out of 10 patients were alive more than 5 years after resection alone for sacral-vertebral chordoma compared with 8 out of 13 after resection and postoperative irradiation (Cohen et al, 1964).

Doses in the order of 4000–5500 cGy are likely to be effective. High doses of radiation using protons (Suit et al, 1982) and helium ions (Saunders et al, 1986) have been given to tumours in the cervical spine and clivus, but meaningful results are not yet available.

## OTHER LESIONS

### Giant cell tumour of bone

Radiotherapy is not the recommended treatment for this condition unless local surgical control fails (see Chapter 6). Then good local control can be seen with doses as low as 4000 cGy in 20 daily fractions over 4 weeks. Radiotherapy is now unfashionable for this treatment and more extensive surgery, often by ablation in the event of soft-tissue involvement, has been preferred. This has largely been due to the high rate of malignant transformation reported after high doses of orthovoltage radiation, both of which are inappropriate (Table 5). These factors probably account for the estimated 70% of malignant giant cell tumours that are generated by local radiotherapy (Campbell and Bonfiglio, 1973).

Lower dose radiation using megavoltage equipment can produce acceptable local tumour control without an unacceptably higher malignant transformation rate, which is inherent in the natural history of this condition (Campanacci et al, 1987).

### Vertebral haemangioma

This is a benign tumour of the dorsal and lumbar vertebrae which causes severe pain. Its radiological appearance is striking and characteristic of

**Table 5.** Recurrent giant cell tumour of bone: further local control and malignant transformation following orthovoltage and megavoltage radiation.

| Reference | Local recurrence no. | Malignant transformation no. |
|---|---|---|
| | *Megavoltage* | |
| Larsson et al (1975) | 0/3 | 0/3 |
| Larsson et al (1975) | 4/14 | 0/14 |
| McGrath et al (1972) | 8/12 | 5/21 |
| Friedman and Pearlman (1968) | 15/45 | 0/45 |
| Bell et al (1983) | 5/15 | 0/15 |
| Chen et al (1986) | 9/35 | 0/35 |
| | 36/133 (27%) | 5/133 (4%) |
| | *Orthovoltage* | |
| Dahlin et al (1970) | 23/43 | 11/43 |
| Mnaymneh (1964) | 15/16 | 2/16 |
| Bradshaw (1964) | 16/50 | 4/50 |
| Walter (1960) | 3/15 | 0/15 |
| | 57/124 (37%) | 17/124 (14%) |

vertebral bony trabeculi between areas of rarefraction, producing a honeycomb pattern (Gramiak et al, 1957). Low doses of 3000 cGy in 15 daily fractions to 4000 cGy in 20 daily fractions to the involved vertebra will produce pain relief without any radiological change. Eight out of nine patients obtained complete pain relief (Faria et al, 1985). Recurrence of symptoms is unusual in less than 5 years. Occasionally, spinal cord compression may be relieved by local irradiation alone (Ferber and Lampe, 1942). Malignant transformation is not a matter of concern since the tumour occurs in the older population.

### Histiocytosis X/eosinophilic granuloma

The decision as to whether the local lesion should be treated with surgical curetting or radiation or left untreated is often based on the severity of symptoms and the localization of disease. Often, spontaneous regression or stabilization of the disease can occur, requiring no further treatment. Radiotherapy may be recommended: (1) in lesions which recur after simple biopsy and curetting, (2) in lesions in which surgical curetting is difficult, such as the orbit or mastoid, and (3) when surgery is contraindicated on other medical grounds.

Radiation dose can be less than 10 Gray and preferably in the range of 5–6 Gy with cobalt-60 irradiation. Higher doses do not appear to be more effective (Smith et al, 1973). Lytic bone defects usually respond to these doses of radiotherapy.

There is no benefit in treating patients with complete diabetes insipidus, manifested as a lack of any osmotic threshold or urinary concentrating ability, but there is a suggestion in patients with residual vasopressin activity (partial diabetes insipidus) that full recovery can be achieved with local radiotherapy doses of 8–12 Gy on cobalt-60 to the hypothalamus/pituitary region (Helbock et al, 1982).

## REFERENCES

Amendola BE, Amendola MA, Oliver E & McCalatchey KD (1986) Chordoma: role of radiation therapy. *Radiology* **158:** 839–843.
Bacci G, Picci P, Gitelis S, Borghi A & Campanacci M (1982) The treatment of localised Ewing's sarcoma. *Cancer* **49:** 1561–1570.
Bacci G, Jaffe N, Emiliani E et al (1986) Therapy for primary non-Hodgkin's lymphoma of bone and a comparison of results with Ewing's sarcoma. *Cancer* **57:** 1468–1472.
Bell RS, Harwood AR Goodman SB & Fornasie VL (1983) Supervital radiotherapy in the treatment of difficult giant cell tumour of bone. *Clinical Orthopaedics and Related Research* **174:** 208–216.
Berry MP, Jenkin DT, Harwood AR et al (1986) Ewing's sarcoma: a trial of adjuvant chemotherapy and sequential half-body irradiation. *International Journal of Radiation Oncology, Biology, Physics* **12:** 19–24.
Bradshaw JD (1964) The values of X-ray therapy in the management of osteoclastoma. *Clinical Radiology* **15:** 70.
Breuer K, Cohen P, Schweisguth O & Hart A (1978) Irradiation of the lungs as an adjuvant therapy in the treatment of osteosarcoma of the limbs. An EORTC randomised study. *European Journal of Cancer* **14:** 461–471.

Cade S (1951)*Malignant Disease and Its Treatment by Radiation*, 2nd edn. Bristol: Wright

Campanacci M, Baldini N, Boriani J & Sudanese A (1987) Giant cell tumour of bone. *Journal of Bone and Joint Surgery* **69a:** 106–114.

Campbell CT & Bonfiglio M (1973) Aggressiveness and malignancy—giant cell tumour of bone. In Price CHG & Ross FGM (eds) *Bone—Certain Aspects of Neoplasia*, pp 15–38. Philadelphia: Butterworths.

Carcelen A, Zaharia M, Carceres E, Morn M & Tejada F (1980) Pulmonary function tests during adjuvant lung irradiation for osteogenic sarcoma. *Cancer Treatment Reports* **64:** 701–703.

Chambers RG & Mahoney WD (1970) Osteogenic sarcoma of the mandible—current management. *American Journal of Surgery* **36:** 463–471.

Chen ZX, Gu DZ, Yu ZH et al (1986) Radiation therapy of giant cell tumour of bone: analysis of 35 patients. *International Journal of Radiation Oncology, Biology, Physics* **12:** 329–334.

Chetiyawardana AD (1984) Chordoma: results of treatment. *Clinical Radiology* **35:** 159–161.

Cohen DM, Dahlin DS & McCarty CS (1964) Apparently solitary tumours of the vertebral column. *Proceedings of the Mayo Clinic* **39:** 509–528.

Coleman M, Saletan S, Wolf D et al (1982) Whole bone marrow irradiation for the treatment of multiple myeloma. *Cancer* **49:** 1328–1333.

Cummings BJ, Hodson ID & Bush RS (1983) Chordoma: the results of megavoltage radiation therapy. *International Journal of Radiation Oncology, Biology, Physics* **9:** 633–642.

Dahlin DC, Cupps RE & Johnson EW (1970) Giant cell tumour: a study of 195 cases. *Cancer* **25:** 1061.

Demeocq F, Oberlin O, Brunat-Mentigny M et al (1984) Primary chemotherapy and tumour resection in Ewing's sarcoma of the ribs. *Report of the French Society of Paediatric Oncology* **84:** 128.

Evans R, Nesbit M, Askin F et al (1984) Local recurrence, rate and sites of metastases and time to relapse as a function of treatment regimen, size of primary and surgical history in 62 patients presenting with non-metastatic Ewing's sarcoma of the pelvic bones. *International Journal of Radiation Oncology, Biology, Physics* **11:** 129–136.

Faria SL, Schlupp WR & Chiminazzo H (1985) Radiotherapy in the treatment of vertebral haemangiomas. *International Journal of Radiation Oncology, Biology, Physics* **11:** 389–390.

Ferber L & Lampe I (1942) Haemangioma of vertebra associated with compression of the cord. Response to radiation therapy. *Archives of Neurology* **74:** 19–29.

Francis KC, Phillips R, Nickson JJ et al (1954) Massive pre-operative irradiation in the treatment of osteogenic sarcoma in children. *American Journal of Roentgenology, Radium Therapy and Nuclear Medicine* **72:** 813.

Friedman M & Pearlman AW (1968) Benign giant cell tumour of bone: radiation dosage for each type. *Radiology* **91:** 1151.

Gobel V, Jurgens H, Etspuler G et al (1987) Prognostic significance of tumour volume in localized Ewing's sarcoma of bone in children and adolescents. *Cancer Research and Clinical Oncology* (in press).

Gramiak R, Ruiz G & Campeti FL (1957) Cystic angiomatosis of bone. *Radiology* **69:** 347–353.

Harwood AR, Krajbich JI & Fornasier VL (1980) Radiotherapy of chondrosarcoma of bone. *Cancer* **45:** 2769–2777.

Heffelfinger MJ, Dahlin DC, MacCarty CS & Babout JW (1973) Chordomas and cartilagenous tumours of the skull base. *Cancer* **32:** 410–420.

Helbock H, Crivit W & Nesbit ME (1982) Patterns of anti-diuretic function in diabetes insipidus caused by histiocytosis X. *Journal of Clinical and Laboratory Medicine* **78:** 194–202.

Jenkin RDT (1970) Ewing's sarcoma—a trial of adjuvant total body irradiation. *Radiology* **96:** 151–155.

Jenkin RDT, Rider WD & Sonley MJ (1976) Ewing's sarcoma, adjuvant total body irradiation, cyclophosphamide and vincristine. *International Journal of Radiation Oncology, Biology, Physics* **1:** 407–413.

Jentzche K, Binder H, Cramer H et al (1981) Leg function after radiotherapy for Ewing's sarcoma. *Cancer* **47:** 1267–1278.

Jereb, Ong RL, Mohan M, Caparros B & Exelby P (1986) Redefined role of radiation in combined treatment of Ewing's sarcoma. *Paediatric Haematology and Oncology* **3**: 111–118.

Kinsella TJ, Gaubiger D, Dressenoth A et al (1983) Intensive combined modality treatment including low dose TBI for high risk Ewing's sarcoma patients. *International Journal of Radiation Oncology, Biology, Physics* **9**: 1955–1960.

Kinsella TJ, Licter AS, Miser J, Gerber L & Glatstein E (1984) Local treatment of Ewing's sarcoma: radiation therapy versus surgery. *Cancer Treatment Reports* **68**: 695–701.

Kliman M, Harwood AR, Jenkin RD et al (1982) Radical Radiotherapy as Primary Treatment for Ewing's sarcoma distal to the elbow and knee. *Clinical Orthopaedics and Related Research* **165**: 233–238.

Krochak R, Harwood AR, Cummings BJ & Quirt IC (1983) Results of radical radiation for chondrosarcoma of the bone. *Radiotherapy and Oncology* **1**: 109–115.

Larsson S, Lorentzon R & Boquist L (1975) Giant cell tumour of bone. *Journal of Bone and Joint Surgery* **57a**: 167.

Lewis RJ, Marcove RC & Rosen G (1977) Ewing's sarcoma—functional effects of radiation therapy. *Journal of Joint and Bone Surgery* **59A**: 325–331.

Martinez A, Goffinet DR, Donaldson SS, Bagshaw MA & Kaplan HS (1985) Intra-arterial infusion of radiosensitive (BU d R) combined with hyperfractionated irradiation and chemotherapy for the primary treatment of osteogenic sarcoma. *International Journal of Radiation Oncology, Biology, Physics* **11**: 123–128.

McGrath PG (1972) Giant cell tumour of bone. *Journal of Bone and Joint Surgery* **54b**: 216.

McNaney D, Lindberg R, Ayala A, Barkley T & Hussey D (1982) Fifteen year radiotherapy experience with chondrosarcoma of bone. *International Journal of Radiation Oncology, Biology, Physics* **8**: 187–190.

Mehta Y & Hendrickson R (1974) C.N.S. involvement in Ewing's sarcoma. *Cancer* **33**: 859–862.

Mendenhall CM, Marcus BB Jr, Enneking WF et al (1983) The prognostic significance of soft tissue extension in Ewing's sarcoma. *Cancer* **51**: 913–917.

Millburn LF, O'Grady L & Hendrickson FR (1986) Radical radiation therapy and total body irradiation in the treatment of Ewing's sarcomas. *Cancer* **22**: 919–925.

Mnaymneh WA, Dudley HR & Mnaymneh LG (1964) Giant cell tumour of bone. *Journal of Bone and Joint Surgery* **46a**: 63.

Nesbit ME, Perez CA, Tefft M et al (1981) Multimodal therapy for the management of primary non metastatic Ewing's sarcoma of bone: an intergroup study. *National Cancer Monograph* **56**: 255–262.

Pearlman AW & Friedman M (1970) Radical radiation therapy of chordoma. *American Journal of Roentgenology* **108**: 333–341.

Perez CA, Tefft M & Nesbitt ME (1981) Radiation therapy in the multimodal management of Ewing's sarcoma of bone: report of the Intergroup Ewing's Sarcoma Study. *National Cancer Institute* **56**: 263–271.

Prurutz LR, Lawson JR, Fleldlander GE, Farber LR & Pezzimenti JF (1981) Avascular necrosis of bone in Hodgkin's disease after previous treatment with combination modality therapy. *Cancer* **49**: 2793–2799.

Rab G, Ivins J, Childs D, Cupps R & Pritchard DJ (1976) Elective whole lung irradiation in the treatment of osteogenic sarcoma. *Cancer* **38**: 939–942.

Rosen G, Wollner N, Tan C et al (1974) Disease free survival in children with Ewing's sarcoma treated with radiation therapy and adjuvant four-drug sequential chemotherapy. *Cancer* **33**: 384–393.

Rosenstock JG, Jones PM, Pearson D, Palmer MK et al (1978) Ewing's sarcoma—adjuvant chemotherapy and pathological fracture. *European Journal of Cancer* **14**: 799–803.

Rostom AY, O'Cathail SM & Folkes A (1984) Systemic irradiation in multiple myeloma: a report on 18 cases. *British Journal of Haematology* **58**: 423–431.

Ryall RD, Bates T, Newton KA & Hellman K (1979) Combination of radiotherapy and razoxane for chondrosarcoma. *Cancer* **44**: 891–895.

Salinas (1980) Experience in fast neutron treatment of locally advanced sarcomas. *International Journal of Radiation Oncology, Biology, Physics* **6**: 267–272.

Saunders WM, Chin GTY, Austin-Seymour M et al (1985) Precision high dose radiotherapy II. Helium ion treatment of tumour adjacent to critical C.N.S. structures. *International Journal of Radiation Oncology, Biology, Physics* **11**: 1339–1347.

Saunders WM, Castrol JR, Chen GTY et al (1986) Early results of ion beam radiation therapy for sacral chordoma. *Journal of Neurosurgery* **64:** 243–247.

Shoji H & Miller TR (1971) Primary reticular cell sarcoma of bone. Significance of clinical features upon prognosis. *Cancer* **28:** 1234–1244.

Smith DG, Nesbit ME, D'Angio GJ & Levitt SH (1973) Histiocytosis X. Role of radiation therapy in management with special reference to dose levels employed. *Radiology* **106:** 419–422.

Springfield DS & Pagliarulo C (1985) Fractures of long bones previously treated for Ewing's sarcoma. *Journal of Bone and Joint Surgery* **67A:** 477–481.

Stokes SH & Waiz BJ (1983) Pathological fracture of radiation therapy for primary non Hodgkin's malignant lymphoma of bone. *International Journal of Radiation Oncology, Biology, Physics* **9:** 1153–1159.

Strong LG, Herson GH, Osborne BM & Sutow W (1979) Risk of radiation related malignant tumour in survivors of Ewing's sarcoma. *Journal of the National Cancer Institute* **62:** 1401.

Suit HD (1975) Role of therapeutic radiology in cancer of bone. *Cancer* **35:** 930–935.

Suit HD, Goitein M & Munzenrider J (1982) Definitive radiation therapy for chordoma and chondrosarcoma of the base of skull and cervical spine. *Journal of Neurosurgery* **56:** 377–385.

Sweetnam R, Knowelden J & Seddon J (1971) Bone sarcoma: treatment by irradiation, amputation or a combination of the two. *British Medical Journal* **ii:** 363.

Tanner HC, Dahlin DC & Childs DS (1961) Sarcoma complicating fibrous dysplasia. Probable role of radiation therapy. *Oral Surgery* **14:** 837–846.

Thomas PRM, Foulkes MA, Gilula L et al (1983) Primary Ewing's sarcoma of the ribs. *Cancer* **51:** 1021–1027.

Thomas PRM, Perez CA, Neff JR, Nesbitt ME & Evans RG (1984) The management of Ewing's sarcoma: role of radiotherapy in local tumour control. *Cancer Treatment Reports* **68:** 703–710.

Walter J (1960) Giant cell lesions of bone. *Radiology* **11:** 14.

Wang & Fleischi DJ (1968) Primary reticulum cell sarcoma of bone, with emphasis on radiation therapy. *Cancer* **22:** 994–998.

Wollner N, Burchnal JH, Lieberman PH et al (1975) Non Hodgkin's lymphoma in children. *Medical and Paediatric Oncology* **1:** 235–263.

Zaharia M, Caceres E, Valdivia S, Moran M & Tejada F (1986) Post-operative whole lung irradiation with or without adriamycin in osteogenic sarcoma. *International Journal Radiation Oncology, Biology, Physics* **12:** 907–910.

# Index

Note: Page numbers of article titles are in **bold** type.

261